AF588035

Health Informatics

This series is directed to healthcare professionals leading the transformation of healthcare by using information and knowledge. For over 20 years, Health Informatics has offered a broad range of titles: some address specific professions such as nursing, medicine, and health administration; others cover special areas of practice such as trauma and radiology; still other books in the series focus on interdisciplinary issues, such as the computer based patient record, electronic health records, and networked healthcare systems. Editors and authors, eminent experts in their fields, offer their accounts of innovations in health informatics. Increasingly, these accounts go beyond hardware and software to address the role of information in influencing the transformation of healthcare delivery systems around the world. The series also increasingly focuses on the users of the information and systems: the organizational, behavioral, and societal changes that accompany the diffusion of information technology in health services environments.

Developments in healthcare delivery are constant; in recent years, bioinformatics has emerged as a new field in health informatics to support emerging and ongoing developments in molecular biology. At the same time, further evolution of the field of health informatics is reflected in the introduction of concepts at the macro or health systems delivery level with major national initiatives related to electronic health records (EHR), data standards, and public health informatics.

These changes will continue to shape health services in the twenty-first century. By making full and creative use of the technology to tame data and to transform information, Health Informatics will foster the development and use of new knowledge in healthcare.

Philip Eappen • Narasimha Rao Vajjhala
Ruiling Guo • Virginia Gunn
Editors

Advancing Healthcare with the Medical Internet of Things

Revolutionizing Patient Care through Connected Devices

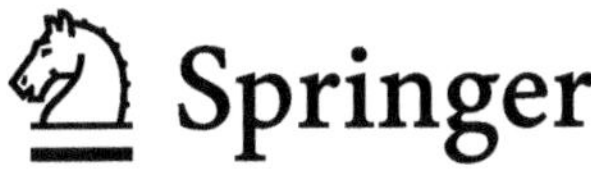

Editors
Philip Eappen
Cape Breton University
Sydney, NS, Canada

Narasimha Rao Vajjhala
Computer Science Department
American University in Bulgaria
Blagoevgrad, Bulgaria

Ruiling Guo
College of Business Healthcare
Administration Program
Idaho State University
Pocatello, ID, USA

Virginia Gunn
School of Nursing
Cape Breton University
Sydney, NS, Canada

ISSN 1431-1917 ISSN 2197-3741 (electronic)
Health Informatics
ISBN 978-3-032-23932-7 ISBN 978-3-032-23933-4 (eBook)
https://doi.org/10.1007/978-3-032-23933-4

This Springer imprint is published by the registered company Springer Nature Switzerland AG
The registered company address is: Gewerbestrasse 11, 6330 Cham, Switzerland

To my beloved dad, Eappen—a pure soul whose unwavering wisdom, profound strength, and boundless compassion continue to illuminate my path even in his absence. He lived with an innocent heart that embraced everyone without prejudice or hatred, seeing only the good in humanity. Though he is no longer with us in body, his cherished values of unconditional love and acceptance breathe life into every page of this work.

This book stands as both a tribute to his enduring spirit and a testament to the countless healthcare professionals, researchers, and advocates around the world who dedicate their lives to advancing patient care and building healthier, more equitable communities for all.

May his legacy of service and love continue to inspire future generations!

Foreword

Has the fantasy of seamless, technology-enabled healthcare finally become reality? It seems like only yesterday that *Star Trek* tantalized us with visions of electronic healing devices and instant diagnostics at the touch of a button. Today, that science fiction has evolved into scientific fact. Smartphones now serve as powerful health monitoring platforms, tracking everything from blood pressure and glucose levels to cardiac rhythms and sleep patterns. Mobile health applications provide instant access to medical information and diagnostic tools, while smartwatches deliver continuous health data streams. Hospitals have embraced smart patient rooms that electronically monitor vital signs, track patient movement, and enhance safety protocols. Patient portals have revolutionized healthcare accessibility, allowing individuals to review their health records, schedule appointments, and manage medications with unprecedented ease.

While the initial costs of these technologies were prohibitive and often excluded from insurance coverage, we are witnessing a rapid democratization of digital health tools that promise to transform healthcare delivery fundamentally.

In *Advancing Healthcare with the Medical Internet of Things: Revolutionizing Patient Care through Connected Devices*, the editors, including Dr. Eappen, and their distinguished contributing authors masterfully navigate this complex landscape of interconnected medical devices and intelligent healthcare systems. This comprehensive collaborative work examines not only the current state of connected health technology but also its profound implications for the future of patient care.

The central question that the editors and contributing authors address is both timely and critical: How will this technological revolution reshape healthcare delivery, and has it already begun to transform the patient-provider relationship? Recent developments in artificial intelligence have led some advocates to claim that AI-powered diagnostic algorithms can outperform human physicians in accuracy and treatment recommendations. Yet this raises fundamental questions about the role of human connection in medicine. Healthcare has always been both a rigorous science and a nuanced art, requiring not only technical expertise but also empathy, cultural sensitivity, and the ability to navigate complex human relationships.

The editors and contributing authors thoughtfully explore this tension between technological capability and human care. While AI offers unprecedented opportunities for personalized diagnosis and treatment based on individual patient data and genetic profiles, the authors examine whether we risk losing something essential if we diminish the human elements of healthcare. The potential for continuously connected patients—linked to their primary care providers and specialists through IoT devices—presents remarkable advantages for monitoring chronic conditions, tracking recovery progress, and predicting health complications before they become critical.

The evolution of wearable technology, which the authors trace from early medical alert systems to today's sophisticated smartwatches and smartphone-integrated health platforms, demonstrates the rapid pace of innovation in this field. The book provides invaluable insight into how these advances are not only becoming more capable but also more affordable and accessible to diverse patient populations.

Advancing Healthcare with the Medical Internet of Things delves deep into whether wearable devices can genuinely strengthen healthcare delivery from both technical and experiential perspectives. The editors and contributing authors examine cutting-edge developments in medical implants—from cardiac monitors to innovative central nervous system devices—while carefully considering both their tremendous potential and important safety considerations. As AI technology becomes increasingly sophisticated in its ability to predict and respond to physiological changes within the body and brain, the book explores how these capabilities might challenge our current understanding of medical practice.

Particularly compelling is the authors' examination of IoT applications in mental healthcare. The book reveals significant opportunities for using AI-enabled wearables to support individuals with various mental health conditions, offering new pathways for monitoring, intervention, and treatment that were previously impossible.

The COVID-19 pandemic accelerated the adoption of telemedicine, opening doors that many thought would remain closed for years. The contributors demonstrate how AI integration is exponentially enhancing telemedicine capabilities, creating new opportunities not only for patients in remote locations but also for improving healthcare access and efficiency in urban environments.

Perhaps most importantly, the editors and contributing authors address the economic realities of implementing AI technology and wearable devices in healthcare systems. The book provides a thorough analysis of how these technologies must ultimately deliver value-based care to achieve sustainable adoption and meaningful impact on patient outcomes.

Advancing Healthcare with the Medical Internet of Things serves as both a comprehensive guide to our current technological capabilities and a thoughtful roadmap for the future of connected healthcare. The editors and contributing authors have assembled a work that will prove invaluable to healthcare professionals, technology developers, policymakers, and anyone seeking to understand how the Internet of Things is revolutionizing patient care while preserving the essential human elements that make healthcare truly healing.

In an era where technology evolves at breakneck speed, this collaborative effort provides the clarity and insight needed to navigate the exciting yet complex intersection of healthcare and connected devices. The editors and contributing authors have created an essential resource for understanding not just what is possible in healthcare technology, but what is practical, beneficial, and ultimately transformative for patient care.

Steven D. Berkshire
Professor Emeritus in Health Administration,
Central Michigan University
Santa Fe, NM, USA

Preface

The Medical Internet of Things in Healthcare Transformation

Healthcare in Transition: A Global Imperative

The contemporary healthcare landscape is experiencing unprecedented transformation driven by converging demographic, technological, and economic pressures. Global health systems confront escalating challenges: aging populations, rising chronic disease prevalence, widening health disparities, and mounting financial constraints. The World Health Organization has consistently emphasized the urgent need for scalable, sustainable, and equitable healthcare delivery approaches that transcend traditional hospital-centered models.

Within this transformative context, digital technologies have emerged as key drivers of innovation, with artificial intelligence, big data analytics, genomics, and cloud computing fundamentally reshaping modern medicine. Among these advances, the Medical Internet of Things (MIoT) occupies a distinctive position as both a technological evolution and a paradigmatic shift in medical philosophy and practice. MIoT encompasses interconnected medical devices, sensors, wearables, implants, and platforms that continuously monitor, collect, and transmit health data, enabling real-time analytics, remote monitoring, and personalized interventions.

The transformative promise of MIoT lies in its capacity to decentralize healthcare delivery, relocating the provision of services from institutional settings into patients' everyday environments. This fundamental reorientation has the potential to reduce dependence on acute care, strengthen primary care systems, empower patient self-management, and redirect health systems toward prevention and proactive health maintenance rather than reactive treatment models. However, realizing these advantages requires addressing significant structural challenges to ensure equitable, sustainable, and patient-centered implementation.

The Evolution and Emergence of MIoT

The origins of MIoT can be traced to the convergence of multiple technological domains over the past two decades. Early telemedicine and mobile health developments demonstrated the feasibility of remote care delivery, while advances in wearable sensors and biomedical engineering enabled continuous measurement of vital signs and physiological parameters. Simultaneously, cloud computing, wireless connectivity, and data analytics created the infrastructure necessary for storing, sharing, and interpreting vast quantities of health-related data.

Research and commercial interest in MIoT has expanded exponentially since 2005, with bibliometric analyses revealing significant growth in publications addressing smart implants, biosensors, and connected healthcare—particularly accelerating after 2015. The wearable device market, encompassing smartwatches, continuous glucose monitors, and fitness trackers, is projected to exceed hundreds of millions of units annually, reflecting both consumer demand and clinical adoption. Governments and health systems are investing heavily in digital health infrastructure, recognizing MIoT's potential to support population health management, reduce costs, and extend care to underserved regions.

Despite remarkable progress, critical gaps persist in the literature. Long-term clinical validation studies remain limited, security and privacy safeguards are often inadequately integrated into device design, and interoperability across platforms and health information systems continues to pose significant barriers. Moreover, the social, ethical, and policy dimensions of MIoT adoption are only beginning to receive sustained scholarly attention, necessitating interdisciplinary approaches to address these multifaceted challenges.

Core Contributions of MIoT to Healthcare Delivery

Strengthening Primary Care Through Wearable Technologies

MIoT's most significant contribution lies in its potential to strengthen primary care and shift health system focus toward prevention. Wearable devices, owing to their accessibility and relatively low cost, enable individuals to monitor health parameters including heart rate, blood pressure, blood oxygen saturation, physical activity, and sleep patterns. When integrated within larger health ecosystems, these data streams support proactive interventions, reduce complications, and minimize requirements for in-person visits. For underserved populations, particularly those in rural or resource-limited settings, wearable technologies can help bridge access gaps and promote health equity by facilitating continuous care beyond hospital walls.

Elder Care and Safety Systems Innovation

The global demographic shift toward aging populations amplifies the importance of connected health solutions. With approximately 727 million people aged 65 or older in 2020—projected to double by 2050—health systems face increasing pressure to respond to the care needs of older adults with complex health conditions, limited mobility, and heightened vulnerability to falls and emergencies. Innovations such as fall-detection devices, GPS-enabled monitoring, and integrated platforms combining wearable sensors, mobile applications, and machine learning algorithms provide real-time safety monitoring. These technologies enhance older adult independence and quality of life while alleviating caregiver burden and reducing avoidable hospitalizations.

Chronic Disease Management Revolution

Chronic conditions including diabetes, cardiovascular disease, and respiratory illness account for the majority of global morbidity and healthcare expenditures. MIoT offers novel strategies for continuous monitoring, early detection, and personalized management of these diseases. Continuous glucose monitors, for instance, enable real-time blood sugar tracking, empowering patients in diabetes self-management while providing clinicians with actionable insights. Similar applications in cardiac and respiratory function monitoring, as well as management of neurological disorders, underscore the versatility of wearable and implantable devices in supporting long-term disease management. Evidence suggests these technologies reduce hospital admissions, improve treatment adherence, and lower overall healthcare costs.

Mental Health and Neuroscience Applications

The global mental health crisis requires equally innovative responses, with MIoT technologies offering promise in providing real-time physiological feedback related to stress, anxiety, and mood. By integrating wearable devices with advances in behavioral neuroscience and neuroplasticity research, connected technologies can foster resilience and adaptive coping strategies. These applications reflect a broader shift toward holistic health models encompassing both physical and psychological dimensions, demonstrating how wearable-based platforms can enhance mental health self-awareness and complement traditional therapeutic modalities.

Precision Medicine and Radiogenomics Integration

The most cutting-edge MIoT applications reside in the domains of precision and personalized medicine. Smart implants, biosensors, and radiogenomics enable the integration of genetic, imaging, and physiological data to tailor therapies to individual patient profiles. Radiogenomics leverages genetic markers and imaging modalities to predict tumor behavior and therapeutic response, offering unprecedented opportunities for individualized cancer treatment. While challenges remain in data standardization, validation, security, and costs, the potential of these technologies to enhance therapeutic precision represents a defining frontier in medical science.

Structural Considerations for Equitable, Sustainable, and Patient-Centered Implementation

Data Governance and Security Imperatives

The collection and transmission of sensitive health data through connected devices necessitates robust privacy and security safeguards. Bibliometric analyses reveal persistent gaps in research explicitly addressing these dimensions, with health data breaches undermining patient trust and posing significant risks to public health infrastructures. Effective governance frameworks must encompass secure data transmission, encryption, interoperability standards, and clear accountability mechanisms to ensure patient privacy, data protection, and system integrity.

Ethical Dimensions and Equity Considerations

While MIoT technologies hold potential to reduce health disparities by extending care to underserved populations, they may inadvertently exacerbate inequities by privileging those with access to digital literacy, connectivity, and financial resources. Ethical frameworks must address issues of consent, autonomy, and inclusivity. Equitable benefit distribution requires cross-sector collaboration and policy support to bridge the digital divide and ensure inclusive healthcare transformation.

Policy and Economic Implications

The economic implications of MIoT adoption are substantial, with wearable technologies potentially reducing costs by preventing complications, minimizing hospital readmissions, and enabling remote care. However, sustainable integration requires healthcare worker training and retraining, alignment of reimbursement models, regulatory compliance, and digital infrastructure investment. Policymakers must balance innovation and cost savings with patient safety, supporting flexible yet rigorous frameworks that encourage technological advancement while protecting public interest and ensuring equitable access to emerging healthcare technologies.

Future Directions and Concluding Reflections

Despite remarkable progress, several challenges persist and require sustained attention. Longitudinal clinical studies validating MIoT intervention efficacy remain limited, device proliferation has led to care fragmentation with unresolved interoperability issues across platforms and electronic health record systems, and data security vulnerabilities pose ongoing threats. Moreover, collaboration among clinicians, engineers, data scientists, and policymakers remains insufficient, limiting the integration of diverse expertise required for holistic solutions.

Future directions must prioritize interdisciplinary research, standardized protocols, robust cybersecurity measures, and equity-focused policies. Integration of artificial intelligence and machine learning with MIoT offers opportunities for predictive analytics, precision dosing, and evidence-informed decision-making, while global standardization remains critical to ensure benefits are widely distributed and ethically aligned with societal values.

The MIoT represents both extraordinary opportunity and profound responsibility in healthcare transformation. Its potential to revolutionize patient care through improved access, continuous monitoring, personalized interventions, and enhanced system sustainability is evident. Yet deployment requires careful navigation of ethical, legal, financial, and social complexities. This volume does not present MIoT as a panacea but as a field of immense potential that must be critically engaged, rigorously studied, and responsibly governed.

By bringing together scholarship from diverse disciplines, this book aims to inform academic discourse, guide research agendas, and support evidence-informed decision-making in healthcare innovation. Through interdisciplinary collaboration and evidence-based approaches, MIoT can contribute to building a healthcare future that addresses contemporary challenges while advancing the fundamental mission of medicine: improving human health and well-being for all populations, regardless of geographic location, economic status, social identity, or demographic characteristics.

The editors express their gratitude to the contributors whose expertise and dedication have made this volume possible. It is our hope that the insights contained herein will inspire further inquiry and collaboration, and support the collective endeavor of building a healthcare future that is not only technologically advanced but also equitable, sustainable, and genuinely patient-centered.

Sydney, NS, Canada — Philip Eappen
Blagoevgrad, Bulgaria — Narasimha Rao Vajjhala
Pocatello, ID, USA — Ruiling Guo
Sydney, NS, Canada — Virginia Gunn

Acknowledgments

We are honored to present *Remote Monitoring and Wearable Devices in Healthcare*, a collaborative effort shaped by the collective expertise, dedication, and vision of an international team of contributors. This book reflects not only technological advancement but also a shared commitment to building a more responsive, inclusive, and intelligent healthcare system for the future.

I would like to express my deepest gratitude to all those who made this project possible. To my fellow editors—*Dr. Narasimha Rao Vajjhala*, *Dr. Ruiling Guo*, and *Dr. Virginia Gunn*—thank you for your collegiality, thoughtful insights, and unwavering support throughout this journey. Your leadership has enriched this work and ensured its relevance across diverse healthcare contexts.

To the contributing authors, your time, knowledge, and scholarship have given this book its substance. I am grateful to each of you for contributing chapters that explore not only technical innovation but also the ethical, social, and clinical dimensions of wearable technologies in healthcare. Your diverse perspectives and rigorous scholarship have created a comprehensive resource that will serve researchers, practitioners, and policymakers alike.

I extend heartfelt appreciation to the institutions and organizations that supported this endeavor. Your encouragement, resources, and belief in the importance of this project were essential to its completion.

Most importantly, I am deeply grateful to my family, whose love and support made this journey possible. To my beloved wife *Figgi*, who stood by me with unwavering patience and understanding during countless hours of writing and research—your strength and encouragement sustained me throughout this process. To my precious son *Evan*, whose innocent questions about "Daddy's book" reminded me daily of the importance of this work for future generations. To my dear mother *Baby*, whose prayers and belief in me have been a constant source of comfort and motivation.

I am thankful to my sister, brothers-in-law, niece, and nephew whose supportive calls and messages provided much-needed encouragement during challenging moments, and to my wonderful in-laws, who embraced this project as their own and offered their blessings at every step. To my cherished niece and nephew, who bring joy and perspective to our family—you remind us that our work in healthcare is ultimately about creating a better world for you and your generation.

This book is lovingly dedicated to the memory of my late father, *Eappen*, whose profound wisdom, unwavering integrity, and compassionate spirit continue to illuminate my path. His belief that knowledge should serve humanity and his dedication to helping others have shaped not only who I am but also the very essence of this work. Through these pages, his legacy lives on, inspiring all of us who strive to advance healthcare and improve the lives of patients and communities around the world.

Philip Eappen

Contents

About the Editors

Philip Eappen is an accomplished healthcare executive, academic, and researcher currently serving as Assistant Professor in the Department of Professional Studies, School of Nursing; Adjunct Faculty in Healthcare Management, Shannon School of Business at Cape Breton University; and Associate Scientist with the Maritime SPOR SUPPORT Unit. With over a decade of experience spanning hospital operations, healthcare education, and strategic leadership, he has consistently advanced innovation and excellence across diverse healthcare systems in Canada, the United States, and internationally.

Dr. Eappen's clinical leadership experience includes progressive roles at the Breton Ability Centre in Sydney, Nova Scotia, where he advanced to Director of Clinical Services and Transition to Community, leading person-centered care initiatives and community transition services. His academic career encompasses appointments at the University of Toronto, Southern Alberta Institute of Technology, and Fanshawe College. Internationally, he served as Director of Health Services and Chief Administrator of Healthcare Operations at the American University of Nigeria, where he spearheaded clinical transformation, emergency preparedness, and inclusive health initiatives, including programs supporting survivors of Boko Haram abductions.

Dr. Eappen holds a Doctorate in Healthcare Administration and Postgraduate Certificate in International Health from Central Michigan University, complemented by an MBA in Healthcare Management and Bachelor of Nursing. He has developed and taught curricula across undergraduate and graduate levels in healthcare leadership, innovation, and health systems analytics, while leading the program development of Cape Breton University's Master of Healthcare Innovation and Leadership program.

An active contributor to national and global health dialogues, Dr. Eappen serves on the boards of the American College of Healthcare Executives, Myeloma Canada, Aplastic Anemia and Myelodysplasia Canada, and the Network of Rare Blood Disorder Organizations (NRBDO). He chairs research and ethics committees, reflecting his commitment to governance, evidence-based practice, and health equity.

Dr. Eappen has published extensively on artificial intelligence in healthcare, digital health transformation, and health workforce development. His recent editorial work includes *Healthcare Informatics Innovation Post COVID-19 Pandemic* (Taylor & Francis). He has presented at major international conferences including ICN 2025, ICIMTH, and INTED. As a Certified Health Executive (CHE) through the Canadian College of Health Leaders and Fellow candidate of the American College of Healthcare Executives (FACHE), Dr. Eappen continues pursuing the highest standards of professional excellence in healthcare leadership. His research agenda focuses on digital innovation, rare diseases, and global workforce integration, continuing to shape policy, practice, and pedagogy in healthcare management.

Narasimha Rao Vajjhala is a distinguished academic and researcher currently serving as Professor and Chair of the Department of Computer Science at the American University in Bulgaria (AUBG). With over two decades of experience in higher education, Dr. Vajjhala has held senior academic leadership positions, including Dean of the Faculty of Engineering and Architecture at the University of New York Tirana (UNYT), Albania, and Chair of Computer Science and Software Engineering programs at the American University of Nigeria (AUN).

Throughout his career, Dr. Vajjhala has taught a comprehensive range of undergraduate and graduate courses in computer science, database systems, and programming across institutions in Europe and Africa. He serves as Editor-in-Chief of the *International Journal of Risk and Contingency Management* (IJRCM) and maintains active membership as a Senior Member of both the Association for Computing Machinery (ACM) and the Institute of Electrical and Electronics Engineers (IEEE), as well as membership in the Project Management Institute (PMI).

Beyond academia, Dr. Vajjhala has provided technology consulting services for various European firms and participated in numerous EU-funded research and innovation projects. He holds a Doctorate in Information Systems and Technology from the United States, an MSc in Computer Science and Applications from India, and an MBA with specialization in Information Systems from Switzerland. His interdisciplinary expertise spans computer science, information systems, and project management, with significant contributions to research, education, and industry practice across international contexts.

Ruiling Guo is a Professor of Healthcare Administration at Idaho State University's College of Business, where she teaches graduate and undergraduate courses in healthcare administration. She holds a graduate faculty appointment in Idaho State University's Graduate School, serving on dissertation and thesis committees for doctoral and graduate students in medicine, health sciences, and health professions.

Dr. Guo earned her Doctor of Health Administration (DHA) from Central Michigan University and brings extensive expertise in healthcare systems and management both domestically and internationally. Her research interests encompass evidence-based management in healthcare decision-making, healthcare policy, health information science and technology, population health, and comparative health systems.

Her professional service includes membership on the Board of Directors of the Association of University Programs in Health Administration (AUPHA) and the Editorial Board of *Healthcare Executive*, published by the American College of Healthcare Executives. Dr. Guo serves as an external reviewer for AUPHA Undergraduate Program Certification, a site reviewer for the Commission on Accreditation of Healthcare Management Education, a Fellow of the Center for Evidence-Based Management, and a Distinguished Member of the Academy of Health Information Professionals. She contributes as a peer reviewer for multiple academic journals in medicine, health sciences, and healthcare administration.

Dr. Guo has received multiple research grants and awards from the National Institutes of Health and the National Library of Medicine. In 2025, she was awarded a Fulbright Specialist grant by the US Department of State and the Fulbright Foreign Scholarship Board, completing her Fulbright research project as Visiting Professor at the University of Malta.

Her scholarly work appears in peer-reviewed journals including the *American Journal of Management*, *International Journal of Healthcare Management*, *Leadership in Health Services*, *Journal of Health Administration Education*, *Journal of Community Health*, *Hospital Topics*, *Journal of American College Health*, *Journal of Medical Informatics*, and the *Chinese Journal of Ophthalmology*. She has co-authored several book chapters and co-edited two books on healthcare systems, healthcare management, and health informatics.

Virginia Gunn is an Associate Professor in the School of Nursing at Cape Breton University and an Affiliate Researcher at the Unit of Occupational Medicine, Institute of Environmental Medicine, Karolinska Institute, Sweden. As a public health researcher with interdisciplinary training in health and social sciences, Dr. Gunn earned her doctoral and master's degrees from the Lawrence Bloomberg Faculty of Nursing and completed a Collaborative Doctoral Specialization in Global Health from the Dalla Lana School of Public Health, University of Toronto.

Dr. Gunn combines her academic background with extensive professional experience as a health practitioner, with expertise spanning public health, acute care, and long-term care settings. She has assumed various leadership roles—including project lead, committee chair, board director, finance officer, and co-founder of interest groups—through which she has spearheaded initiatives to improve health systems and promote evidence-informed decision-making.

As a dedicated researcher, Dr. Gunn maintains an active record of engagement in international, national, and regional projects and collaborations. Her established research program examines the intersection of advanced technologies, including artificial intelligence, with social determinants of health—particularly employment, migration, and gender—and their role in shaping health inequities. Through this work, she contributes to understanding how technological advancement can address or exacerbate existing health disparities in diverse populations.

Chapter 1
Wearable Devices in Healthcare: Transforming Healthcare and Facilitating Personalized Patient-Centered Care Delivery

Philip Eappen, Virginia Gunn, Narasimha Rao Vajjhala, and Ruiling Guo

Introduction

Wearable devices have emerged as vital tools in healthcare provision, enabling personalized monitoring and proactive care management within and outside hospitals [21]. These technologies, ranging from simple consumer smartwatches to sophisticated biomedical sensors, offer continuous monitoring of physiological parameters, facilitating preventive healthcare measures and early intervention strategies [13, 15, 22]. Moreover, the increasing prevalence of chronic diseases [24] and aging populations across the globe [36] requires innovative healthcare solutions that advance patient engagement, enhance patient outcomes, improve care accessibility, and manage healthcare costs effectively. Wearable devices, equipped with advanced sensors capable of tracking diverse health metrics including heart rate, activity levels, sleep patterns, glucose levels, and more, provide invaluable data for patients and healthcare providers [43]. Their potential to empower patients through self-monitoring and active health engagement represents a fundamental shift from traditional reactive healthcare models toward proactive, personalized care approaches [33]. This chapter explores the complex landscape of wearable technology in healthcare,

P. Eappen (✉) · V. Gunn
Cape Breton University, School of Nursing, Sydney, NS, Canada
e-mail: philip_eappen@cbu.ca; virginia_gunn@cbu.ca

N. R. Vajjhala
American University in Bulgaria, Blagoevgrad, Bulgaria

University of New York Tirana, Tirana, Albania
e-mail: narasimharao@unyt.edu.al

R. Guo
Idaho State University, Business Administration, Pocatello, ID, USA
e-mail: ruilingguo@isu.edu

P. Eappen et al. (eds.), *Advancing Healthcare with the Medical Internet of Things*, Health Informatics, https://doi.org/10.1007/978-3-032-23933-4_1

analyzing device functionality, applications across various health contexts, implementation and user challenges, and future potential in reshaping healthcare delivery. Special attention is given to wearables' transformative role in enabling personalized care delivery and revolutionizing chronic disease management, patient-provider communication, and care delivery models.

Definition and Classification of Wearable Devices

Wearable devices range from simple to sophisticated electronic technologies designed for comfortable, continuous body-worn use. These devices have gained widespread adoption across healthcare domains due to their ability to collect real-time health data, enabling personalized healthcare management and evidence-informed clinical decision-making. The classification of wearable devices is based on their functionalities, target applications, and degree of technological sophistication.

Types of Wearable Devices

Fitness Trackers: These consumer-grade devices serve different purposes including the monitoring of physical activities, sleep patterns, and general fitness metrics. They are valuable in promoting healthy lifestyles and encouraging physical activity through gamification and goal-setting features [21]. Modern fitness trackers incorporate advanced algorithms for activity recognition, providing users with comprehensive insights into their daily movement patterns and exercise habits.

Smartwatches: Beyond basic fitness tracking capabilities, smartwatches provide integrated communication features, including notifications, calls, and convenient application access that enhance daily activity management. Contemporary smartwatches often include sophisticated health-monitoring features such as pulse monitoring, single lead electrocardiogram (ECG) readings designed to detect certain irregular heart rhythms, and blood oxygen saturation measurement, positioning them as valuable health monitoring tools [48, 51], notwithstanding several limitations regarding the type of hearth conditions they can detect and consistent measurement accuracy [48].

Medical-Grade Wearables: These promising and revolutionary specialized technological devices are specifically designed for clinical applications; they are equipped with advanced noninvasive, on-body sensors for monitoring or interpreting (i) specific health conditions, including cardiovascular disease, diabetes, and neurological disorders and (ii) other data related to health status and symptom patterns

[54]. Medical wearables can take many forms; examples include continuous glucose monitors (CGMs) for diabetes management, wearable ECG monitors for cardiac arrhythmia detection, and ambulatory blood pressure monitors for hypertension management [4].

Smart Clothing: This innovative category incorporates sensors directly into textile materials, offering comfortable, unobtrusive continuous health monitoring. Smart clothing is particularly valuable for applications requiring long-term monitoring, especially in elderly care, rehabilitation settings, and sports medicine, where traditional devices might be cumbersome or restrictive [46].

Biosensors: These advanced technological devices measure specific biological signals or biomarkers, including glucose levels, lactate concentrations, and various metabolites. They provide real-time physiological insights crucial for chronic disease management and clinical decision support [49]. Advanced biosensors can detect multiple biomarkers simultaneously, showing potential to offer a comprehensive health status assessment.

The Transformative Impact of Wearable Devices in Healthcare and Role in Facilitating Personalized Patient-Centered Care Delivery

Wearable devices hold significant potential for revolutionizing healthcare delivery through improved patient engagement, real-time monitoring capabilities, and data-driven clinical insights. Their applications extend across diverse health contexts, offering unique advantages for patients, healthcare providers, and health systems.

Given a wide range of wearable devices available to choose from, it is becoming easier for health workers to personalize their care delivery and center it around the needs of their patients. For instance, the selection of monitoring devices used is often done to fit patient preferences, lifestyles, and budgets. Similarly, since wearables allow for certain health symptom monitoring and follow-up to be done outside of health settings and outside of prescribed health institution or health worker schedules, such health-related activities are now increasingly centered on patients' convenience and availability. Moreover, a high number of user-friendly applications are available to users to enable patients' convenient access to recorded metrics and sharing of such data with health providers. Further, patients' active engagement with wearable technologies increases the likelihood that they will participate alongside health professionals in the development of personalized care plans, and, as a result, find it easier to adhere to such plans in the long term.

Empowering Patients Through Active Engagement

Wearable devices transform the patient experience by enabling individuals to have increased control over their health through continuous self-monitoring and engagement. By providing users with real-time feedback on health metrics, these devices have potential to enhance adherence to treatment regimens and motivate sustainable lifestyle changes [33]. This capability is vital for achieving health-related behavior modifications, encouraging users to maintain healthier lifestyles, and effectively manage chronic conditions. Furthermore, the psychological benefits of health-monitoring devices are profound, providing users with a sense of control and ownership over their health conditions [5, 18]. This empowerment is crucial for enhancing treatment compliance, particularly among older adults who may feel disconnected from traditional healthcare processes [19]. Modern wearable devices incorporate intelligent recommender frameworks—a type of information organizing system based on algorithms that use synthesized data about previous behaviors and outcomes—that support individuals in making informed health decisions, ensuring patients and healthcare providers benefit from personalized recommendations and insights [39]. In addition, wearable devices can detect early signs of health deterioration, thus, possibly enabling timely interventions and preventing complications. The continuous monitoring allows for identifying subtle changes in health status that might otherwise be missed during periodic clinical visits, supporting proactive healthcare management. Despite fewer in-person interactions, improved patient-provider rapport is achieved through seamless data sharing, which provides healthcare professionals with critical insights into patient behaviors and health-related needs [10].

Enhancing Healthcare Delivery and Clinical Practice

Integrating wearable devices into patient care workflows in clinical settings enables healthcare providers to continue to monitor patients remotely, even after they complete their stay in a health setting or follow-up with a health professional, thus potentially enhancing care quality and delivery efficiency. Real-time health data facilitates more informed clinical decision-making, thus improving patient outcomes and enabling personalized treatment approaches [38]. Moreover, wearable devices facilitate enhanced communication between patients and healthcare providers, particularly as healthcare delivery increasingly incorporates telehealth solutions. These devices generate actionable health data that enhances telehealth consultation quality, providing healthcare professionals with comprehensive insights into patient behaviors, adherence patterns, and health trends between visits. Integration of this data into electronic health records allows for comprehensive tracking of patient health, which is vital for proactive care management. For instance, wearable ECG monitors can detect cardiac arrhythmias in high-risk patients, prompting timely medical interventions and potentially reducing emergency department visits and hospitalizations [32, 51]. Furthermore, as demonstrated during the COVID-19 pandemic, remote monitoring solutions have become essential in enabling healthcare delivery while minimizing in-person interactions [4].

Transforming Chronic Disease Management

Wearable devices are pivotal in managing chronic conditions such as diabetes, cardiovascular disease, and respiratory disorders. Ongoing research demonstrates that continuous glucose monitors and heart rate trackers significantly enhance self-management capabilities among patients with chronic illnesses [10, 21, 38, 45, 49, 53]. Devices monitoring heart rates and physical activity levels foster proactive health management, with potential to enable individuals to adjust behaviors in real time based on physiological feedback. Furthermore, data from systematic reviews highlight wearable devices' effectiveness in disease management, noting their role in facilitating timely medical interventions [27, 28]. Wearables equipped with heart rhythm monitoring functions demonstrate potential for reducing hospital admissions among patients with atrial fibrillation through early detection of irregular rhythms and prompt medical response [40, 53]. Unsurprisingly, wearable devices are valuable for managing chronic conditions and preventing the onset of additional complications associated with these diseases.

Cost Reduction and Healthcare Economics

Through proactive monitoring and early intervention capabilities, wearable devices can significantly reduce healthcare costs by decreasing hospital visits, admissions, and readmissions [43]. By enabling continuous monitoring, healthcare providers can proactively manage chronic conditions, and thus, contribute to fewer disease complications and reduced healthcare expenditures. In addition, early identification and self-management of health issues by individuals, facilitated by wearables, shows strong potential for improved health outcomes, ultimately reducing the economic burden on healthcare systems [1, 2, 6, 29, 31, 35]. The shift from reactive to proactive care models supported by wearable technology represents a fundamental change in healthcare economics, supporting prevention and earlier intervention over costly emergency interventions.

Implementation Challenges and Barriers

Despite the numerous advantages of wearable technology in healthcare, several significant challenges can hinder widespread adoption and effective implementation across diverse healthcare settings.

Data Privacy and Security Concerns

Data privacy and security are paramount concerns in healthcare, especially with the increasing use of wearable devices that continuously collect sensitive health information. The risk of data breaches poses threats not only to patient confidentiality but also to trust in healthcare providers and technology adoption rates [4]. Adherence to regulatory frameworks such as the Health Insurance Portability and Accountability Act (HIPAA) protects patient data against unauthorized access and misuse [11]. Healthcare providers must implement robust cybersecurity measures to safeguard patient information stored and transmitted through wearable devices. Ensuring adequate storage solutions, such as fog computing architectures, can better handle massive health data influxes while preserving patient privacy, which is critical for sustainable implementation [56]. Furthermore, artificial intelligence (AI) can play a multifaceted role in fortifying healthcare cybersecurity, focusing on safeguarding patient data, ensuring regulatory compliance, and maintaining operational stability [13–16].

Integration into Clinical Practice

Integrating wearable devices into existing healthcare systems presents significant challenges due to infrastructural and logistical limitations. Healthcare professionals often lack the necessary training to interpret wearable-generated data and incorporate it effectively into clinical practices [11], reflecting a larger health informatics training deficit in healthcare that negatively impacts health workers' capacity to capitalize on existing health technologies [14]. Clear protocols and guidelines are needed to assist practitioners with using data collected through wearable devices in clinical decision-making. Established clinical workflows may require substantial redesign to accommodate the continuous data streams produced by wearable devices. Healthcare systems must evolve to ensure providers are adequately trained to utilize and protect captured data effectively, requiring significant investments in education, infrastructure, and workflow optimization [34]. Standard operating protocols and appropriate reimbursement models must be established to manage data generated from wearable devices effectively [44].

Patient Acceptance and Usability Barriers

Patient acceptance of wearable technology is influenced by multiple factors, including associated cost, ease of use, perceived value, trust in technology, and demographic characteristics [8]. Higher costs associated with more sophisticated wearable devices or the upfront investments required could act as a deterrent to their acceptance by certain population groups [50]. Elderly or less technologically savvy individuals may resist adopting wearable devices due to apprehension about new technologies or anxiety surrounding their use [7]. Furthermore, the complexity of wearable devices could deter older adults from engaging with technology that could significantly benefit their health [19]. Companies developing wearable devices must prioritize user-centered designs and conduct extensive usability testing to ensure products are accessible and engaging for all demographic groups, particularly vulnerable populations who might benefit most from continuous monitoring [43].

Regulatory and Reimbursement Challenges

Existing regulatory frameworks covering consumer devices may not adequately address the rapid evolution of wearable technology. Depending on their classification as medical devices or consumer electronics, wearables face varying levels of scrutiny before market approval [33]. Regulatory bodies must develop guidelines specific to wearable technologies that ensure safety and efficacy while fostering innovation. Standard operating protocols and appropriate reimbursement models need to be established to manage data generated from wearable devices effectively. The healthcare—including health insurance—payment systems must evolve to recognize and compensate (i) patients buying wearable devices for health purposes and (ii) health workers and institutions for remote monitoring services and data interpretation, thus, creating sustainable business models for widespread adoption [9, 41].

Healthcare Provider Resistance

Resistance among healthcare providers to integrate new technologies into practice presents significant barriers to the increased use of health informatics, including wearable devices, thus requiring a clear understanding of contributing factors [14]. A common reason mentioned by health workers is insufficient training [14]. It is essential that healthcare workers must be equipped with the necessary resources and training to be able to embrace technological advancements, ensuring they can maximize potential patient benefits [12, 14]. Other reasons explaining health workers' resistance often stem from concerns about increased workload, data interpretation challenges, fear of privacy breaches and the unethical use of collected data, or disruption to established practice patterns [14]. Further, the consequences of the increased use of wearable devices for patient care for health workers' health, well-being, and working conditions are not yet well understood [22]. Additionally, while the literature discussing the potential of wearables to improve health outcomes is constantly expanding, the body of empirical evidence linking the use of wearable devices to improved patient and health system outcomes is currently in its early stages [38], partly due to a range of methodological, legal, and operational challenges faced by researchers studying this field [30].

Future Directions and Emerging Trends

The future of wearable devices in healthcare appears promising, with technological advancements paving the way for enhanced applications and greater integration into clinical practice across diverse healthcare settings.

Enhanced Capabilities Through Artificial Intelligence and Machine Learning

AI and machine learning (ML) offer exciting prospects not only for the strengthening of cybersecurity in healthcare [13] but also for augmenting wearable device capabilities [35]. By employing advanced algorithms to analyze health data, providers can gain deeper insights into patient conditions, which is crucial for early detection of health problems and early planning or implementation of intervention strategies [3]. Furthermore, machine learning models can identify patterns and correlations in patient data that human providers might overlook, ultimately leading to improved health outcomes and personalized health management approaches [42]. AI integration enables predictive analytics, allowing for anticipatory care interventions before clinical symptoms manifest. For instance, ML models can predict survival outcomes using wearable actigraphy data among end-stage cancer patients [27, 28, 55].

Expanding Uses and Applications

As health technologies evolve, the breadth of uses and applications for wearable devices continues expanding across healthcare domains. For instance, wearables are increasingly utilized in mental health monitoring, rehabilitation medicine, new types of chronic disease management, and elderly care [49]. They provide versatile platforms for healthcare professionals to monitor patients in diverse settings, thus enabling the adoption of novel proactive care strategies across the continuum of care.

Wearables have the potential to provide care for underserved populations, expand care delivery in low-resource settings, and reduce disparities in healthcare access [25]. Developing cost-effective, culturally appropriate wearable solutions can democratize health-monitoring capabilities globally. Additionally, wearables show promising potential in specialized areas such as cancer care delivery and prognostic assessment among hospice patients [27, 28].

Telehealth Integration and Remote Care

Integrating telehealth and wearable devices redefines healthcare service delivery models [46]. Specifically, remote patient monitoring through wearables enhances telehealth consultations, allowing providers to access real-time data during virtual visits. In turn, this integration enables more comprehensive assessments and informed clinical decisions during remote encounters. Empowering patients to share wearable-generated data with healthcare teams leads to better informed clinical decisions and greater patient satisfaction. The synergy between telehealth and wearable technologies has potential to create more efficient and effective healthcare delivery models, particularly valuable for managing chronic conditions and providing care to geographically dispersed populations. The COVID-19 pandemic has accelerated this integration, demonstrating the essential role of remote monitoring in maintaining healthcare continuity [4].

Interoperability and Standardization

Future developments must focus on improving interoperability between different wearable devices and healthcare systems. Standardization of data formats, communication protocols, and integration standards will facilitate seamless data exchange and comprehensive health record maintenance [47]. The development of universal health data standards will enable better coordination between multiple wearable devices, electronic health records, and clinical decision support systems, creating comprehensive digital health ecosystems. This includes integrating IoT-based health monitoring systems for real-time monitoring and control capabilities [17, 26].

Conclusion

Wearable devices represent a transformative force in modern healthcare, fundamentally altering patient management and care delivery through continuous monitoring and data-driven insights. Their ability to empower patients, enhance healthcare quality, and reduce costs marks a significant global health management shift within healthcare systems. Successful implementation and integration of wearables into healthcare practices depend on systematically addressing challenges related to data privacy, clinician training, patient acceptance, regulatory compliance, and reimbursement structures. As healthcare systems evolve to accommodate these technologies, the focus must remain on ensuring equitable access, maintaining privacy and security, and optimizing clinical workflows to maximize benefits for all stakeholders.

Furthermore, wearable technology with artificial intelligence, telehealth platforms, and integrated care models promise to create more personalized, efficient, and proactive healthcare delivery systems [37]. Future research into effective integration strategies, ethical frameworks, and user engagement will be pivotal in leveraging the full potential of wearable devices to improve health outcomes across diverse populations [47].

As technology advances, the potential applications of wearable devices in healthcare will likely expand further, enabling innovative care approaches that are more efficient, patient-centered, and anticipatory. The transformation of healthcare through wearable technology represents not just technological advancement, but a fundamental reimagining of the relationship between patients, providers, and health data in pursuit of optimal health outcomes for individuals and populations worldwide [52]. The future of healthcare lies in the seamless integration of wearable technology into comprehensive care models that prioritize prevention, early intervention, and patient empowerment. By addressing current challenges and capitalizing on emerging opportunities, wearable devices will continue to play an increasingly central role in creating sustainable, effective, and accessible healthcare systems for the twenty-first century and beyond.

References

1. Al-Khafajiy M, Baker T, Chalmers C, Asim M, Kolivand H, Fahim M, Waraich A. Remote health monitoring of elderly through wearable sensors. Multimed Tools Appl. 2019;78(17):24681–706. https://doi.org/10.1007/s11042-018-7134-7.
2. Almansour HAH, Almanajam FA, Alyami MA, Al-Mahamad AHS, Al Zabid NHS, Al-Mahamad MSH, Al Hammam HNY, Al Matif MY, Almansour MA, Almansour AHM, Al Mansour SMS. Evaluating the impact of wearable health devices on mental health outcomes: a collaborative study between psychologists, social workers, and nursing staff. J Int Crisis Risk Commun Res. 2024;7(S9):103. https://doi.org/10.63278/jicrcr.vi.282.
3. Arueyingho O, Al-Taie A, McCallum C. Scoping review: machine learning interventions in the management of healthcare systems. Digital Health. 2024;10. https://doi.org/10.1177/20552076221144095.

4. Azodo I, Williams R, Sheikh A, Cresswell K. Opportunities and challenges surrounding the use of data from wearable sensor devices in health care: qualitative interview study. J Med Internet Res. 2020;22(10):e19542. https://doi.org/10.2196/19542.
5. Babar F, Cheema A, Ahmad Z, Sarfraz A, Sarfraz Z, Ashraff H, et al. Sensitivity and specificity of wearables for atrial fibrillation in elderly populations: a systematic review. Curr Cardiol Rep. 2023;25(7):761–79. https://doi.org/10.1007/s11886-023-01898-3.
6. Beniczky S, Wiebe S, Jeppesen J, Tatum WO, Brazdil M, Wang Y, et al. Automated seizure detection using wearable devices: a clinical practice guideline of the international league against epilepsy and the International Federation of Clinical Neurophysiology. Clin Neurophysiol. 2021;132(5):1173–84.
7. Chen J, Wang T, Fang Z, Wang H. Research on elderly users' intentions to accept wearable devices based on the improved UTAUT model. Front Public Health. 2023;10. https://doi.org/10.3389/fpubh.2022.1035398.
8. Chong K, Guo J, Deng X, Woo B. Consumer perceptions of wearable technology devices: retrospective review and analysis. JMIR Mhealth Uhealth. 2020;8(4):e17544. https://doi.org/10.2196/17544.
9. Coye MJ, Haselkorn A, DeMello S. Remote patient management: technology-enabled innovation and evolving business models for chronic disease care. Health Aff. 2009;28(1):126–35. https://doi.org/10.1377/hlthaff.28.1.126.
10. Dias D, Cunha JPS. Wearable health devices—vital sign monitoring, systems and technologies. Sensors. 2018;18(8):2414. https://doi.org/10.3390/s18082414.
11. Dinh-Le C, Chuang R, Chokshi S, Mann D. Wearable health technology and electronic health record integration: scoping review and future directions. JMIR Mhealth Uhealth. 2019;7(9):e12861. https://doi.org/10.2196/12861.
12. Doekhie KD, Buljac-Samardžić M, Strating MMH, Paauwe J. Elderly patients' decision-making embedded in the social context: a mixed-method analysis of subjective norms and social support. BMC Geriatr. 2020;20(1). https://doi.org/10.1186/s12877-020-1458-7.
13. Eappen P, Gunn V, Brar HS, Stedman I. Capitalizing on the transformative role of AI and human capital to strengthen cybersecurity in healthcare: safeguarding patient data and advancing regulatory compliance. In: AI-enabled threat intelligence and cyber risk assessment. CRC Press; 2025. p. 112–25. https://doi.org/10.1201/9781003504979-7.
14. Eappen P, Parker Davidson K, MacLeod M, Cousins A, Gunn V. Global healthcare informatics – structural considerations and workforce training challenges and solutions. In: Eappen P, Vajjhala NR, editors. Healthcare informatics innovation post Covid-19 pandemic. 1st ed. Routledge, Taylor and Francis & CRC Press; 2025.
15. Eappen P, Stedman I, Gunn V. Transforming healthcare: the role of health informatics and provider perspectives. In: Vajjhala NR, Martiri E, Dalipi F, Yang B, editors. Artificial intelligence in healthcare information systems—security and privacy challenges. Springer; 2025. p. 205–22. https://doi.org/10.1007/978-3-031-84404-1_11.
16. Eappen P, Vajjhala NR, Zikos D, Davidson KP, editors. Remote monitoring and wearable devices in healthcare. Springer; 2025.
17. Elias JR, Chard R, Libera JA, Foster I, Chaudhuri S. The manufacturing data and machine learning platform: enabling real-time monitoring and control of scientific experiments via IoT. In: 2020 IEEE 6th world forum on internet of things (WF-IoT); 2020. p. 1–2. https://doi.org/10.1109/wf-iot48130.2020.9221078.
18. Elkefi S, Asan O. Wearable devices' use in geriatric care between patient-centeredness and psychology of patients. Proc Int Symp Hum Factors Ergon Health Care. 2022;11(1):125–8. https://doi.org/10.1177/2327857922111025.
19. Farivar S, Abouzahra M, Ghasemaghaei M. Wearable device adoption among older adults: a mixed-methods study. Int J Inf Manag. 2020;55:102209. https://doi.org/10.1016/j.ijinfomgt.2020.102209.
20. Grote T, Berens P. On the ethics of algorithmic decision-making in healthcare. J Med Ethics. 2020;46(3):205–11. https://doi.org/10.1136/medethics-2019-105586.

21. Guk K, Han G, Lim J, Jeong K, Kang T, Lim E, Jung J. Evolution of wearable devices with real-time disease monitoring for personalized healthcare. Nanomaterials. 2019;9(6):813. https://doi.org/10.3390/nano9060813.
22. Gunn V, Eappen P, Brar HS, Brulin E, Muntaner C. Integration of wearable devices in healthcare: the need to examine their implications for health workers. In: Eappen P, Vajjhala NR, Zikos D, Davidson KP, editors. Remote monitoring and wearable devices in healthcare. Springer; 2025. p. 101–18. https://doi.org/10.1007/978-3-031-98897-4_6.
23. Guo R, Zhu J, Cai M, He W, Yang Q. Toward privacy-preserving directly contactable symptom-matching scheme for IoT devices. Electronics. 2023;12(7):1641. https://doi.org/10.3390/electronics12071641.
24. Hacker K. The burden of chronic disease. Mayo Clin Proc Innov Qual Outcomes. 2024;8(1):112–9. https://doi.org/10.1016/j.mayocpiqo.2023.08.005.
25. Hawley S, Haymart M. The potential of wearable devices in cancer care delivery. JAMA Oncol. 2024;10(5):573. https://doi.org/10.1001/jamaoncol.2024.0001.
26. Ho C, Hana J, Park S. IoT based health monitoring system - recent trends and directions. Geron. 2022;21:1–1. https://doi.org/10.4017/gt.2022.21.s.524.pp1.
27. Huang Y, Kabir M, Upadhyay U, Dhar E, Uddin M, Syed-Abdul S. Exploring the potential use of wearable devices as a prognostic tool among patients in hospice care. Medicina. 2022;58(12):1824. https://doi.org/10.3390/medicina58121824.
28. Huang Y, Upadhyay U, Dhar E, Kuo L, Syed-Abdul S. A scoping review to assess adherence to and clinical outcomes of wearable devices in the cancer population. Cancer. 2022;14(18):4437. https://doi.org/10.3390/cancers14184437.
29. Islam MM, Mahmud S, Muhammad LJ, Islam MR, Nooruddin S, Ayon SI. Wearable technology to assist the patients infected with novel coronavirus (COVID-19). SN Comput Sci. 2020;1:1–9. https://doi.org/10.1007/s42979-020-00335-4.
30. Izmailova ES, Wagner JA, Perakslis ED. Wearable devices in clinical trials: hype and hypothesis. Clin Pharmacol Ther. 2018;104(1):42–52. https://doi.org/10.1002/cpt.966.
31. Jo A, Coronel BD, Coakes CE, Mainous AG III. Is there a benefit to patients using wearable devices such as Fitbit or health apps on mobiles? A systematic review. Am J Med. 2019;132(12):1394–400. https://doi.org/10.1016/j.amjmed.2019.06.018.
32. Kamga P, Mostafa R, Zafar S. The use of wearable ECG devices in the clinical setting: a review. Curr Emerg Hosp Med Rep. 2022;10(3):67–72. https://doi.org/10.1007/s40138-022-00248-x.
33. Kang H, Exworthy M. Wearing the future—wearables to empower users to take greater responsibility for their health and care: scoping review. JMIR Mhealth Uhealth. 2022;10(7):e35684. https://doi.org/10.2196/35684.
34. Laplante PA, Kassab M, Laplante N, Voas J. Building caring healthcare systems in the internet of things. IEEE Syst J. 2018;12(3):3030–7. https://doi.org/10.1109/jsyst.2017.2662602.
35. Lu L, Zhang J, Xie Y, Gao F, Xu S, Wu X, Ze Z. Wearable health devices in health care: narrative systematic review. JMIR Mhealth Uhealth. 2020;8(11):e18907. https://doi.org/10.2196/18907.
36. Maresova P, Javanmardi E, Barakovic S, Barakovic Husic J, Tomsone S, Krejcar O, Kuca K. Consequences of chronic diseases and other limitations associated with old age–a scoping review. BMC Public Health. 2019;19(1):1431.
37. Margam R. The promising future of wearable technology in healthcare industry. Rev Contemp Sci Acad Stud. 2023;3(7). https://doi.org/10.55454/rcsas.3.07.2023.006.
38. Mattison G, Canfell O, Forrester D, Dobbins C, Smith D, Töyräs J, et al. The influence of wearables on health care outcomes in chronic disease: systematic review. J Med Internet Res. 2022;24(7):e36690. https://doi.org/10.2196/36690.
39. Nia M, Kazemi M, Valmohammadi C, Abbaspour G. Wearable IoT intelligent recommender framework for a smarter healthcare approach. Libr Hi Tech. 2021;41(4):1238–61. https://doi.org/10.1108/lht-04-2021-0151.
40. Nuvvula S, Ding E, Saleeba C, Shi Q, Wang Z, Kapoor A, et al. Nexus-heart: novel examinations using smart technologies for heart health—data sharing from commercial wearable devices and telehealth engagement in participants with or at risk of atrial fibrillation. Cardiovasc Digit Health J. 2021;2(5):256–63. https://doi.org/10.1016/j.cvdhj.2021.08.001.

41. Oderanti FO, Li F, Cubric M, Shi X. Business models for sustainable commercialisation of digital healthcare (eHealth) innovations for an increasingly ageing population. Technol Forecast Soc Chang. 2021;171:120969. https://doi.org/10.1016/j.techfore.2021.120969.
42. Rahmani A, Yousefpoor E, Yousefpoor M, Mehmood Z, Haider A, Hosseinzadeh M, Ali Naqvi R. Machine learning (ML) in medicine: review, applications, and challenges. Mathematics. 2021;9(22):2970. https://doi.org/10.3390/math9222970.
43. Ranganathan C, Katthula V, Moustakas E. Patterns of use and key predictors for the use of wearable health care devices by US adults: insights from a national survey. J Med Internet Res. 2020;22(10):e22443. https://doi.org/10.2196/22443.
44. Rosman L, Lampert R, Zhuo S, Li Q, Varma N, Burg MM, et al. Wearable devices, health care use, and psychological well-being in patients with atrial fibrillation. J Am Heart Assoc. 2024;13(15). https://doi.org/10.1161/jaha.123.033750.
45. Sharma A, Mahajan P, Singh A, Arya S. Detection of physiological markers via wearable devices for human healthcare. ECS Trans. 2022;107(1):20265–74. https://doi.org/10.1149/10701.20265ecst.
46. Sivaraman H. IoT-enabled healthcare monitoring: a systematic review of wearable devices. Inf Technol Indus. 2019;7(3):78–86. https://doi.org/10.17762/itii.v7i3.815.
47. Smuck M, Odonkor C, Wilt J, Schmidt N, Swiernik M. The emerging clinical role of wearables: factors for successful implementation in healthcare. NPJ Digit Med. 2021;4(1). https://doi.org/10.1038/s41746-021-00418-3.
48. Strik M, Ploux S, Weigel D, van der Zande J, Velraeds A, Racine HP, Ramirez FD, Haïssaguerre M, Bordachar P. The use of smartwatch electrocardiogram beyond arrhythmia detection. Trends Cardiovasc Med. 2024;34(3):174–80. https://doi.org/10.1016/j.tcm.2022.12.006.
49. Tam W, Alajlani M, Abd-Alrazaq A. An exploration of wearable device features used in UK hospital Parkinson disease care: scoping review. J Med Internet Res. 2023;25:e42950. https://doi.org/10.2196/42950.
50. Tanaka M, Ishii S, Matsuoka A, Tanabe S, Matsunaga S, Rahmani A, Dutt N, Rasouli M, Nyamathi A. Perspectives of Japanese elders and their healthcare providers on use of wearable technology to monitor their health at home: a qualitative exploration. Int J Nurs Stud. 2024;152:104691. https://doi.org/10.1016/j.ijnurstu.2024.104691.
51. Tran H, Urgessa N, Geethakumari P, Kampa P, Parchuri R, Bhandari R, et al. Detection and diagnostic accuracy of cardiac arrhythmias using wearable health devices: a systematic review. Cureus. 2023. https://doi.org/10.7759/cureus.50952.
52. Venn R, Khurshid S, Grayson M, Ashburner J, Al-Alusi M, Chang Y, et al. Characteristics and attitudes of wearable device users and nonusers in a large health care system. J Am Heart Assoc. 2024;13(1). https://doi.org/10.1161/jaha.123.032126.
53. Wang L, Nielsen K, Goldberg J, Brown JR, Rumsfeld JS, Steinberg BA, et al. Association of wearable device use with pulse rate and health care use in adults with atrial fibrillation. JAMA Netw Open. 2021;4(5):e215821. https://doi.org/10.1001/jamanetworkopen.2021.5821.
54. Xu S, Kim J, Walter JR, Ghaffari R, Rogers JA. Translational gaps and opportunities for medical wearables in digital health. Sci Transl Med. 2022;14(666):eabn6036.
55. Yang T, Kuo P, Huang Y, Lin H, Malwade S, Lu L, et al. Deep-learning approach to predict survival outcomes using wearable actigraphy device among end-stage cancer patients. Front Public Health. 2021;9. https://doi.org/10.3389/fpubh.2021.730150.
56. Yousefpour A, Fung C, Nguyen TN, Kadiyala K, Jalali F, Niakanlahiji A, et al. All one needs to know about fog computing and related edge computing paradigms: a complete survey. J Syst Archit. 2019;98:289–330. https://doi.org/10.1016/j.sysarc.2019.02.009.

Chapter 2
Could Wearable Devices Strengthen the Provision of Primary Care?

Virginia Gunn, Philip Eappen, Hikmat Singh Brar, Emma Brulin, and Carles Muntaner

Introduction

The continuous development and refinement of health technologies in recent years has the potential to restructure the provision of health care [19, 34, 37, 42, 76, 80]. Wearable devices, an example of health technologies, could empower individuals to enjoy better health through (i) improved monitoring of health data and real-time ongoing feedback [68, 72, 78], which could facilitate healthier lifestyle choices, speedier diagnoses, and earlier treatments, (ii) increased engagement and ownership of health symptom tracking and proactive health issue management [9, 52, 60, 72], and (iii) better care and enhanced access to health services considering that care could be offered more conveniently to those in remote locations [4, 53, 85].

V. Gunn (✉)
Cape Breton University, Sydney, NS, Canada

Unit of Occupational Medicine, Institute of Environmental Medicine, Karolinska Institute, Stockholm, Sweden
e-mail: Virginia_gunn@cbu.ca

P. Eappen · H. S. Brar
Cape Breton University, Sydney, NS, Canada
e-mail: Philip_Eappen@cbu.ca; hikmat_brar@cbu.ca

E. Brulin
Unit of Occupational Medicine, Institute of Environmental Medicine, Karolinska Institute, Stockholm, Sweden
e-mail: emma.brulin@ki.se

C. Muntaner
Lawrences F. Bloomberg Faculty of Nursing & Dalla Lana School of Public Health, University of Toronto, Toronto, ON, Canada
e-mail: carles.muntaner@utoronto.ca

P. Eappen et al. (eds.), *Advancing Healthcare with the Medical Internet of Things*, Health Informatics, https://doi.org/10.1007/978-3-032-23933-4_2

Wearable devices could enhance disease management through improvements in the consistency and accuracy of health indicator monitoring across a variety of health contexts including (i) primary care, including community care settings, as detailed in this chapter, (ii) acute and urgent care [6, 39, 55, 56], and (iii) long-term, elderly, or palliative care [5, 70, 78]. Within primary care, wearables are used for a variety of reasons. For instance, individuals use wearables to keep track of health metrics, which, in turn, enables them to better self-manage signs and symptoms of diseases such as diabetes, respiratory and cardiovascular illnesses, brain disorders (e.g., epilepsy), or mental health problems [5, 12, 47, 55]. Another application of wearables in primary care is for activity recognition and classification, which refers to the identification of activities performed by individuals (e.g., walking, ascending stairs, eating, brushing teeth, washing hands, crawling, kneeling), possible through interpreting the combination of actions they perform [25]. Unsurprisingly, this function is especially valuable in supporting health monitoring and assistance for the elderly in community settings [25]. A more advanced technical use consists of IoT-enabled wearables used to facilitate remote management of patients through enabling the capturing and transmitting of real-time health monitoring data to caregivers, both professional workers and family members, to ensure uninterrupted care even when individuals are not attending clinical facilities [6, 56].

The purpose of this chapter is to discuss the potential for wearable devices to strengthen primary care. Specifically, the chapter answers the following questions: (i) Could the use of wearable devices in health care strengthen primary care? and (ii) In what ways do wearable devices reshape the provision of primary care?

Background

While there is no widely accepted definition of *primary care* [8, 50], this concept is commonly used to refer to a model of care provision that involves easily accessible, continuous, wide-ranging, comprehensive, and coordinated care that is person-centered [3, 50, 92]. Primary care is considered essential for accomplishing universal health coverage, improving health equity, and reducing health care costs [3, 7, 50]. Primary care, discussed in this chapter, is distinct from the concept of *primary health care*, which is an approach to the provision of care based on key principles such as social equity, inclusive coverage, intersectoral collaboration, and individual or community involvement and empowerment [18, 61, 90]. The concepts of primary care and primary health care are inconsistently utilized in the extant literature and, in some occasions, are used interchangeably [8].

Primary care is typically provided in primary care practices, including nurse-led clinics, which are settings serving as entry points or first points of contact into the health care system for individuals seeking initial health-related services or resources [7, 13, 50, 79]. Primary care practices could include health offices, inpatient or outpatient units, critical or long-term care, home care, or telehealth [7], along with community settings such as schools, colleges or universities, workplaces, assisted living for the elderly or others needing support with daily activities, churches, prisons, or individuals' homes [15, 25, 54, 86]. Community settings are defined by the Ottawa Charter as the places or contexts where individuals participate in everyday activities, situated at the intersection of diverse factors that affect an individual's health and wellbeing [15, 88, 89]. The provision of primary care could be done by various health professionals including (i) primary care physicians with training in health disciplines such as family medicine, internal medicine, or general pediatrics; (ii) non-primary care physicians focusing on health maintenance, disease prevention, acute or chronic care, or rehabilitation; (iii) nurse practitioners; or (iv) other clinicians providing interprofessional care as part of collaborative health care teams [7, 66]. Such clinicians could involve nurses, physician assistants, or allied health professionals such as dieticians, social workers, councilors, or physiotherapists [21, 66].

Primary care practitioners (e.g., physicians, nurse practitioners, etc.) address a wide range of issues including undiagnosed health concerns along with a focus on health promotion and maintenance, illness prevention, health counselling, patient education, diagnosis, treatment, referrals, and advocacy [7, 64]. There are many specific examples of primary care provision including preventive care, the provision of routine care, urgent care for minor or common health issues, mental health care, prenatal care, child care, home care, psychosocial services, nutrition counselling, or end-of-life care [21, 84]. In addition to being available in person, most primary care services are increasingly offered virtually via phone, email, application messaging, or other communication technologies [21, 31], thus, potentially increasing service accessibility for individuals benefiting from access to such technologies and decreasing costs for health systems and individual users [23]. An additional advantage of primary care services is their potential to support individuals and health systems with avoiding unscheduled visits to emergency departments for health conditions that could be addressed in the community through primary care, in person, or virtual [22]. Given its numerous advantages including its potential to support the achieving of universal health coverage, improved health equity, and health cost reduction [3, 7], a wide range of strategies to strengthen the provision of primary care are commonly explored and implemented [23, 35], and numerous health systems around the world [11, 14, 75] as well and international institutions, including the World Health Organization, are committed to improving primary care [88, 90, 92].

Wearable devices are commonly referred to as non-invasive technological devices that are designed to be worn by individuals either on a continuous or a sporadic basis [52]. Sometimes called wearables, they serve a large range of purposes as reviewed earlier [6, 10, 28], could take many forms [41, 44], and represent varying degrees of technological development, from basic devices [55, 60] to highly advanced ones [69, 74]. Examples of wearable devices include glucose sensors, smartwatches, smart glasses, sensor-based skin patches, fitness trackers, or bodily sensors. Within health care, most wearable devices are currently designed for patient use; however, the number of devices designed for health worker use is steadily increasing [42]. Unsurprisingly, the increased availability of wearable devices, their relatively low cost, and very wide range of applications all have the potential to transform the provision of health care by increasing the use of health services outside of acute care settings such as hospitals. In turn, reducing the use of acute health services and strengthening the provision of primary care may enhance the sustainability of health systems and improve population health through facilitating increased access to care for underserved individuals and populations including those living in rural areas or other areas with insufficient availability of basic or specialized health services.

Potential of Wearable Devices to Strengthen Primary Care

A continuously increasing body of evidence examining wearable devices suggests that wearable devices present great potential to strengthen primary care. Specifically, as summarized next, wearable devices could do so through (i) improved access to care when integrated as components of a larger health ecosystem; (ii) enhanced opportunities for engagement in health promotion and maintenance activities; (iii) modernized and streamlined data collection when data is accurate, reliable, and relevant; (iv) better data sharing and integration across individuals seeking care, health professionals, and services; and (v) cost savings through prevention, early intervention, reduced complications, or limited need for in-person visits.

Improved Access to Care When Integrated as Components of a Larger Health Ecosystem

Several studies investigating the role of wearables and provision of remote health services in strengthening primary care focus explicitly on access to care [4, 6, 20, 38, 53, 68, 85], showing positive outcomes through reduced wait times [20] and elimination of physical barriers (e.g., distance to facilities) [6, 38], which used to disadvantage individuals living in remote locations or in locations with low density of health centers. There is generally a sense of optimism that the widespread adoption of wearables in primary care may facilitate the quicker achievement of the Sustainable Development Goal 3, aimed at enabling *healthy lives and well-being* for individuals and populations across the whole age spectrum [48].

As expected, given that typically access to wearables is not equal among individuals and groups [1, 81], improvements in access to care will also be unequal, which could, in turn, worsen health inequities [27]. Additionally, despite numerous advantages, wearables on their own could not make up for insufficient health settings (e.g., hospitals, clinics), limited financial resources to run them, or shortages of qualified health workers. A sufficient supply of workers is needed to support people maintain or regain their health [43, 46, 91]. Consequently, wearables should not be seen as a replacement for well-funded health systems that provide access to expert health professionals and services; instead, they should be planned and integrated as components of a larger health ecosystem [73]. Further, as is the case with other health technologies, their actual impact should be properly evaluated to assess if they are indeed improving health care outcomes [59] and access to care.

Enhanced Opportunities for Engagement in Health Promotion and Maintenance Activities

Wearables are believed to enhance opportunities for engaging in health promotion and maintenance through enabling the (i) monitoring of modifiable risk factors commonly linked to chronic diseases [45] and (ii) earlier diagnosis and treatment among at risk individuals and groups, which could, in turn, prevent a vast range of health issues and complications linked to premature morbidity and mortality [83]. Additionally, cost-effective wearables are deemed to enhance opportunities for individuals with less resources to connect not only with health care providers but with their social networks, including families, friends, and informal caregivers, who could support their health promotion and maintenance activities (information about healthy lifestyles, diagnosis, treatment, and recovery) [83]. Equally important is the affordable cost of many commonly used wearables, which are produced on a large scale and are often reusables, thus, making it easier for populations who do not benefit from high incomes or universal health systems to access such health tools [83].

While engagement in health promotion and maintenance activities is obviously important, a preoccupation with certain health metrics without placing them in the larger health or wellbeing context could inadvertently minimize the importance of providing holistic patient care. Additionally, the social determinants of health (e.g., income, employment, housing, or access to food), known as the root causes of ill health and health inequities, require high-level intervention [62, 63, 87] and are, thus, not improved through the use of wearables. Consequently, wearable devices remain limited in the role they could play in improving individual and population health. Placing the onus of responsibility on individuals to stay healthy through the use of improved monitoring and health behaviors resembles behavioral approaches to health and victim blaming [49].

Modernized and Streamlined Data Collection When Data Is Accurate, Reliable, and Relevant

The non-invasive design, widespread applications, relative ease of use, often-affordable cost, along with their capacity to collect and store data remotely and conveniently (either continuously or intermittently), according to individual need, make wearables a modern and streamlined tool of real-time data collection for individuals who need to monitor their health metrics outside of traditional health settings such as clinics or hospitals [27, 53, 67, 69, 93]. As a result, individuals are able to gain insight into a wider range of health indicators than ever before which may, in turn, enable them an easier engagement in preventative care, health maintenance, and health treatments, all with potential to improve health outcomes [67].

Needless to say, not all individuals have access to steadfast Internet connections or benefit from access to health systems equipped with cutting-edge technological infrastructures and sufficient integration of wearables within digital networks [24]. Accordingly, this modern method of health metric monitoring or collection may not be equally available across individuals and groups. Additionally, unless wearables provide consistently accurate readings and recordings of health metrics (Gonçalves et al.), they could not be considered reliable health tools [67] and may cause more harm than benefits. Another consideration must be given to the amount of data collected by wearables, which could be difficult to handle, interpret, or protect by individuals or health professionals alike, thus requiring comprehensive collection, interpretation, ethical storage, and use of standards and guidelines [2, 30, 40].

Better and Protected Data Sharing and Integration Across Individuals Seeking Care, Health Professionals, and Services

Given that wearables are often integrated with electronic health records, they have the potential to facilitate better data sharing among health professionals and across services throughout the continuum of care, which could, in turn, improve accuracy of health monitoring and decision-making [26] and, thus, improve health outcomes. Additionally, the integration of data collected by wearable devices with electronic health records and other digital platforms could provide health professionals with opportunities to proactively identify health issues and increase communication with individuals seeking care and their families to devise and implement personalized care plans that take advantage of primary care services [73].

However, the enhanced sharing and integration of data brings several challenges and requires stringent strategies to ensure protection of data privacy and improved system interoperability to avoid burdening workers with solving technical data transfer issues [2, 26, 29, 33]. Furthermore, wearable devices that are not user-centric or designed with input from those they target may result in poor user experiences and incorrect or inconsistent usage of these health tools, which may limit their benefits [55, 73, 82]. Closely related, enough resources must be allocated to the training of health workers to improve the consistent and correct application of health technologies [16, 32, 58], including wearables. Additionally, while there is evidence that the use of wearables may decrease health workers' workloads [65, 71], the vast amount of data collected may also increase the workload due to the added time involved in reviewing, documenting, or interpreting the data, or in some cases, helping the individuals using wearables make sense of the monitoring results [17, 36].

Cost Savings Through Prevention, Early Intervention, Reduced Complications, or Limited Need for In-Person Visits

There are several ways in which the use of wearable devices in primary care could contribute to cost cutting for individuals seeking care and for the health institutions delivering such care. First, the ongoing tracking of health metrics (e.g., pulse, blood pressure, blood glucose, etc.) and the real-time feedback afforded by such tracking may motivate individuals to engage in prevention activities including opting for healthier lifestyle behaviors or be more invested in health and well-being goals [9, 60, 72]. Second, the early identification of health problems could facilitate early intervention, reduced complications, and better outcomes, all of which could contribute to cost savings [4, 51]. Last but not least, in-person visits needed solely for the measuring of health metrics by health providers may now be eliminated, which constitutes another way of sparing resources and freeing up time for professionals to focus on other tasks. Several studies estimate that, when compared with in-person monitoring of care, remote patient monitoring for the management of chronic conditions through the use of wearables facilitates savings with comparable results [20, 57].

By and large, while there is potential for cost savings in the long run, the initial investments required by individuals and health institutions to purchase the wearable devices, the digital platforms needed for their health system integration, and the resources required to train the health professionals who will be using these devices could be significant and should not be ignored, especially since it could act as a barrier to the adoption of wearables and remote monitoring [77]. Moreover, health systems looking for cost cutting should avoid placing the responsibility for health outcome monitoring on to individuals without ensuring that such individuals have the required technologies, Internet infrastructure, and skill set to take on such tasks. Equally important is that decision-makers responsible for allocating health system budgets do not falsely assume that the costs for health metric monitoring previously needed by primary care settings can be now reduced or eliminated.

Conclusion

The increased availability of wearable devices, their relatively low cost, and very wide range of applications all have the potential to transform the provision of health care by increasing the use of health services outside of acute care settings such as hospitals. In turn, reducing the use of acute health services and strengthening the provision of primary care may enhance the sustainability of health systems and improve population health through facilitating increased access to care for underserved individuals and populations including those living in rural areas or other areas with insufficient availability of basic or specialized health services. A continuously expanding body of evidence examining wearable devices indicates that, under the right circumstances, wearable devices present great potential to strengthen primary care. Specifically, wearable devices could do so through (i) improved access to care when integrated as components of a larger health ecosystem; (ii) enhanced opportunities for engagement in health promotion and maintenance activities; (iii) modernized and streamlined data collection when data is accurate, reliable, and relevant; (iv) better data sharing and integration across individuals seeking care, health professionals, and services; and (v) cost savings through prevention, early intervention, reduced complications, or limited need for in-person visits.

References

1. Adepoju O, Dang P, Nguyen H, Mertz J. Equity in digital health: assessing access and utilization of remote patient monitoring, medical apps, and wearables in underserved communities. INQUIRY J Health Care Organ Prov Financ. 2024;61:00469580241271137.
2. Ahammed MF, Labu MR. Privacy-preserving data sharing in healthcare: advances in secure multiparty computation. J Med Health Stud. 2024;5(2):37–47.
3. Akman M, Ayhan Başer D, Usanma Koban B, Marti T, Decat P, Lefeuvre Y, Miller R. Organization of primary care. Prim Health Care Res Dev. 2022;23:e49, Article e49. https://doi.org/10.1017/S1463423622000275.
4. Al-Khafajiy M, Baker T, Chalmers C, Asim M, Kolivand H, Fahim M, Waraich A. Remote health monitoring of elderly through wearable sensors. Multimed Tools Appl. 2019;78(17):24681–706. https://doi.org/10.1007/s11042-018-7134-7.
5. Almansour HAH, Almanajam FA, Alyami MA, Al-Mahamad AHS, Al Zabid NHS, Al-Mahamad MSH, Al Hammam HNY, Al Matif MY, Almansour MA, Almansour AHM, Al Mansour SMS. Evaluating the impact of wearable health devices on mental health outcomes: a collaborative study between psychologists, social workers, and nursing staff. J Int Crisis Risk Commun Res. 2024;7(S9):103. https://doi.org/10.63278/jicrcr.vi.282.
6. Albahri OS, Albahri AS, Mohammed KI, Zaidan AA, Zaidan BB, Hashim M, Salman OH. Systematic review of real-time remote health monitoring system in triage and priority-based sensor technology: taxonomy, open challenges, motivation and recommendations. J Med Syst. 2018;42:1–27.
7. American Academy of Family Physicians. Primary care. n.d. Retrieved 21 April 2025 from https://www.aafp.org/about/policies/all/primary-care.html. Accessed 21 Apr 2025.
8. Amisi J, Downing R. Primary care research: does it defy definition? Prim Health Care Res Dev. 2017;18(6):523–6. https://doi.org/10.1017/S1463423617000652.
9. Asensio-Cuesta S, Sánchez-García Á, Conejero JA, Saez C, Rivero-Rodriguez A, García-Gómez JM. Smartphone sensors for monitoring cancer-related quality of life: app design, EORTC QLQ-C30 mapping and feasibility study in healthy subjects. Int J Environ Res Public Health. 2019;16(3):461.
10. Azodo I, Williams R, Sheikh A, Cresswell K. Opportunities and challenges surrounding the use of data from wearable sensor devices in health care: qualitative interview study. J Med Internet Res. 2020;22(10):e19542.

11. Barkley S, Starfield B, Shi L, Macinko J. Barbara Starfield and colleagues on the contribution of primary care to health systems and health (2005). In: Kidd M, Heath I, Howe A, editors. Family medicine: the classic papers, vol. 10. London: CRC Press; 2016. p. 9781315365305.
12. Beniczky S, Wiebe S, Jeppesen J, Tatum WO, Brazdil M, Wang Y, et al. Automated seizure detection using wearable devices: a clinical practice guideline of the International League Against Epilepsy and the International Federation of Clinical Neurophysiology. Clin Neurophysiol. 2021;132(5):1173–84.
13. Bispo GMB, Rodrigues EMD, Carvalho AC d O, Lisboa KW d SC, Freitas RWJF, Damasceno MMC. Assessment of access to first contact in the perspective of professionals. Rev Bras Enferm. 2020;73:e20180863.
14. Bitton A, Ratcliffe HL, Veillard JH, Kress DH, Barkley S, Kimball M, Secci F, Wong E, Basu L, Taylor C. Primary health care as a foundation for strengthening health systems in low-and middle-income countries. J Gen Intern Med. 2017;32(5):566–71.
15. Bloch P, Toft U, Reinbach HC, Clausen LT, Mikkelsen BE, Poulsen K, Jensen BB. Revitalizing the setting approach – supersettings for sustainable impact in community health promotion. Int J Behav Nutr Phys Act. 2014;11(1):118. https://doi.org/10.1186/s12966-014-0118-8.
16. Braun R, Catalani C, Wimbush J, Israelski D. Community health workers and mobile technology: a systematic review of the literature. PLoS One. 2013;8(6):e65772.
17. Bruno E, Simblett S, Lang A, Biondi A, Odoi C, Schulze-Bonhage A, Wykes T, Richardson MP, RADAR-CNS Consortium. Wearable technology in epilepsy: the views of patients, caregivers, and healthcare professionals. Epilepsy Behav. 2018;85:141–9.
18. Bryar R. Primary health care: does it defy definition? Prim Health Care Res Dev. 2000;1(1):1–2. https://doi.org/10.1191/146342300669830843.
19. Buntin MB, Jain SH, Blumenthal D. Health information technology: laying the infrastructure for national health reform. Health Aff. 2010;29(6):1214–9.
20. Campbell K, Greenfield G, Li E, O'Brien N, Hayhoe B, Beaney T, Majeed A, Neves AL. The impact of remote consultations on the quality of primary care: a systematic review. medRxiv. 2023:2023–2005.
21. Canadian Institute for Health Information. Primary care. n.d.. Retrieved 14 April 2025 from https://www.cihi.ca/en/topics/primary-care. Accessed 14 Apr 2025.
22. Canadian Institute for Health Information. Visits to the emergency department for conditions that could be managed in primary care (in person and virtual). n.d.. Retrieved 22 April 2025 from https://www.cihi.ca/en/indicators/visits-to-the-emergency-department-for-conditions-that-could-be-managed-in-primary-care-in-person. Accessed 22 Apr 2025.
23. Chapman JL, Zechel A, Carter YH, Abbott S. Systematic review of recent innovations in service provision to improve access to primary care. Br J Gen Pract. 2004;54(502):374.
24. Charkviani M, Barreto EF, Pearson KK, Amberg BM, Amundson RH, Bell SJ, Cleveland EJ, Daniels CE, Kohler CM, Leuenberger AM. Development and implementation of an acute kidney injury remote patient monitoring program. Can J Kidney Health Dis. 2023;10:20543581231192746.
25. Chaurasia SK, Reddy SRN. State-of-the-art survey on activity recognition and classification using smartphones and wearable sensors. Multimed Tools Appl. 2022:1–32.
26. Dinh-Le C, Chuang R, Chokshi S, Mann D. Wearable health technology and electronic health record integration: scoping review and future directions. JMIR Mhealth Uhealth. 2019;7(9):e12861.
27. Dobson R, Stowell M, Warren J, Tane T, Ni L, Gu Y, McCool J, Whittaker R. Use of consumer wearables in health research: issues and considerations. J Med Internet Res. 2023;25:e52444.
28. Dunn J, Runge R, Snyder M. Wearables and the medical revolution. Pers Med. 2018;15(5):429–48.
29. Eappen P, Gunn V, Brar HS, Stedman I. Capitalizing on the transformative role of AI and human capital to strengthen cybersecurity in healthcare: safeguarding patient data and advancing regulatory compliance. In: AI-enabled threat intelligence and cyber risk assessment. CRC Press; 2025. p. 112–25.

30. Eappen P, Gunn V, Stedman I. Transforming healthcare: the role of health informatics and provider perspectives. In: Vajjhala NR, Martiri E, Dalipi F, Yang B, editors. Artificial intelligence in healthcare information systems—security and privacy challenges, vol. 34. 1st ed. Springer Nature; 2025. p. 203–16. https://doi.org/10.1007/978-3-031-84404-1_11.
31. Eappen P, Olujinmi TD. Telemedicine and digital public health in pandemic times. In: Vajjhala NR, Eappen P, editors. Health informatics and patient safety in times of crisis. IGI Global; 2023. p. 118–37.
32. Eappen P, Parker Davidson K, MacLeod M, Cousins A, Gunn V. Global healthcare informatics – structural considerations and workforce training challenges and solutions. In: Eappen P, Vajjhala NR, editors. Healthcare informatics innovation post Covid-19 pandemic. 1st ed. Routledge, Taylor and Francis & CRC Press; 2025.
33. Eappen P, Stedman I, Gunn V. Transforming healthcare: the role of health informatics and provider perspectives. In: Vajjhala NR, Martiri E, Dalipi F, Yang B, editors. Artificial intelligence in healthcare information systems—security and privacy challenges. Springer Nature Switzerland; 2025. p. 203–16. https://doi.org/10.1007/978-3-031-84404-1_11.
34. Eappen P, Vajjhala NR. Healthcare informatics innovation post-Covid-19: lessons, challenges, and opportunities. In: Eappen P, Vajjhala NR, editors. Healthcare informatics innovation post Covid-19 pandemic. 1st ed. Routledge, Taylor and Francis & CRC Press; 2025.
35. Endalamaw A, Erku D, Khatri RB, Nigatu F, Wolka E, Zewdie A, Assefa Y. Successes, weaknesses, and recommendations to strengthen primary health care: a scoping review. Arch Public Health. 2023;81(1):100.
36. Fridolfsson J, Arvidsson D, Doerks F, Kreidler TJ, Grau S. Workplace activity classification from shoe-based movement sensors. BMC Biomed Eng. 2020;2:1–8.
37. Geisler E. Technology and innovation in the restructuring of healthcare delivery. Int J Healthc Technol Manag. 2001;3(2–4):111–22. https://doi.org/10.1504/IJHTM.2001.001111.
38. Glasby J, Litchfield I, Parkinson S, Hocking L, Tanner D, Roe B, Bousfield J. New and emerging technology for adult social care–the example of home sensors with artificial intelligence (AI) technology. Health Soc Care Deliv Res. 2023;11:1.
39. Gluck S, Lee-anne SC, Chapman MJ, Iwashyna TJ, Deane AM. A scoping review of use of wearable devices to evaluate outcomes in survivors of critical illness. Crit Care Resusc. 2017;19(3):197–204.
40. Goodyear VA. Social media, apps and wearable technologies: navigating ethical dilemmas and procedures. Qual Res Sport, Exerc Health. 2017;9(3):285–302.
41. Guk K, Han G, Lim J, Jeong K, Kang T, Lim E-K, Jung J. Evolution of wearable devices with real-time disease monitoring for personalized healthcare. Nanomaterials. 2019;9(6):813.
42. Gunn V, Eappen P, Singh Brar H, Brulin E, Muntaner C. Integration of wearable devices in healthcare: the need to examine their implications for health workers. In: Eappen P, Rao Vajjhala N, Zikos D, Parker Davidson K, editors. Remote monitoring and wearable devices in healthcare. Springer Nature; 2025. p. 103–21. https://link.springer.com/chapter/10.1007/978-3-031-98897-4_6.
43. Gunn V, Somani R, Muntaner C. Health care workers and migrant health: pre- and post-COVID-19 considerations for reviewing and expanding the research agenda. J Migr Health. 2021;4(100048):1–8. https://doi.org/10.1016/j.jmh.2021.100048.
44. Hariharan U, Rajkumar K, Akilan T, Jeyavel J. Smart wearable devices for remote patient monitoring in healthcare 4.0. In: Internet of medical things: remote healthcare systems and applications. Springer Nature; 2021. p. 117–35.
45. Harris MT. Addressing gaps in equity through wearables. PhD thesis. Urbana: University of Illinois at Urbana-Champaign; 2022. https://www.ideals.illinois.edu/items/126800.
46. International Council of Nurses. Policy brief – the global nursing shortage and nurse retention. Geneva: International Council of Nurses; 2021.
47. Islam MM, Mahmud S, Muhammad LJ, Islam MR, Nooruddin S, Ayon SI. Wearable technology to assist the patients infected with novel coronavirus (COVID-19). SN Comput Sci. 2020;1:1–9. https://doi.org/10.1007/s42979-020-00335-4.

48. Izu L, Scholtz B, Fashoro I. Wearables and their potential to transform health management: a step towards Sustainable Development Goal 3. Sustainability. 2024;16(5):1850.
49. Jancey J, Barnett L, Smith J, Binns C, Howat P. We need a comprehensive approach to health promotion. Health Promot J Austr. 2016;27(1):1–3.
50. Jimenez G, Matchar D, Koh GCH, Tyagi S, van der Kleij RMJJ, Chavannes NH, Car J. Revisiting the four core functions (4Cs) of primary care: operational definitions and complexities. Prim Health Care Res Dev. 2021;22:e68, Article e68. https://doi.org/10.1017/S1463423621000669.
51. Jo A, Coronel BD, Coakes CE, Mainous AG III. Is there a benefit to patients using wearable devices such as Fitbit or health apps on mobiles? A systematic review. Am J Med. 2019;132(12):1394–400. https://doi.org/10.1016/j.amjmed.2019.06.018.
52. Kang HS, Exworthy M. Wearing the future—wearables to empower users to take greater responsibility for their health and care: scoping review. JMIR Mhealth Uhealth. 2022;10(7):e35684.
53. Levine JA. The application of wearable technologies to improve healthcare in the world's poorest people. Technol Invest. 2017;8(2):83–95.
54. Leviton LC, Raczynski JM. Interventions in community settings. In: Boll TJ, Frank RG, Baum A, Wallander JL, editors. Handbook of clinical health psychology: models and perspectives in health psychology, vol. 3. American Psychological Association; 2004. p. 501–48. https://doi.org/10.1037/11590-015.
55. Lu L, Zhang J, Xie Y, Gao F, Xu S, Wu X, Ye Z. Wearable health devices in health care: narrative systematic review. JMIR Mhealth Uhealth. 2020;8(11):e18907. https://doi.org/10.2196/18907.
56. Mao P, Li H, Yu Z. A review of skin-wearable sensors for non-invasive health monitoring applications. Sensors. 2023;23(7):3673.
57. Marques A, Bosch P, de Thurah A, Meissner Y, Falzon L, Mukhtyar C, Bijlsma JWJ, Dejaco C, Stamm TA. Effectiveness of remote care interventions: a systematic review informing the 2022 EULAR Points to Consider for remote care in rheumatic and musculoskeletal diseases. RMD Open. 2022;8(1):e002290.
58. Mastellos N, Tran T, Dharmayat K, Cecil E, Lee H-Y, Wong CCP, Mkandawire W, Ngalande E, Wu JT-S, Hardy V. Training community healthcare workers on the use of information and communication technologies: a randomised controlled trial of traditional versus blended learning in Malawi, Africa. BMC Med Educ. 2018;18(1):61.
59. Mattison G, Canfell O, Forrester D, Dobbins C, Smith D, Töyräs J, Sullivan C. The influence of wearables on health care outcomes in chronic disease: systematic review. J Med Internet Res. 2022;24(7):e36690. https://doi.org/10.2196/36690.
60. Mirmomeni M, Fazio T, von Cavallar S, Harrer S. From wearables to THINKables: artificial intelligence-enabled sensors for health monitoring. In: Wearable sensors. Elsevier; 2021. p. 339–56.
61. Muldoon LK, Hogg WE, Levitt M. Primary care (PC) and primary health care (PHC) what is the difference? Can J Public Health. 2006;97(5):409–11. https://doi.org/10.1007/BF03405354.
62. Muntaner C, Benach J. Why social (political, economic, cultural, ecological) determinants of health? Part 1: background of a contested construct. Int J Soc Determinants Health Health Serv. 2023;53(2):117–21.
63. Muntaner C, Finn Mahabir D, Gunn V. Social determinants of health. In: Oxford bibliographies in public health; 2017. https://doi.org/10.1093/OBO/9780199756797-0150.
64. Oswald N, Bateman H. Treating individuals according to evidence: why do primary care practitioners do what they do? J Eval Clin Pract. 2000;6(2):139–48.
65. Pavithra LS, Khurdi S. Impact of remote patient monitoring systems on nursing time, healthcare providers, and patient satisfaction in general wards. Cureus. 2024;16(6):e61646.
66. Peters AL. The changing definition of a primary care provider. Ann Intern Med. 2018;169(12):875–6. https://doi.org/10.7326/M18-2941.
67. Piwek L, Ellis DA, Andrews S, Joinson A. The rise of consumer health wearables: promises and barriers. PLoS Med. 2016;13(2):e1001953.

68. Prieto-Avalos G, Cruz-Ramos NA, Alor-Hernandez G, Sánchez-Cervantes JL, Rodriguez-Mazahua L, Guarneros-Nolasco LR. Wearable devices for physical monitoring of heart: a review. Biosensors. 2022;12(5):292.
69. Sakphrom S, Limpiti T, Funsian K, Chandhaket S, Haiges R, Thinsurat K. Intelligent medical system with low-cost wearable monitoring devices to measure basic vital signals of admitted patients. Micromachines. 2021;12(8):918.
70. Sandic Spaho R, Uhrenfeldt L, Fotis T, Kymre IG. Wearable devices in palliative care for people 65 years and older: a scoping review. Digit Health. 2023;9:20552076231181212.
71. Serrano LP, Maita KC, Avila FR, Torres-Guzman RA, Garcia JP, Eldaly AS, Haider CR, Felton CL, Paulson MR, Maniaci MJ. Benefits and challenges of remote patient monitoring as perceived by health care practitioners: a systematic review. Perm J. 2023;27(4):100.
72. Sharma A, Badea M, Tiwari S, Marty JL. Wearable biosensors: an alternative and practical approach in healthcare and disease monitoring. Molecules. 2021;26(3):748.
73. Smuck M, Odonkor CA, Wilt JK, Schmidt N, Swiernik MA. The emerging clinical role of wearables: factors for successful implementation in healthcare. NPJ Digit Med. 2021;4(1):1–8.
74. Sreenilayam SP, Ahad IU, Nicolosi V, Brabazon D. MXene materials based printed flexible devices for healthcare, biomedical and energy storage applications. Mater Today. 2021;43:99–131.
75. Starfield B, Shi L, Macinko J. Contribution of primary care to health systems and health. Milbank Q. 2005;83(3):457–502. https://doi.org/10.1111/j.1468-0009.2005.00409.x.
76. Stoumpos AI, Kitsios F, Talias MA. Digital transformation in healthcare: technology acceptance and its applications. Int J Environ Res Public Health. 2023;20(4):3407.
77. Tanaka M, Ishii S, Matsuoka A, Tanabe S, Matsunaga S, Rahmani A, Dutt N, Rasouli M, Nyamathi A. Perspectives of Japanese elders and their healthcare providers on use of wearable technology to monitor their health at home: a qualitative exploration. Int J Nurs Stud. 2024;152:104691. https://doi.org/10.1016/j.ijnurstu.2024.104691.
78. Teixeira E, Fonseca H, Diniz-Sousa F, Veras L, Boppre G, Oliveira J, Pinto D, Alves AJ, Barbosa A, Mendes R. Wearable devices for physical activity and healthcare monitoring in elderly people: a critical review. Geriatrics. 2021;6(2):38.
79. Terry D, Hills D, Bradley C, Govan L. Nurse-led clinics in primary health care: a scoping review of contemporary definitions, implementation enablers and barriers and their health impact. J Clin Nurs. 2024;33(5):1724–38. https://doi.org/10.1111/jocn.17003.
80. Vajjhala NR, Eappen P. Smart health: advancements in machine learning and the Internet of Things solutions. In: Samui P, Sekhar Roy S, Zhang W, Taguchi YH, editors. Machine learning and IoT applications for health informatics. CRC Press; 2024. p. 31–51.
81. Venn RA, Al-Alusi M, Ashburner JM, Atlas S, Chang Y, Ellinor PT, Foulkes A, Grayson M, Khurshid S, McManus D. The WATCH-IT study: wearable device use among primary care and cardiology patients in a large healthcare system. Circulation. 2022;146(Suppl_1):A11018.
82. Volpato L, del Río Carral M, Senn N, Santiago Delefosse M. General practitioners' perceptions of the use of wearable electronic health monitoring devices: qualitative analysis of risks and benefits. JMIR Mhealth Uhealth. 2021;9(8):e23896.
83. Walter JR, Xu S, Rogers JA. From lab to life: how wearable devices can improve health equity. Nat Commun. 2024;15(1):123.
84. Way D, Jones L, Baskerville B, Busing N. Primary health care services provided by nurse practitioners and family physicians in shared practice. CMAJ: Can Med Assoc J = journal de l'Association medicale canadienne. 2001;165(9):1210–4.
85. West DM. Improving health care through mobile medical devices and sensors. Brookings Inst Policy Rep. 2013;10(9):1–13.
86. Whitelaw S, Baxendale A, Bryce C, MacHardy L, Young I, Witney E. 'Settings' based health promotion: a review. Health Promot Int. 2001;16(4):339–53. https://doi.org/10.1093/heapro/16.4.339.

87. WHO Commission on Social Determinants of Health & World Health Organization. Closing the gap in a generation: health equity through action on the social determinants of health: Commission on Social Determinants of Health final report. World Health Organization; 2008. https://www.who.int/publications/i/item/9789241563703.
88. World Health Organization. The Ottawa charter for health promotion: first international conference on health promotion, Ottawa, 21 November 1986. Geneva: World Health Organization; 1986.
89. World Health Organization. Health promotion glossary. Geneva: World Health Organization; 1998.
90. World Health Organization. Implementing the primary health care approach: a primer. World Health Organization; 2024.
91. World Health Organization. Health and care workforce planning tools: a rapid review (9240106278). 2025. https://www.who.int/publications/i/item/9789240106277.
92. World Health Organization. Integrated primary care for universal health coverage (UHC). n.d. Retrieved 21 April 2025 from https://www.who.int/teams/integrated-health-services/clinical-services-and-systems/primary-care. Accessed 21 Apr 2025.
93. Yang L, Amin O, Shihada B. Intelligent wearable systems: opportunities and challenges in health and sports. ACM Comput Surv. 2024;56(7):1–42.

Chapter 3
Stay-Safer: An IoT-Based On-Demand Monitoring System for Elderly Assistance

Abhik Ghosh, Kaankaana Bag, Arnab Mitra, Kamalesh Karmakar, and Satyabrata Maity

Introduction

Elderly individuals are a major concern for society when they are staying or moving alone in and outside of the home. Keeping them safe is extremely important in today's world, whether they live in cities or the countryside, with or without their families. Sadly, issues like medical emergencies, falling, physical assault, theft, kidnapping, and molestation are still prevalent problems faced by weak and vulnerable individuals. Changing people's mindsets might be challenging, but technology can significantly improve the safety of these people by transmitting the information to the authorities or family members who can take necessary actions. In many of the cases, timely response is very crucial for the recovery of the people. For instance, the probability of recovering from a cardiac arrest is inversely proportional to the time taken to start the treatment from the event occurred. Henceforth, information propagation is extremely necessary for safety. Figure 3.1 describes a few instances of emergencies that may be faced by elderly people, like an elderly person requiring help during daily exercise, may require medical assistance after feeling unwell in/outside the home, may forget the way to reach the destination, or may require some assistance after falling. *Stay-Safer* is a solution that propagates the information to the required authority on-demand basis to preserve the privacy of every individual. The user is given the liberty to select the assistant like family members, neighbors, government offices like a police station or hospital, etc. With this in mind, *Stay-Safer* has been specially developed to

A. Ghosh · K. Bag · A. Mitra · K. Karmakar · S. Maity (✉)
Department of Information Technology, Techno International New Town, Kolkata, West Bengal, India
e-mail: dr.arnab.mitra@tint.edu.in; kamalesh.karmakar@tint.edu.in; dr.satyabrata.maity@tint.edu.in

P. Eappen et al. (eds.), *Advancing Healthcare with the Medical Internet of Things*, Health Informatics, https://doi.org/10.1007/978-3-032-23933-4_3

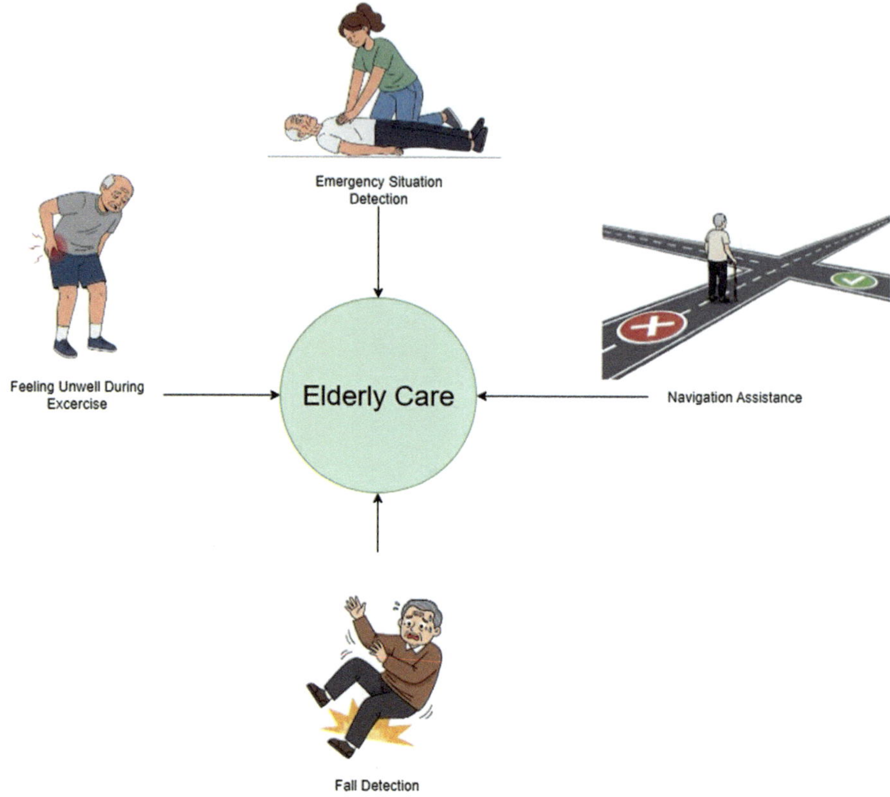

Fig. 3.1 Problems faced by elderly people during their daily activities

focus on the care the protection of the elderly, so that they do not fall victim to catastrophic accidents and crimes. The urgency of ensuring the safety and well-being of the aged individuals cannot be overstated.

Let us consider some alarming statistics about vulnerable elders to understand the need to *Stay-Safer*. In India, the senior population, aged above 60 years, is expected to rise from 137.9 million in 2021 to nearly 193.8 million by 2031, that is, a spike of almost 56 million in a decade, accounting for nearly 14% of the nation's total population, where elderly females are expected to outnumber the elderly males [1]. The seniors are reportedly experiencing a high number of medical emergencies, with a vast majority indicating that they find it difficult to access timely medical services because they have mobility problems or no immediate support. Moreover, urbanization and changes in family structure have also brought about more loneliness for the elderly, which makes them more vulnerable to mental illnesses and delayed emergency services. Over 26,110 crimes against the elderly were reported in 2021 alone, including theft, assault, and fraud—a 5.3% rise from the previous year [2]. It is very evident from the horrifying statistics that there is a greater need for a better elderly care mechanism.

While taking care of the elderly is the primary concern of *Stay-Safer*, it can be easily customized to meet the safety needs of both women and children. These two vulnerable groups are also victims of several crimes and accidents, making their security a very important issue in today's world, as already stated earlier. In major metropolitan cities like Delhi, Mumbai, Bengaluru, Hyderabad, Kolkata, Pune, and Chennai, around 70% of working women face safety concerns and yet are unable to report their problems [3]. Even as India's economy grows, incidents of sexual offenses and kidnappings remain troublingly frequent. The global Safe Cities initiative underscores the critical need to invest in local data and evidence to develop participatory safe city strategies, engaging women and girls, especially those facing multiple forms of discrimination and violence. In India, the need for better child safety measures is very clear from several important statistics. Unintentional injuries make up nearly 7.2% of all deaths among children under 14 years old [4]. In 2021 alone, there were 149,404 reported cases of crimes against children, which is about 17 crimes every hour—a 16.2% increase from the previous year. Sexual offenses are a major concern, with 36.1% of these crimes under the Protection of Children from Sexual Offenses (POCSO) Act [5]. UNICEF has played a big role in promoting childcare reforms, benefiting approximately 375,000 children in 14 states by strengthening childcare services and preventing family separation [6].

To address these issues, *Stay-Safer* plays a crucial role in capturing the crucial information from the user, assessing it to check the level of emergency, and propagating the same to the corresponding authorities, when necessary. *Stay-Safer* assures to improve current safety measures by using advanced technology for data collection, processing, and follow-up actions, a safer and smarter solution for elderly people and the society. There are a few safety applications available in the related domain as discussed below.

A. *HABITAT Project*: A smart home platform equipped with RFID, wearable electronics, and wireless sensor networks to allow the elders to live independently while also ensuring their safety and that their medical emergencies are taken care of [7].
B. *Ally Cares*: An AI-based solution that keeps track of the elder user's movements (mainly at night) and keeps the staff informed at the care homes/old age homes in England [8].
C. *Adinberri Project*: A teleassistance project, which is an initiative by the Basque Government in Pasaia, that uses IoT along with other technologies combined to predict and identify fall risks, cognitive decline, and other medical issues of the elderly individuals, who need proper attention and care [9].

Stay-Safer makes location tracking better with GPS, geofencing, and indoor positioning systems for better accuracy and precision. It uses deep learning algorithms to spot unusual patterns in travel and alert users and emergency services quickly. Additionally, it also monitors audio to detect screams or emergency words like "help" to trigger alerts automatically. *Stay-Safer* further leverages motion sensors like accelerometers and gyroscopes to detect sudden changes in the user's motion and trigger the alarm. It also provides a window of 10–20 s (user-customizable) to prevent any false alerts.

Although we found a focus on staying safe, it has been observed no such device/system is present to monitor and generate alerts in real-time for staying safe and avoiding falls. Keeping in mind all these tragic mishaps, *Stay-Safer* can actively work for the betterment of all vulnerable groups. Although designed primarily to take care of senior individuals, with its multimodal sensing and other cutting-edge technologies, *Stay-Safer* stands out as an all-rounder, coming in handy for all vulnerable groups of society.

The major contributions of this chapter are as follows.

1. IoT-Based Support and Assistive Monitoring System Design for the Elderly
2. Intelligent Emergency Detection through Multimodal Sensors and Machine Learning Approaches
3. Navigation Assistance for the Elderly with Wayfinding Challenges
4. Sound-based Abnormality Detection
5. Motion-based Abnormality Detection
6. An Extensive Safety Solution for All Vulnerable Groups

The rest of the chapter organization is as follows: a literature review is presented in section "Related Literature," the proposed solution is presented in section "Proposed Solution," the results are presented in section "Results," a brief discussion section is presented in section "Discussions" that focuses on the comparative studies on the performance of the proposed model with reference to a few existing models and the conclusions are presented in section "Conclusions."

Related Literature

A number of research works have been proposed in the related research domain to address the elderly monitoring issue to assure their safety employing the use of wearable devices, IoT framework, and machine learning model. It has been observed that with advancements in technology, caring for the elderly is now more effective with the application of smart devices with multimodal facilities. There is an increasing dependency on wearable gadgets that measure various medical parameters and give feedback in real time, ensuring that any dangerous situation is detected and taken care of promptly. Heart rate measurement, body temperature measurement, global positioning system (GPS) tracking, and fall detection are some of the common features of a modern foster care wristband.

In a recent study, as discussed in [10], the authors developed a novel wearable device comprising IoT sensors for tracking heart rate, temperature, and movement activity. An alert is sent to the caregiver's phone when any of the monitored parameters cross the preset limits. The reliability of any system in a life-threatening situation is strongly related to its ability to provide important real-time data. Also, the system has GPS tracking functionality to help find elderly patients who tend to wander away and get lost or disoriented, which is a frequent problem for dementia patients. This solution integrates cloud storage to record user data, allowing caregivers and healthcare professionals to track trends and intervene preemptively if symptoms deteriorate.

Baig et al. developed a comprehensive smart wearable solution that integrates ECG monitoring with fall detection [11]. In [11], the device employs sophisticated algorithms to distinguish between accidental falls and normal movements, significantly reducing false alarms. This innovation ensures elderly individuals maintain independence while reducing the risk of unnoticed emergencies. Furthermore, their system records past fall data to help caregivers assess risk patterns and make informed healthcare decisions. Additional features include step count analysis and oxygen level monitoring, further enhancing its applicability for comprehensive elderly care.

The HABITAT project of [7] introduced to the limelight an adaptive digital platform for smart homes that integrated IoT technologies such as Radio Frequency Identification (RFID), wearable electronics, and wireless sensor networks. In [7], an online system focused on streamlining the support of elderly citizens to enable them to live at home by incorporating smart elements into their daily use of commodities. With interoperability and adjustability of the system, uninterrupted monitoring and care can be implemented to maintain healthcare costs low while a high quality of life for users can be ensured.

Padikkapparambil et al. introduced an IoT-driven monitoring system that utilizes machine learning algorithms to analyze collected data [12]. In [12], the system predicts potential health risks by examining patterns in the elderly's daily routines and physiological trends. The caregivers can anticipate issues beforehand, which enables them to take action to minimize relevant critical incidents. In addition, healthcare professionals can supervise the patient's medical condition by accessing patient data from anywhere through cloud storage. Additionally, this system can be customized to address particular conditions, such as hypertension or cardiac risk management due to its modular structure.

An IoT-based healthcare system to improve medication adherence was developed by Awadalla et al. [13]. In [13], the system employs the use of smart pill dispensers that not only remind elderly patients to adhere to medication but also alert caregivers when doses are missed. Motion sensors also incorporate additional behavioral patterns, such as a patient being abnormally still for an extended period, and automatically notify the caregivers. This feature combination guarantees that proper proactive interventions can be made use of, thus improving elderly care outcomes. For comfort and safety purposes, the system also has smart lights and a smart heating-cooling power control system. It has become essential to utilize machine learning models in predicting behavior patterns of the elderly, fall likelihood, and critical health issues. Healthcare monitoring and early warning systems have significantly benefited from predictive analytics using machine learning technology.

Cheng et al. designed a fall detection system that uses wearable devices along with IoT-based sensors to facilitate safety monitoring for elderly people [14]. In

[14], the Motion analysis was performed with sensors like accelerometers, and gyroscopes packaged in the wearable devices themselves. It also adds the use of advanced ML algorithms like decision trees and support vector machines (SVM) for motion data analysis, where daily activities such as sitting and walking are analyzed and grouped, and falls are figured out from other activities. The system limits false alarms by analyzing the speed, angle of impact, and the length of time a person is motionless after a movement that suddenly ceases. After a fall is confirmed, notifications are sent to caregivers or emergency responders to provide necessary assistance immediately. Furthermore, the system improves over time by learning user movement patterns, so fewer corrective actions are needed.

A wide survey carried out by Karar et al. investigated IoT-fall detection systems with an emphasis on various sensors and methods employed to identify the falling of the elderly [15]. In [15], the study indicated the challenge of achieving high precision and eliminating false positives and urged for better algorithms and sensor fusion techniques in a bid to make it more reliable.

AI-oriented fall detection and motion pattern recognition system for eldercare, based on the work of Wang et al., uses accelerometers and gyroscopes combined with SVM and CNN [16]. In [16], the technology monitors live motion patterns, signaling those anomalous ones consistent with falls and notifying the caregiver of such an event. They trained the model on different sets to lower false positive amounts and accrued accuracy above the 90% mark. Research brought to light the need for personalized motion data, proposing that concerted efforts be put into increasing detection accuracy through the use of deep learning models.

Rucco et al. studied and analyzed the contribution of AI in promoting successful aging and an independent lifestyle of older adults by keeping a check on gait and balance through inertial sensors and neural networks [17]. Their solution successfully spotted early signs of imbalance and fall-prone behavior while achieving an incident prediction accuracy of 84%. The adaptive learning model personalized the gait patterns and thereby reduced misclassifications and increased predictive accuracy. It was established in [17] that falls can be prevented, and elderly community mobility enhanced through the combination of machine learning and wearable technology.

Joshi et al. created a smart home ecosystem that includes an RFID system, temperature regulators, and voice-activated emergency systems [18]. In [18], the device dynamically adjusts ambient variables to meet the elderly's comfort needs while also improving security through automated alarms and surveillance features. The system also includes door and window sensors to detect movement patterns and protect against potential invasions. The system also includes smart locks with remote control features, allowing family members to manage entrance permits for visitors and caregivers.

Saguna et al. proposed a smart home system that relies on AI for senior citizen care. They used machine learning algorithms to track day-to-day activities and identify patterns that indicate health problems or accidents in their model [19]. In [19], the system enabled real-time alerts to caregivers and offered predictive insights about deteriorating health. Their study particularly cited that system scalability and adaptability to individual health profiles were essential.

According to Abidi, the efficient system that uses multimodal data for human activity recognition with a special application of elderly care has three components: a video diagnostics unit, a sensor-based noise unit, and, finally, an artificial-intelligence-based-sensing unit for activities performed in the daily life of people [20]. Besides, artificial intelligence (AI) within care homes for the elderly is also a focus among researchers. For instance, a UK care home employed an AI system called Ally Cares, which monitors the movement of residents and notifies staff of potential health issues [8]. PainChek is another such technology that utilizes AI to detect pain in non-verbal residents through facial micro-expressions. These innovations aim to address problems such as undetected falls and varying interpretations of care, thereby enhancing the safety and welfare of older residents [21].

In Spain, the Adinberri project introduced a predictive teleassistance program aimed at the early detection of risk indicators among the elderly. With the use of AI, IoT, and big data, the project aims to detect cognitive impairment, loneliness, and fall risk, thereby improving the quality of life, autonomy, and safety of older adults at home [9]. This visionary approach is aligned with strategies that promote personalized and preventive care for the elderly.

These studies and initiatives highlight the pivotal role of IoT and AI technologies in transforming care for the elderly. They signal a trend towards preventive, personalized, and technology-driven responses to the aging population, ensuring safety and enhancing the quality of life. The summary of the state-of-the-art works with timeline, primary objectives, and the limitations are included in the Table 3.1.

The major considerations to develop a smart and effective solutions toward elderly monitoring as escalated from the study of the state-of-the-art methodologies are listed below.

- *Addressing the Elders' Requirement for Security*: The system has the objective of negating the very critical figures about safety among elderly citizens, i.e., the extremely high rate of falls and medical emergencies among individuals over the age of 65 years. Various studies have proven that nearly 26–37% of older Indians at least fall every year, leading to extended disability and even fatal injury [22, 23].
- *Smooth Integration with Wearable and Mobile Technology*: The wearable unit has GPS, motion sensors, and an audio sensing mechanism that together track the user's movement, activity, and body motion in real-time [10–14, 24]. These pieces of information are also transmitted to the mobile app in real-time, where machine learning algorithms predict and infer trends to detect probable urgencies like falls, atypical or unnatural movement, or distress calls.
- *Automated and Non-intrusive Emergency Response*: Unlike other security systems that depend on manual activation (e.g., SOS buttons), *Stay-Safer* is used automatically. In case of necessity, they alert registered emergency contacts, caregivers, or medical professionals automatically. Additionally, geofencing also keeps elderly users away from hazardous/unknown areas, thus giving them a further safety element.

Table 3.1 Summary of the state-of-the-art methodologies for elderly monitoring

System/study	Objectives	Limitations
Ally Cares (UK Care Home AI System 2025) [8]	Monitors resident movement and notifies staff of potential health issues	Reliance on accurate sensor data; potential for false alarms
Abidi (2024)—Multimodal Human Activity Recognition [20]	Combines video analysis, sensor data, and AI motion tracking; identifies activities and detects abnormalities; adapts to patterns	Requires significant processing power; potential for bias in video analysis; privacy concerns
Adinberri Project (Spain Predictive Teleassistance 2024) [9]	Detects cognitive impairment, loneliness, and fall risk; Aims to improve quality of life, autonomy, and safety	Data privacy concerns; accuracy depends on data quality and quantity
Karar et al. (2022)—IoT Fall Detection Systems (General) [15]	Aims to detect falls using various sensors and methods	Challenge of high precision; potential for false positives; needs better algorithms and sensor fusion
Awadalla et al. (2021)—IoT Medication Adherence [13]	Smart pill dispensers with reminders and missed dose alerts; motion sensors detect abnormal stillness; smart lights and heating/cooling control	Subject to malfunction, power outages, or patient override (inferred)
Joshi et al. (2014)—Smart Home Ecosystem [18]	RFID, temperature regulators, voice-activated emergency systems; dynamic adjustment of ambient variables; security (alarms, sensors, and smart locks)	Dependence on power/network; potential system failures; user training needed
Padikkapparambil et al. (2020)—IoT-Driven Monitoring System [12]	Uses machine learning to predict health risks; allows proactive intervention; remote access to data for professionals; customizable for specific conditions	Potential for algorithmic bias in predictions; reliance on accurate data input (inferred)
Saguna et al. (2020)—AI-Based Smart Home System [19]	Monitors daily activities and detects abnormal patterns; real-time alerts and predictive insights; scalable and adaptable	Potential for privacy breaches, algorithmic bias, over-reliance
Cheng et al. (2020)—Fall Detection System [14]	Accelerometers and gyroscopes track motion; machine learning distinguishes falls from daily activities; considers multiple parameters; sends alerts; adapts to user patterns	Potential for false negatives; reliance on consistent device wear
HABITAT Project (2019)—Adaptive Digital Platform for Smart Homes [7]	Integrates IoT technologies (RFID, wearables, and wireless sensors); streamlines support for elderly at home; interoperable and adjustable; maintains healthcare costs and high quality of life	Potential technology dependence; privacy concerns (inferred)

(continued)

Table 3.1 (continued)

System/study	Objectives	Limitations
Baig et al. (2019)—Smart Wearable Solution [11]	ECG monitoring and fall detection; distinguishes falls from normal movements (fewer false alarms); records past fall data for caregiver assessment; step count and oxygen level monitoring	Potential for device dependence; data privacy considerations (inferred)
Wang et al. (2019)—AI-Based Fall Detection and Motion Pattern Analysis [16]	Accelerometers and gyroscopes with SVM/CNN; real-time motion monitoring; alerts caregivers; high accuracy	Requires personalized motion data; potential for false positives; computationally expensive deep learning
Rucco et al. (2018)—AI Gait and Balance Monitoring [17]	Identifies early signs of imbalance and fall risk; adaptive learning model; predicts incidents in 84% of cases	84% accuracy leaves margin for error; requires consistent monitoring
Al Hossain et al. (2015)—Wearable Device [10]	Tracks heart rate, temperature, movement activity; alerts caregiver to out-of-range parameters; GPS tracking; cloud storage for data	System reliability depends on providing real-time data in critical situations
PainChek (AI Pain Detection System 2015) [21]	Detects pain in non-verbal residents via facial micro-expressions	Accuracy depends on facial recognition quality; may not capture all pain types

- *Enhanced Motion Sensing and Fall Alarm*: The traditional fall alarm systems use accelerometers alone, which trigger false alarms (e.g., detecting normal movement as falls).
- *Audio-Based Emergency Identification*: The intelligent device has an audio identification module that identifies calls for assistance, such as shouting out words like "help" or "danger" [25].
- *Adjustable False Alarms Prevention Alarm System*: The system allows its owner to specify an adjustable delay time interval between alarms (e.g., 10–20 s) before it triggers a panic alarm to emergency numbers. When the user cancels the alarm within a configurable time, the system considers it a false alarm. Such a system facilitates reliability without neglecting to provide attention to actual emergencies.
- *Extension to other safety issues*:
  - Women's Safety: The majority of women who reside in urban and rural areas are threatened by security daily, especially in their mobility. *Stay-Safer* can safeguard women with its geofencing, location tracking, and default SOS notifications to save emergency contacts and authorities like the police [26, 27]. The system even foresees unusual travel patterns with machine learning algorithms and sends an alert to the woman users and in case needed, her emergency numbers, if anyone is following her as a potential threat or if she is making any off-path travels.
  - Child Safety Monitoring: Parents can be assured that *Stay-Safer* will be tracking the location of the ward whenever it is convenient for them to do so that they never end up outside the pre-set safe areas (e.g., school, school-to-home

path or play area) [28]. The device would alert parents automatically on pre-defined distress signals such as abnormal motion profiles or familiar cries for help under emergent situations.

- Comparison with Other Safety Apps: The chapter is aware of the limitations of the other safety solutions for all the vulnerable groups including Ally Cares, HABITAT project, Adinberri project, We-Care and works [29]. They have some disadvantages like faulty location tracking, incapability of reaching timely response rates, and being dependent on manual activation.

Proposed Solution

Stay-Safer, an innovative and smart Internet of Things (IoT)-based system, has been designed in this chapter to improve the safety and well-being of elderly individuals or older citizens. The system combines a wearable device with a mobile application, thus offering continuous, real-time monitoring and active safety interventions. The main features in *Stay-Safer* include the following features.

- *Stay-Safer* is designed to eliminate the threats by creating a smart, automated safety system that does not need human intervention during moments of crisis.
- *Stay-Safer* includes multimodal sensing unit like GPS and motion sensors (accelerometers and gyroscopes), and an audio recognition system—to accurately identify and classify emergencies. *Stay-Safer* provides a smart and adaptive emergency detection solution through the integration of multi-modal sensing devices with advanced machine learning, which distinguishes it from existing safety solutions based mainly on human-initiated triggers and prone to generating false alarms or missing actual emergencies.
- *Stay-Safer* uses motion sensor information in conjunction with deep learning models that have been trained on real-life motion patterns. This is more precise since it identifies normal/abnormal activities, like walking, sitting, or bending, and real emergencies like sudden falls or extended periods of immobility.
- *Stay-Safer* can very well be configured to extend security protection from security threats to women and children as well and thus become a multi-purpose protection product.
- As *Stay-Safer* has machine learning-based speaker diarization and voice verification, it ensures that alerts are sent only when the user's voice is identified and not any nearby voice/sound, eliminating false alarms.
- *Stay-Safer* beats these alternatives with its promise of:
  - Enhanced location identification with GPS, geofencing, and indoor positioning
  - Enhanced detection of emergencies with intelligent motion and sound understanding
  - Hands-free automatic emergency alarms that are automatically activated without the need for the user to activate them manually

Stay-Safer is a single solution for safeguarding all vulnerable populations such as elderly people, women, and children and makes a huge contribution to public safety initiatives since it integrates multiple safety features into a single system.

Stay-Safer is a mobile-based application comprising a three-stage approach as discussed in Fig. 3.2. In the first stage, *Stay-Safer* uses location tracking and geo-fencing using a mobile GPS sensor for tracking the user. However, due to low connectivity in some regions, this may not be effective. The second stage, the application uses the motion sensor, accelerometer, and gyroscope of the mobile device to maintain the orientation of the device as well as to determine the current state of the user whether the user is walking or running, or doing some activity using deep learning. This is also used for automatic alert generation if a sudden change of movement is detected. It also increases the precision of location tracking in low-networked areas.

Stage three of the application uses the audio sensor and the mic of the mobile device to detect any emergency words like "help," etc. as well as detect screaming to trigger an alert. To avoid false alarms, the speaker voice recognition method is

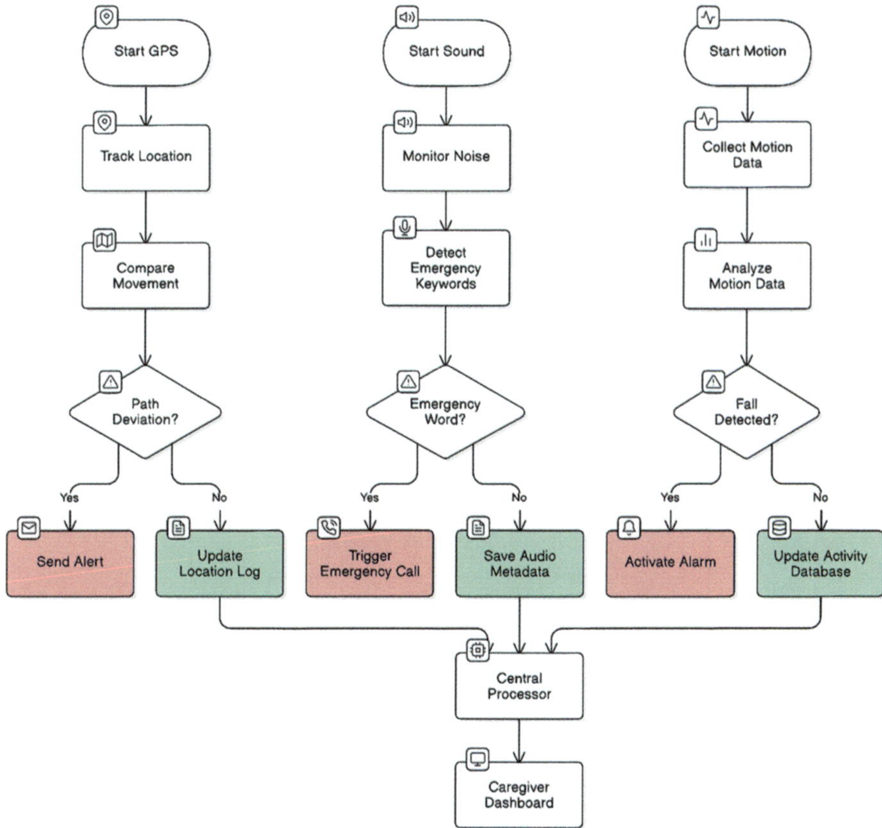

Fig. 3.2 Process flow diagram of *Stay-Safer* system architecture

also implemented so that alerts are only triggered when the app recognizes its user's voice, and it also helps in detecting multiple users in a crowd or any congested areas.

Figure 3.2 shows the flow of the IOT device for intelligent emergency detection for elderly people. The diagram is inspired by the diagram of the Smart Home System. It shows first that the sensors are initialized, then the data is collected through the sensors. A channel of communication is established between the IoT device and the phone, where all the data processing will be done. After the connection is established, the data is passed to the phone, where the data is analyzed using machine learning algorithms. If an emergency is detected, then it generates an alert to all the emergency contacts for immediate help. If no emergency is detected, then the data is updated in the system interface for future monitoring purposes.

A diagram of the system architecture follows, which describes the proposed solution and methodology in brief detail:

Stay-Safer is broadly divided into three modules: Sections "Location Information Tracker Module," "Distress Sound Detection Module," and "Abnormal Movement or Fall Detection Module," as discussed in Fig. 3.3.

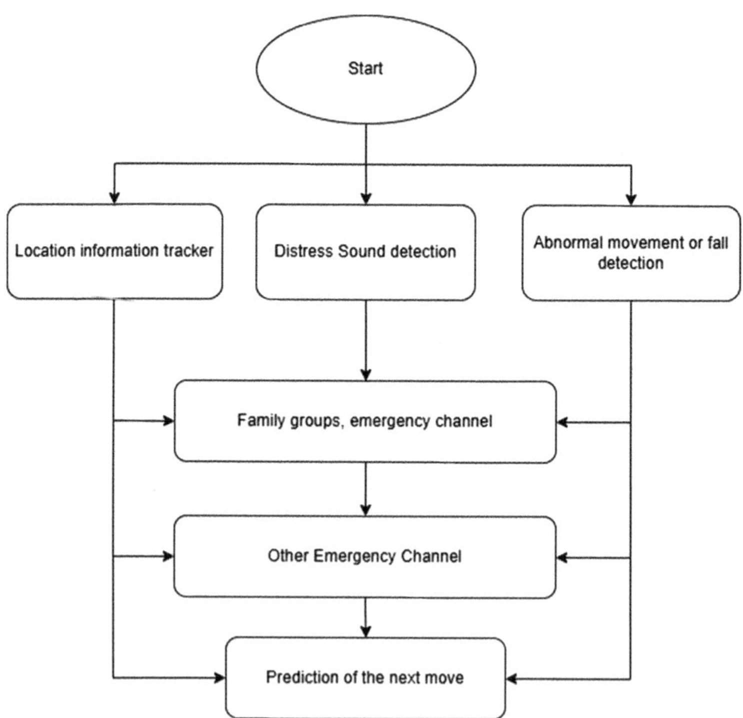

Fig. 3.3 Modular diagram of *Stay-Safer*

Location Information Tracker Module

The first module uses GPS Technology for location information tracking as shown in Fig. 3.3. It is a huge necessity for elderly care as the elderly people in our families tend to have very restricted movement, and they tend to walk down the same path for morning walks, evening walks, or grocery shopping. Hence, using GPS technology, we can easily monitor and learn from their movements, which later allows us to predict their movement after the training period is over. It uses a Long Short-Term Memory (LSTM) neural network to predict future movements based on historical GPS and motion sensor data. Initially, GPS data containing timestamps, latitude, and longitude coordinates alongside accelerometer and gyroscope data are loaded. Preprocessing is done to normalize latitude and longitude values using MinMax scaling, ensuring uniformity across the dataset. This step is pivotal for LSTM, a specialized architecture adept at handling sequential data.

For path prediction, the LSTM model takes a sequence of input positions consisting of GPS coordinates and motion data over time $t - n, t - n + 1, \ldots, t$ and predicts the position at future time steps $t + 1, t + 2, \ldots, t + k$. The output can be expressed as:

$$y_{t+k} = f\left(x_{t-n},;x_{t-n+1},;\ldots,;x_t,;W\right) \tag{3.1}$$

where:

- $x_{t-n}, \ldots, x_t$ Input sequence (e.g., past positions or features like velocity and acceleration).
- W: Trainable weight parameters of the LSTM model.
- $f(\cdot)$: Function learned by the LSTM network during training.
- y_{t+k} : Predicted position at future time step $t + k$.

The data is then fed to train the LSTM model, and sequences of historical data points are created, defined by a sequence length parameter (`SEQ_LENGTH`). The data pattern acts as input for the model. It allows the model to learn the temporal patterns as well as the dependencies in the data. The LSTM architecture of the model is comprised of two layers. Each of the layers is followed by a dropout layer to remove the overfitting from the data. Adam Optimizer is used to optimize the model. Adam Optimizer iteratively adjusts the model parameters to minimize the mean square error (MSE) loss.

Mean Squared Error (MSE) Loss Function:

$$L = \frac{1}{N}\sum_{i=1}^{N}\left(y_i - y_i\right)^2 \tag{3.2}$$

where

- N: Total number of samples.
- y_i: Actual value at time step i.
- y_i : Predicted value at time step i.

This equation minimizes the squared difference between the predicted and actual values, making it suitable for regression tasks such as path prediction.

Next, the model is trained. During the training, the LSTM model learns from historical sequences to predict the next given number of steps of latitude and longitude coordinates. The training process involves forward propagation, where input sequences propagate through the network to produce predictions. Backpropagation then computes gradients of the MSE loss for model parameters, facilitating weight updates to enhance prediction accuracy over successive epochs.

Distress Sound Detection Module

The second module is used for distress sound detection which employs speaker classification as well as speaker verification to generate an emergency alert. Speaker Diarization is a computational technique aimed at automatically identifying and dividing different speakers within an audio recording based on different features using Eq. 3.3. This is an important process during emergencies, which distinguishes and identifies the user in crowded areas and identifies the number of people around to understand the importance of the situation and the surroundings. The algorithm uses two primary methods to achieve the task. The initial segmentation uses pyAudioAnalysis and the Hidden Markov Models (HMM). Initially, the algorithm uses the pyAudioAnalysis, a tool used to analyze the audio signals. This tool examines the speech patterns within the input audio file to classify the audio file into distinct sections to represent different speakers. Then, these sections are labeled with unique identifiers with their corresponding speakers identified in the recording. It uses a powerful model trained on lots of different voices of the user to understand what makes the voice unique—things like how fast the user talks, the pitch of their voice, and other subtle details. Then, it extracts these important features to identify the user to be able to recognize whenever a new audio clip is given to the system for recognition using Eq. 3.7.

To understand the algorithm in depth, the audio sequence $O = (o_1, o_2, \ldots, o_T)$ is considered, which typically consists of feature vectors extracted from audio signals, such as Mel-Frequency Cepstral Coefficients (MFCCs). The likelihood of this sequence given the model parameters $\lambda = (A, B, \pi)$ can be expressed as:

$$P(O|\lambda) = \sum_{Q} P(O|Q,\lambda) P(Q|\lambda) \tag{3.3}$$

where

- $Q = (q1, q2, \ldots, qT)$: A sequence of hidden states representing phonemes or other linguistic units in speech recognition tasks.
- o_t: Feature vector extracted from audio data at time t.

Using the *Forward Algorithm,* the likelihood can be computed iteratively using the forward variable $\alpha_t(i)$, which represents the probability of observing the partial sequence $o_1, o_2, \ldots, o_t$ and ending in state i at time t:

$$\alpha_t(i) = P(o_1, o_2, \ldots, o_t, q_t = i | \lambda) \tag{3.4}$$

The recursive computation is:

$$\alpha_{t+1}(j) = \left[\sum_{i=1}^{N} \alpha_t(i) a_{ij}\right] b_j(o_{t+1}) \tag{3.5}$$

where:

- $a_{ij} = P(q_{t+1} = j | q_t = i)$: State transition probability.
- $b_j(o_{t+1}) = P(o_{t+1} | q_{t+1} = j)$: Observation probability, typically modelled as a Gaussian mixture model (GMM) for audio features.

Initialization:

$$\alpha_1(i) = \pi_i b_i(o_1) \tag{3.6}$$

Finally, the likelihood of the observation sequence is:

$$P(O|\lambda) = \sum_{i=1}^{N} \alpha_T(i) \tag{3.7}$$

Abnormal Movement or Fall Detection Module

The third module is employed for abnormal movement and fall detection of the user. Apart from that, it is also employed to learn the user's motion patterns and to detect falls to generate the automatic alert signal in emergencies. The data is then processed using Eqs. 3.8 and 3.9 to understand and classify various movements of the user and also helps the device to learn about the user's movement for future analysis using Eqs. 3.10, 3.11, and 3.12. Next, a machine learning algorithm, Random Forest Classifier, is used, which makes predictions based on multiple decision trees to detect the user's motion and also helps in fall detection. Hence, it is a very vital feature employed for elderly care. The algorithm with detailed equations has been discussed below.

Acceleration Magnitude:

$$A_{\text{res}} = \sqrt{A_x^2 + A_y^2 + A_z^2} \tag{3.8}$$

Angular Velocity Magnitude:

$$\omega_{\text{res}} = \sqrt{\omega_x^2 + \omega_y^2 + \omega_z^2} \tag{3.9}$$

Fall Detection:
Lower Fall Threshold:

$$\mathrm{LFT}_{\mathrm{acc}} = \min\left(A_{\mathrm{res}}\right) \tag{3.10}$$

Upper Fal Thresholds:

$$\mathrm{UFT}_{\mathrm{acc}} = \max\left(A_{\mathrm{res}}\right), \quad \mathrm{UFT}_{\mathrm{gyro}} = \max\left(\omega_{\mathrm{res}}\right) \tag{3.11}$$

Fall Detected if:

$$\left(A_{\mathrm{res}} < \mathrm{LFT}_{\mathrm{acc}}\right)\mathrm{and}\left(A_{\mathrm{res}} > \mathrm{UFT}_{\mathrm{acc}}\right) \wedge \left(\omega_{\mathrm{res}} > \mathrm{UFT}_{\mathrm{gyro}}\right) \tag{3.12}$$

Results

The LSTM model is developed for predicting future geographical coordinates (latitude and longitude) when elderly people go out for evening walks, morning walks or grocery shopping by learning from the historical data of the user. Using historical movement data, the model attempts to forecast the next location based on the previous historical data. This technique is used to check whether the user is taking the correct path or not.

First, we present Audio Recording Segmentation for Speaker Labelling in Table 3.2.

After the audio is divided into segments and the speakers are labeled, as we can see in Table 3.2, where the segments are categorized according to the specific speakers, the algorithm counts the number of distinct speakers detected in the audio file. This step has a huge impact as it is the foundation of knowledge of the data that is going to be used for the model. After the speaker count is done, the algorithm initializes and trains the Hidden Markov Model, which is a statistical model that learns from the divided audio data to capture the patterns in speaker transitions and the characteristics of the speech over time.

Then the output of the algorithm is included in the visual representation, in Fig. 3.4, for both the segmented initial speaker data and the learned speaker dynamics, like, pitch, speaking rate, or pronunciation, modeled by the Hidden

Table 3.2 Audio recording segmentation for speaker labelling

Speaker	Start time(s)	End time(s)
1	0	0.04644
0	0.04644	0.301859
1	0.301859	0.603719
0	0.603719	0.824308
1	0.824308	0.870748

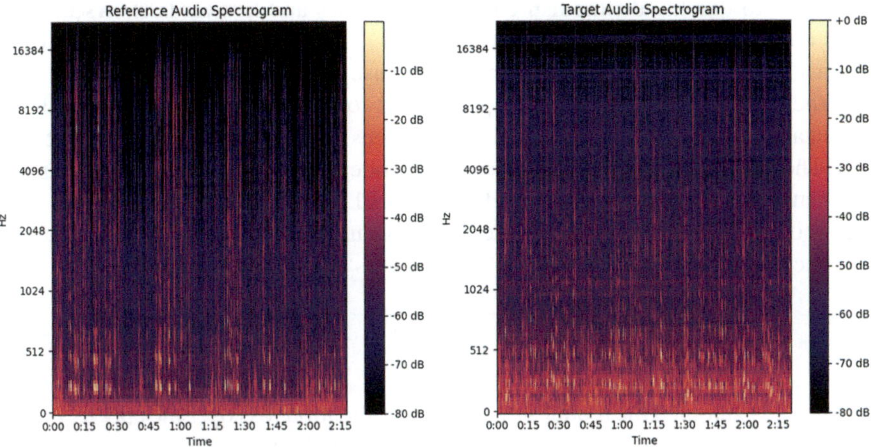

Fig. 3.4 Speaker verification process

Markov Model. These visualizations provide valuable insights on how the user is identified from the audio. The speaker verification algorithm works like a digital detective for voices. It can be considered as a super-smart system that listens to two audio clips: one it already knows well, like a voice password set by the user, and another it checks to see if it matches the voice password. When it is time to verify, the algorithm compares these features from the two clips as seen in Fig. 3.4. It calculates a score that shows how much they sound alike. If the score is high enough, it means the clips are likely from the same per-son. This is useful not just for recognizing voices but also for quickly spotting emergency words or phrases. For instance, if someone says a specific emergency word, the system can instantly sound an alarm or send an alert. It is all about using voice to make sure the right person is speaking and acting fast when needed.

Two models were evaluated for speaker diarization [30] and speaker recognition. The speaker diarization model, which combines pyAudioAnalysis for initial audio segmentation and Hidden Markov Models (HMM) for advanced analysis, proved to be quite effective. The pyAudioAnalysis tool successfully segmented the audio into distinct sections, each representing different speakers. This segmentation is crucial in complex scenarios, such as crowded or emergencies, where it is essential to identify and distinguish between various speakers. Following segmentation, the HMM was employed to analyze speaker transitions and speech patterns over time. This model's ability to accurately segment and label different speakers indicates its effectiveness in managing and understanding dynamic auditory environments. The speaker recognition model also demonstrates strong performance in comparing two audio clips to check their similarity. The model uses dynamic features like the pitch and speaking rate of the audio clip to establish a unique vocal profile for the users. This profile is later used to compare with new audio clips to identify the speakers. The model's accuracy in comparing audio samples demonstrates that it can accurately authenticate the speakers and correctly identify who is speaking. Its capability to quickly distinguish emergency phrases and keywords shows it has a huge impact in real-time emergencies. Overall, both models are highly effective in the task, which makes them a valuable tool to use in emergencies.

When we compared the model's predictions to the actual next coordinates from the dataset, we found that the model's predictions were generally close but not perfect. The prediction error, measured as the Euclidean distance between the predicted and actual coordinates, is shown in Eq. 3.13 and gives us a sense of how accurate the model is. A smaller error indicates better accuracy, but there was still some discrepancy, suggesting that the model's predictions are not always spot-on.

$$\text{Prediction Error} = \sqrt{\left(\text{predicted}_{\text{lat}} - \text{actual}_{\text{lat}}\right)^2 + \left(\text{predicted}_{\text{lon}} - \text{actual}_{\text{lon}}\right)^2} \quad (3.13)$$

We also examined the model's training and validation loss over the epochs shown in Fig. 3.5. The training loss shows how well the model fits the training data, and a decrease over time suggests that the model is learning effectively. On the other hand, the validation loss indicates how well the model performs on unseen data. Ideally, both losses should decrease and stabilize, which would indicate that the model is learning well and not overfitting.

Figure 3.5 provides more insights into the model's performance. The plot comparing predicted and actual latitude/longitude values helped us to see how closely the model's predictions matched the actual path.

The map visualization in Fig. 3.6. was particularly useful; it displayed the entire movement path in blue color, which shows the path traveled by the user, and the

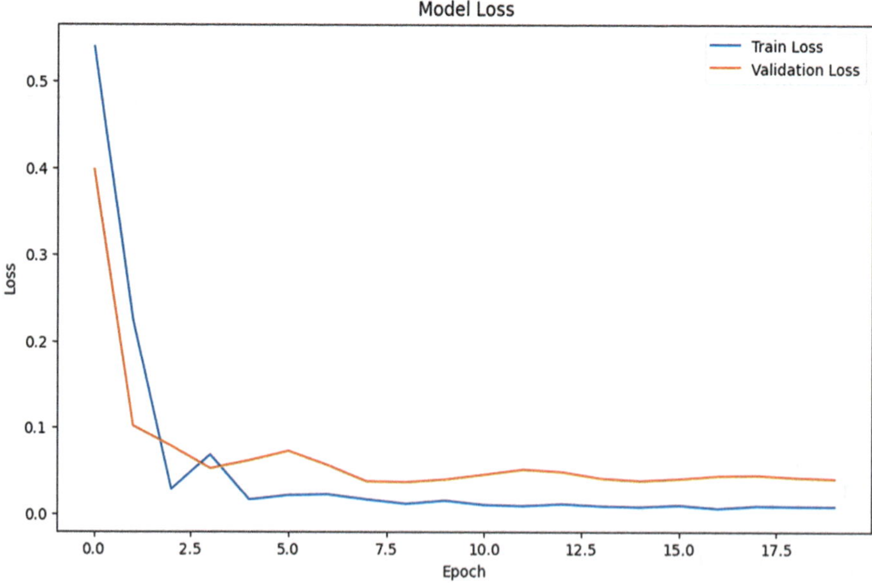

Fig. 3.5 Trajectory prediction loss analysis

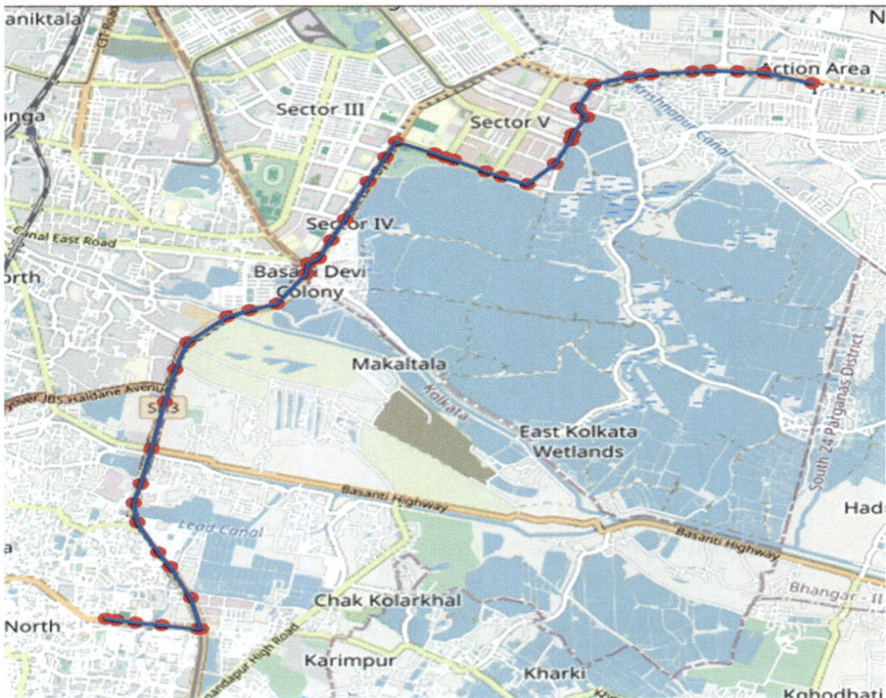

Fig. 3.6 Travelled path and next movement prediction for *Stay-Safer*

highlighted path in red is the predicted point, which shows what the next steps of the user should be. This map gave us a clear picture of how we can monitor the beloved elderly people of our family outside of the home.

As the third module of *Stay-Safer*, we employed a Random Forest Classifier to classify various activities based on sensor data. The dataset consists of features like the orientation of the device in three-dimensional space, the gravitational components that are acting on the device, the rotation rates to determine the rotation speed of the device, and the acceleration components to check the acceleration experienced by the device. The dataset is divided into a train set and a test set for the algorithm to use. Normalization functions are used to normalize the data. Then the training set is used on a Random Forest Classifier Model to train. The performance of the model is later evaluated using the test subset.

The model's performance is evaluated primarily on its accuracy as seen in Fig. 3.7. During the training, it is observed that the model achieves a high accuracy, which indicates that the model is effectively learning to differentiate between different activities based on the dataset features. It is observed that the accuracy curve shows a steady improvement, which means that the model is learning very well during its training period. However, it is important to check that the performance of the validation curve is slightly fluctuating, which could show the inherent variability in the data or the complexity of the activity classification.

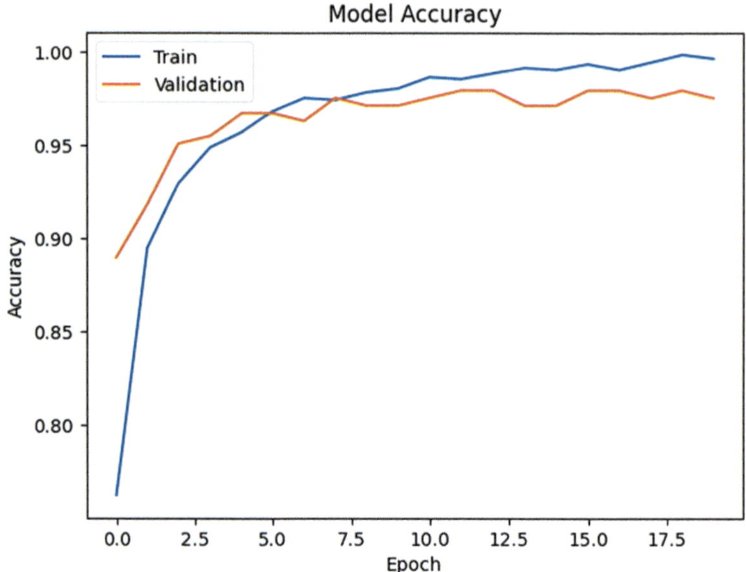

Fig. 3.7 Random forest classifier performance for activity recognition using inertial sensor data

To correctly understand the model's performance, we see the accuracy in Fig. 3.7 and the loss in Fig. 3.8 metrics across different epochs of the model training. The accuracy curve shows the consistency improvement with some fluctuations. The loss curve shows the general decrease, which reflects the model's ability to minimize the error prediction over time. The curves are important to visualize to understand how well the model uses generalization for the unseen data. Overall, the model proved to be efficient for distinguishing various activities based on the sensor dataset. This demonstrated good performance evaluation. Future works can explore tuning the parameters or adding more features to improve the model's performance.

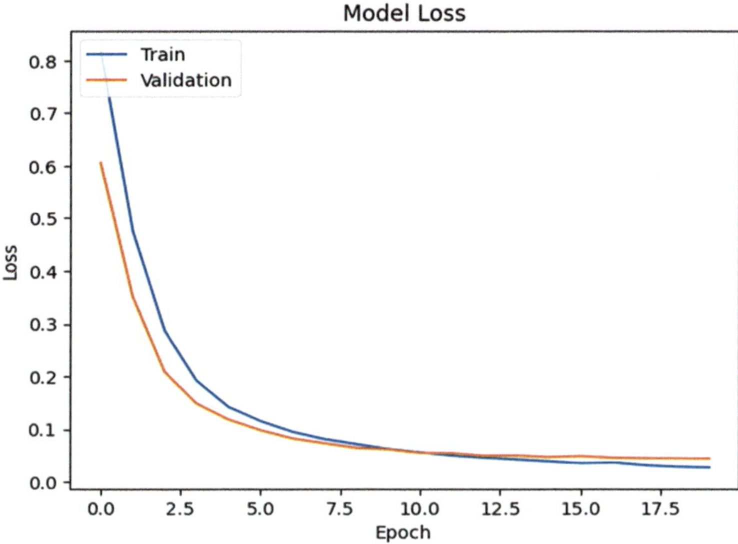

Fig. 3.8 Loss curve required to assess model error minimization

Discussions

Detailed results and their performance as achieved with our system were presented and discussed in section "Results." We further compared the performance of our system with a few existing systems. The detailed comparative discussion is presented in Table 3.3.

In Table 3.3, a comparative analysis of *Stay-Safer* with reference to other *state-of-the-art* methods was presented. In the presented comparison of Table 3.3, availability or scope for different useful parameters like multimodal sensing, GPS-based location tracking, Fall Detection, Emergency Alert system, Predictive monitoring, On-Demand Solution, and Outdoor monitoring was considered. In Table 3.3, the corresponding ✗ mark denotes unavailability and ✓ mark denotes availability. From the comparative results of Table 3.3, it might be observed that in the case of the HABITAT Project and Adinberri Project included a total of six and five, respectively, out of nine parameters were included; others dealt with very few parameters. Only *Stay-Safer* includes all nine parameters to make the system more effective and smarter. Moreover, *Stay-Safer* includes a sound-based triggering method to make the system more purposeful and smarter.

Thus, it might be concluded that *Stay-Safer* performs better with reference to several existing methods (refer to Table 3.3).

Table 3.3 Comparative study of *Stay-Safer* with state-of-the-art approaches

System/Paper Name	Multimodal Sensing	GPS Tracking	Fall Detection	Emergency Alerts	Predictive Analytics	On-Demand Solution	Outdoor Protection	Motion Abnormality Detection	Sound Abnormality Detection
Al Hossain et al. (2015) [10]	✗	✓	✗	✓	✗	✗	✗	✗	✗
HABITAT Project (2019) [7]	✓	✓	✓	✓	✓	✓	✗	✗	✗
Baig et al. (2019) [11]	✗	✗	✓	✓	✗	✗	✗	✓	✗
Padikkapparambil et al. (2020) [12]	✗	✓	✗	✓	✓	✓	✗	✗	✗
Karar et al. (2022) [15]	✗	✗	✓	✓	✗	✗	✗	✓	✗
Adinberri Project (2024) [9]	✗	✓	✗	✓	✓	✓	✓	✗	✗
Stay-Safer (our proposed)	✓	✓	✓	✓	✓	✓	✓	✓	✓

Conclusions

It can be concluded that *Stay-Safer* is an innovative and effective solution designed to enhance the safety and security of all vulnerable groups of society, initiated for senior citizens and can be molded for the use of women and children, by integrating technologies like GPS tracking, motion sensors, machine learning, and some essential sensors. By taking care of challenges such as accuracy in locating the user, automatic SOS alert generation, and on-time emergency responses, *Stay-Safer* creates a safe space for every vulnerable individual both indoors and outdoors.

Despite the use of all these innovations, *Stay-Safer* has additional reasons for improvement. Future refinements could make the GPS and machine learning algorithms more accurate in order to increase the efficiency of the application. Searching for means to handle privacy concerns more effectively, and streamlining the solution for various environments could also enhance its influence and usability further. Its audio recognition can majorly be used to identify the surroundings of vulnerable people when a distress signal is sent by the device to help the user. It will allow the rescuer to identify the location based on the environment sounds more easily where pinpointing using GPS technology is difficult.

In total, *Stay-Safer* has the potential to revolutionize safety measures by offering an efficient, real-time solution that protects the elderly, women, and children. With ongoing development and evolution, *Stay-Safer* may become an essential tool for enhancing personal security and safety.

Acknowledgments The authors sincerely acknowledge that the anonymous review comments received from the anonymous reviewers have helped to enhance the quality of the final manuscript. The authors also declare that there is no known conflict of interest, and no funding was received from any organization to carry out the research and to write the chapter manuscript.

References

1. Ministry of Statistics and Programme Implementation, National Statistical Office. Elderly in India 2021. n.d. Retrieved from https://mospi.gov.in/sites/default/files/publication_reports/Elderly%20in%20India%202021.pdf. Accessed on 13 Mar 2025.
2. Gupte Y. Data shows rise in crime against senior citizens in India: a look at steps taken by the government to protect the elderlies. India Tracker. Retrieved from https://www.indiatracker.in/story/data-shows-rise-in-crime-against-senior-citizens-in-india-a-look-at-steps-taken-by-the-government-to-protect-the-elderlies. Accessed 13 Mar 2025.
3. Chachra A. 70% women don't report workplace sexual harassment, employers show poor compliance. Hindustan Times. Retrieved from https://www.hindustantimes.com/india-news/70-women-don-t-report-workplace-sexual-harassment-employers-show-poor-compliance/story-40pcb35iu328VSLjjjpotL.html. Accessed on 13 Dec 2024.
4. Ashok Kumar P, Seth R, Varghese AD, editors. Safe childhood: right of every child. Indian Child Abuse, Neglect & Child Labour (ICANCL) Group of Indian Academy of Pediatrics. Retrieved from https://iapindia.org/pdf/n7iZwdjf5QBy23m_Safe-Childhood-27012025.pdf. Accessed on 13 Dec 2024.

5. iLearnCANA. Child protection in India. Retrieved from https://ilearncana.com/details/CHILD-PROTECTION-IN-INDIA/3629. Accessed on 13 Dec 2024.
6. UNICEF. Child protection. UNICEF India. Retrieved from https://www.unicef.org/india/what-we-do/child-protection. Accessed on 13 Dec 2024.
7. Borelli E, Giacomo P, Francesco A, Barbiroli M, Benassi F, Chesani F, Chiari L. HABITAT: an IoT solution for independent elderly. Sensors. 2019;19(5):1258.
8. Cares A. Transform night-time care. Retrieved from https://www.allycares.com/. Accessed on 13 Mar 2025.
9. Sebastián RS. Teleasistencia predictiva: El proyecto pionero de Adinberri para identificar situaciones de emergencia en las personas mayores [Predictive telecare: Adinberri's pioneering project to identify emergency situations in older people]. Cadena SER. https://cadenaser.com/euskadi/2024/12/12/teleasistencia-predictiva-el-proyecto-pionero-de-adinberri-para-identificar-situaciones-de-emergencia-en-las-personas-mayores-radio-san-sebastian/. Accessed on 12 Dec 2024.
10. Al Hossain MN, Pal A, Hossain SA. A wearable sensor based elderly home care system in a smart environment. In: 2015 18th international conference on computer and information technology (ICCIT). IEEE; 2015. p. 329–34.
11. Baig MM, Afifi S, GholamHosseini H, Mirza F. A systematic review of wearable sensors and IoT-based monitoring applications for older adults–a focus on ageing population and independent living. J Med Syst. 2019;43:1–11.
12. Padikkapparambil J, Ncube C, Singh KK, Singh A. Internet of Things technologies for elderly health-care applications. In Emergence of pharmaceutical industry growth with industrial IoT approach. Academic Press. 2020:217–43.
13. Awadalla M, Kausar F, Ahshan R. Developing an IoT platform for the elderly health care. Int J Adv Comput Sci Appl. 2021;12(4). https://doi.org/10.14569/IJACSA.2021.0120453.
14. Cheng BJ, Jamil MMA, Ambar R, Wahab MHA, Ma'radzi AA. Elderly care monitoring system with IoT application. In: Recent advances in intelligent information systems and applied mathematics. Springer International Publishing; 2020. p. 525–37.
15. Karar ME, Shehata HI, Reyad O. A survey of IoT-based fall detection for aiding elderly care: sensors, methods, challenges and future trends. Appl Sci. 2022;12(7):3276.
16. Wang G, Li Q, Wang L, Zhang Y, Liu Z. Elderly fall detection with an accelerometer using lightweight neural networks. Electronics. 2019;8(11):1354.
17. Rucco R, Sorriso A, Liparoti M, Ferraioli G, Sorrentino P, Ambrosanio M, Baselice F. Type and location of wearable sensors for monitoring falls during static and dynamic tasks in healthy elderly: a review. Sensors. 2018;18(5):1613.
18. Joshi GP, Acharya S, Kim CS, Kim BS, Kim SW. Smart solutions in elderly care facilities with RFID system and its integration with wireless sensor networks. Int J Distrib Sens Netw. 2014;10(8):713946.
19. Saguna S, Åhlund C, Larsson A. Experiences and challenges of providing IoT-based care for elderly in real-life smart home environments. In: Handbook of integration of cloud computing, cyber physical systems and internet of things. Cham: Springer; 2020. p. 255–71.
20. Abidi MH. Multimodal data-based human motion intention prediction using adaptive hybrid deep learning network for movement challenged person. Sci Rep. 2024;14(1):30633.
21. PainChek. Our story. Retrieved from https://www.painchek.com/about/our-story/. Retrieved on 14 Mar 2025.
22. Kaur R, Sirohi A, Goswami AK, Mani K, Nongkynrih B, Gupta SK. Magnitude and risk factors for falls among elderly in India: a systematic review. J Family Med Prim Care. 2019;8(6):1875–9. https://doi.org/10.4103/jfmpc.jfmpc_248_19.
23. Sari CWM, Rahayu U, Fauziah N. Overview of falling and risk factors of falling in the elderly in Bandung, West Java, Indonesia. J Crit Rev. 2021;7(19):7777.
24. Dengler S, Awad A, Dressler F. Sensor/actuator networks in smart homes for supporting elderly and handicapped people. In: 21st international conference on advanced information networking and applications workshops (AINAW'07), vol. 2. IEEE; 2007. p. 863–8.

25. Dosbayev Z, Abdrakhmanov R, Akhmetova O, Nurtas M, Iztayev Z, Zhaidakbaeva L, Shaimerdenova L. Audio surveillance: detection of audio-based emergency situations. In: International conference on computational collective intelligence. Cham: Springer International Publishing; 2021. p. 413–24.
26. Mishra V, Shivankar N, Gadpayle S, Shinde S, Khan MA, Zunke S. Women's safety system by voice recognition. In: 2020 IEEE international students' conference on electrical, electronics and computer science (SCEECS). IEEE; 2020. p. 1–5.
27. Wagh NR, Sutar SR, Yadav AS. Smart security solution for women and children using wearable IOT systems. Wirel Pers Commun. 2024;138(2):701–15.
28. Joyal Isac S, Ulagammai M, Shanmugakani J. Child safety wearable device using Raspberry Pi. Solid State Technol. 2020;63(2s):6350–8.
29. Pinto S, Cabral J, Gomes T. We-care: an IoT-based health care system for elderly people. In: 2017 IEEE international conference on industrial technology (ICIT). IEEE; 2017. p. 1378–83.
30. Anguera X, Bozonnet S, Evans N, Fredouille C, Friedland G, Vinyals O. Speaker diarization: a review of recent research. IEEE Trans Audio Speech Lang Process. 2012;20(2):356–70.

Chapter 4
Machine Learning Models in Wearable Health Data Processing: An Illustration Using Older Adult Data

Rafiqul Chowdhury and Sahand Ashtab

Introduction

The development and use of wearable devices to capture data on humans, the environment, and other areas are increasing rapidly. Various statistical and mathematical models are typically used to analyze this data and derive operational information. According to the United Nations 2023 report on the aging of the world population, most LDCs had a young age structure [1]. The proportion of older people (aged 65 years or older) was 3.7%, compared with 9% in other developing countries and 20% in developed countries. This figure is anticipated to increase noticeably in LDCs and elsewhere over the next several decades. Digital healthcare, enabled by the Internet of Medical Things (IoMT) and wearable devices with built-in sensors, is used to monitor human activity and vital signs, and to detect disease, among other applications [2, 3]. It is well known that older adults are more likely to have frequent clinical visits and to experience changes in their health status. It has already proven its potential for various wearable health devices in effectively managing chronic diseases [4]. For instance, continuous glucose monitors (CGMs) have transformed diabetes management by providing real-time glucose readings, leading to more precise insulin dosing and improved glycemic control [5]. Wearable devices are well-suited for monitoring older adults because they display up-to-date health information and track health metrics longitudinally. For example, fall-detection devices are worn all day and can detect unexpected falls and dispatch warning notifications. Similarly, wearable devices that monitor heart rate (HR), blood pressure (BP), and pulse during moderate exercise can aid in managing cardiovascular diseases by identifying arrhythmias, monitoring BP, and promoting critical cardiovascular function through exercise [6, 7]. Additionally, wearable medical devices can collect data

R. Chowdhury (✉) · S. Ashtab
Shannon School of Business, Cape Breton University, Sydney, NS, Canada
e-mail: Rafiqul_Chowdhury@cbu.ca

P. Eappen et al. (eds.), *Advancing Healthcare with the Medical Internet of Things*, Health Informatics, https://doi.org/10.1007/978-3-032-23933-4_4

on a range of health parameters, including heart rate, blood oxygen saturation, body temperature, physical activity, sleep, blood pressure, daily activity, and other metrics. Rapid growth in wearable technology is expected in the coming years. Various companies that provide services to the users of these devices collect real-time data and store it in their databases.

Despite their potential benefits, various challenges impede the widespread adoption of wearable devices in medicine. The accuracy and reliability of the data collection are a concern [8]. Additionally, integrating wearable device data with existing health records poses operational challenges [9]. Also, data privacy and security are major concerns for wearable healthcare devices. The effectiveness of these devices depends on their continuous use. The continuous data stream from wearable devices will gradually generate big data, and a new modeling framework may be needed to analyze these data and provide feedback to users to improve their conditions. This will be a significant challenge to analyze such data in real time to identify risks, trends, and patterns and to provide online, automated feedback to the user. Despite these challenges, healthcare data stored in wearable devices is a valuable source of information for feeding into machine learning algorithms to detect patterns and identify and predict diseases. In recent years, Machine Learning (ML) algorithms/models have proven effective for disease prediction. For instance, heart-related conditions and heart disease are among the leading causes of death. In [10], a supervised machine learning algorithm (i.e., classification and regression tree) is used to predict heart disease, whereas in [11] a random forest classifier is employed. Other applications of machine learning algorithms in the healthcare domain include predictive analytics models for mental illness [12] and liver cancer diagnosis [13]. Researchers in several papers presented the application of ML models to predict the activities of daily living problem (ADL) among the elderly. Han and Wang [14] found that ML models can accurately evaluate the risk of disability in healthy older adults. The authors of a recent paper used ML models to predict modifiable risk factors and found some activities that significantly reduce the ADL problems [15]. Chen et al. developed a predictive model using ML algorithms (RF, XGBoost) to assess the disability risk in older adults [16]. Jafari-Koulaee et al. [17] found that single older adults who are depressed with more chronic conditions are more likely to have ADL problems.

In this chapter, we will use a dataset of older adults from the Health and Retirement Study in the USA. We will discuss the data analysis methodology, present step-by-step scenarios, and demonstrate various machine learning algorithms with illustrations to provide readers with a comprehensive understanding and enable them to apply their knowledge to solve real-life problems.

Methods

Data

Databases used in health care delivery systems store various types of risk factors (features) collected from wearable devices. The variables may be qualitative, quantitative, or both. These new data sources can be analyzed to augment personalized insights into health risk trajectory and areas for improvement. We will use follow-ups (time points) of six to eleven waves of data from HRS in the USA, which is repeatedly measured and mimics the data collected repetitively from wearable devices for illustration. These datasets are publicly available from the HRS website: https://hrs.isr.umich.edu/data-products. The outcome variables considered are the Activity of Daily Living (ADL) Index, denoted by $y1$, $y2$, $y3$, $y4$, $y5$, $y6$, and $y7$, where $y1$ to $y7$ are binary outcomes (0 = No ADL problem, 1 = ADL problem). These outcome variables are constructed by recategorizing the ADL index (ranging from 0 to 5). The original ADL score reflects whether respondents had difficulty walking, dressing, bathing, eating, or getting in/out of bed. The datasets used are complex and high-dimensional, collected longitudinally. For this presentation, a selected set of features (independent variables) is presented for illustration purposes. For details on the many other available features, see the HRS codebooks (https://hrs.isr.umich.edu/documentation/codebooks).

The following list presents the features used for illustration purposes. Table 4.1 presents the frequency distribution of outcomes for y_1 to y_7. For simplicity, we used the complete cases from each repeated measure.

For the illustration, the risk factors considered are:	
1.	Age in years (X1)
2.	Marital status (Mstat: married/partnered = 1, single/separated = 0) (X2)
3.	Whether they drink alcohol (yes = 1, no = 0) (X3)
4.	Gender (male = 1, female = 2) (X4)
5.	The health conditions ever had (Ncond) range from 0 to 8 (X5)
6.	Race (White/Caucasian = 1, Black/African American/others = 0) (X6)
7.	Education in years (X7)
8.	Veteran status (1 = yes, 0 = no) (X8)
9.	Body mass index (BMI) (X9)
10.	Mental health index (CESD) ranging from 0 to 8 (X10)
11.	Large muscle index (Lmuscle) ranging from 0 to 4 (X11)
12.	Total income (Income) (X12)
13.	Self-rated memory (Memory) ranging from 1 to 5 (1 = excellent, 2 = very good, 3 = good, 4 = fair, 5 = poor) (X13)
14.	Word recall score (Wrecall) ranging from 0 to 20 (X14)

Table 4.1 Distribution of the activity of daily living (ADL) Index across follow-ups

Value	y_1	y_2	y_3	y_4	y_5	y_6	y_7
No ADL (0)	5660	5165	4667	4290	3733	3417	2906
ADL (1)	770	714	740	671	696	640	656
Total	6431	5881	5410	4965	4434	4063	3569

Longitudinal data on adverse health conditions (e.g., IADL, ADL) or chronic diseases can be used to predict the risk of adverse health trajectories. These trajectories can be visualized graphically, which may provide an in-depth understanding of disease progression (paths) [18]. Additionally, this longitudinal data is useful for analyzing events (outputs) of interest in life-course research. The most important advantage of using longitudinal data is that it enables the study of individual disease course development over time [19, 20]. In other words, we can study the individual trajectories (path). Healthcare providers would be interested in analyzing disease progression over time and identifying the causes that drive the disease toward a particular trajectory. Among others, the following naturally arising questions may be asked and are essential:

(i) What is the risk of a specific output for a patient at a particular point in time given the features and the history of any previous outputs?
(ii) Estimates of the risk of specific output over a range of time points given the features and the past conditions/disease history
(iii) Predicting the output for the next time point given the features and the history (i.e., predicting the future path of the disease)

Answering the above questions and predicting risk at a particular point in time along trajectories enables healthcare professionals to screen individuals and recommend appropriate therapy and preventive measures. Furthermore, this helps a patient's awareness of the future course of the disease [21] and compliance with healthcare providers' suggestions. For example, Figs. 4.1 and 4.2 present trajectory risk using conditional and joint probabilities of several patients' Activity of Daily Living (ADL) problems across different time points. Note that, in this context, the conditional probabilities quantify risk within the subgroup defined by conditioning (stratifying) on disease status at the previous time point(s), whereas the joint probabilities quantify the risk among the full sample.

The estimated joint probabilities for each trajectory in Fig. 4.1 can be shown mathematically as follows

$$\hat{P}\left(Y_1 = y_1,\, Y_2 = y_2,\, Y_3 = y_3,\, Y_4 = y_4,\, Y_5 = y_5,\, Y_6 = y_6,\, Y_7 = y_7, \middle| \mathbf{X} = x\right) =$$
$$\hat{P}\left(Y_1 = y_1 \text{ and } Y_2 = y_2 \text{ and } Y_3 = y_3 \text{ and } Y_4 = y_4 \text{ and } Y_5 = y_5 \text{ and } Y_6 = y_6 \text{ and } Y_7 = y_7 \middle| \mathbf{X} = x\right)$$

where $Y_1, \ldots, Y_7$ are random variables and $y_1, \ldots, y_7$ are variates, i. e. specific value of each random variables.

For example, $\hat{P}\left(Y_1 = 1 \text{ and } Y_2 = 1 \text{ and } Y_3 = 1 \text{ and } Y_4 = 1 \text{ and } Y_5 = 1 \text{ and } Y_6 = 1 \text{ and } Y_7 = 1 \middle| \mathbf{X} = x\right)$ is the joint probability of a person with the ADL problem at all seven time points for given values of covariate vectors.

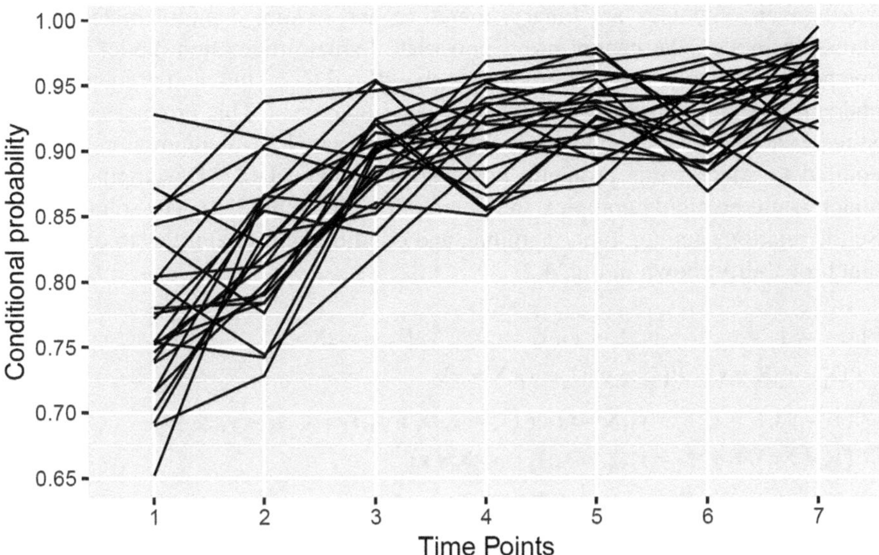

Fig. 4.1 Trajectories of risk for conditional probabilities of several patients' Activities of Daily Living problems

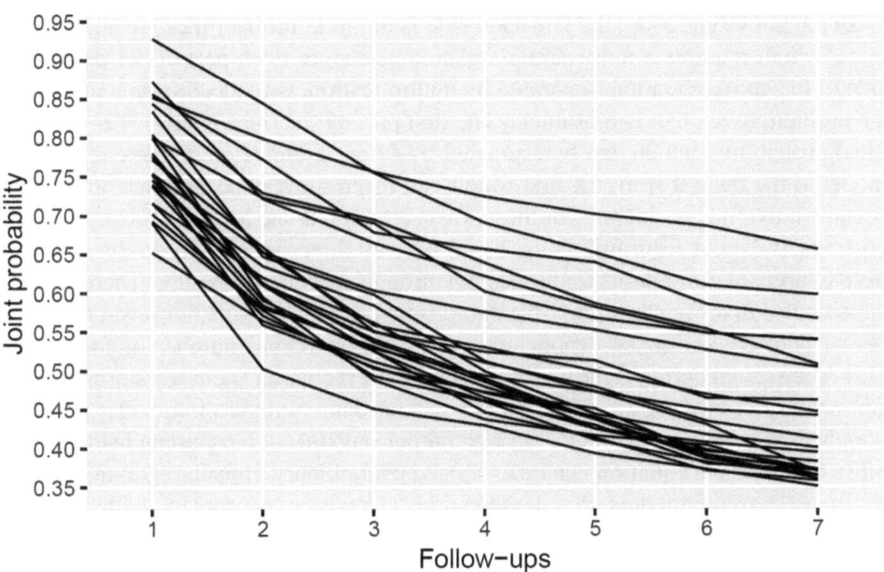

Fig. 4.2 Trajectories of risk for joint probability of several patients' Activities of Daily Living problems

All seven outcomes are binary; therefore, we require a multivariate logistic regression model. We cannot use a univariate logistic regression model for each time point separately, because this approach will fail to capture and account for the inherent temporal dependence among repeated outcomes. This produces distorted estimates and, hence, wrong inferences. A multivariate logistic regression model is required to address this problem; however, it is unavailable. Developing such a model would be highly complex and potentially intractable [22]. The solution is to use the relations among joint, marginal, and conditional probabilities to obtain the joint probability shown in Fig. 4.2.

$$
\begin{aligned}
&\hat{P}\left(Y_1 = y_1, Y_2 = y_2, Y_3 = y_3, Y_4 = y_4, Y_5 = y_5 Y_6 = y_6, | Y_7 = y_7, | \mathbf{X} = x\right) \\
&= \hat{P}\left(Y_1 = y_1 | \mathbf{X} = \mathbf{x}\right) \times \hat{P}\left(Y_2 = y_2 | ; Y_1 = y_1 | ; \mathbf{X} = \mathbf{x}\right) \\
&\times \hat{P}\left(Y_3 = y_3 | ; Y_1 = y_1 ; Y_2 = y_2 ; \mathbf{X} = \mathbf{x}\right) \times \hat{P}\left(Y_4 = y_4 | ; Y_1 = y_1 ; Y_2 = y_2 ; Y_3 = y_3 ; \mathbf{X} = \mathbf{x}\right) \\
&\times \hat{P}\left(Y_5 = y_5 | ; Y_1 = y_1 ; Y_2 = y_2 ; Y_3 = y_3 ; Y_4 = y_4 ; \mathbf{X} = \mathbf{x}\right) \\
&\times \hat{P}\left(Y_6 = y_6 | ; Y_1 = y_1 ; Y_2 = y_2 ; Y_3 = y_3 ; Y_4 = y_4 ; Y_5 = y_5 ; \mathbf{X} = \mathbf{x}\right) \\
&\times \hat{P}\left(Y_7 = y_7 ; Y_1 = y_1 ; Y_2 = y_2 ; Y_3 = y_3 ; Y_4 = y_4 ; Y_5 = y_5 ; Y_6 = y_6 ; \mathbf{X} = \mathbf{x}\right)
\end{aligned}
\tag{4.1}
$$

where $y_1, \ldots, y_7 = 0, 1$ and $\mathbf{X} = [X_1, X_2, \ldots, X_p]$ is vector of covariates (features).

In the above equation, the left-hand side is the joint probabilities we aim to estimate, which requires a multivariate logistic regression. Each part of the right-hand side of the above equation, separated by multiplication, is reduced from a multivariate problem to a univariate problem. The first part on the right-hand side is the marginal probability, which can be estimated by fitting a univariate logistic regression model to the dataset from the first follow-up. From the second onward, others also became univariate problems. For these, we can fit univariate logistic regression models to each dataset from follow-up 2 to follow-up 7, separately. To do this, we first need to prepare the datasets for the second through seventh follow-ups. There are two approaches: first, we can stratify the datasets by prior follow-ups; however, the number of datasets will grow exponentially with the increased number of follow-ups [22]. The second option is the use of the regressive modeling framework proposed by Chowdhury et al. [18, 22, 23]. Using a special data configuration, using previous output(s) as a covariate from the second output onward each right-hand side probability of the above equation can be estimated using binary logistic regression or any machine learning models for classifications. However, a problem with machine learning models is their lack of interpretability, which prevents us from performing hypothesis testing. If the objective is to predict trajectory risk, we can readily employ machine learning algorithms using a regression modeling approach. We can then estimate the marginal and conditional risks on the right-hand side of the equation and, hence, obtain the joint probability of the left-hand side. For some machine learning algorithms, we can compute variable importance, but not for all. Table 4.2 presents the data structure for fitting models within the regression modeling framework.

Machine Learning Models

We apply various machine learning (ML) models and compare their performances, for example, neural network (NN) [24–28], random forest (RF) model [29, 30], Decision tree [31], support vector machine (SVM) [32, 33], and Lasso [34, 35]. Lasso improves models by applying L1 regularization to shrink coefficient estimates toward zero, thereby performing automatic feature selection and reducing model complexity. Lasso, by eliminating irrelevant features, prevents overfitting. Of course, there are many other machine learning models for classification, and those can also be used using this framework. However, to keep the manuscript concise, we did not evaluate certain learning algorithms that have recently gained popularity. The goal is to demonstrate that data collected from wearable devices can be analyzed within a regression modeling framework using machine learning models to address some of the questions posed earlier. As noted earlier, the proposed framework requires fitting one model per repeated response, incorporating previous responses and the feature vector (as shown in Table 4.2).

Table 4.2 Data structure to fit models using a regressive modeling framework

ID	Y1	X1	X2	X3	X4	X5	X6
10	0	62	0	0	0	1	1
10	0	64	0	0	0	1	1
10	0	66	0	0	0	1	1
10	0	69	0	0	1	1	1
10	0	71	0	0	0	1	1
10	0	72	0	0	0	1	1
10	0	74	0	0	0	1	1
X7	X8	X9	X10	X11	X12	X13	X14
12	0	24.4	1	0	6276	0	10
12	0	22.4	1	0	9588	0	12
12	0	21.7	1	0	10,188	1	13
12	0	22.3	1	0	10,260	1	12
12	0	21.3	1	0	14,400	0	11
12	0	20.2	1	0	12,000	1	11
12	0	20.9	0	0	12,000	0	12
Y1	Y2	Y3	Y4	Y5	Y6	Follow-ups	
NA	NA	NA	NA	NA	NA	1	
0	NA	NA	NA	NA	NA	2	
0	0	NA	NA	NA	NA	3	
0	0	0	NA	NA	NA	4	
0	0	0	0	NA	NA	5	
0	0	0	0	0	NA	6	
0	0	0	0	0	0	7	

Data Pre-processing

The data were divided for each follow-up. From the second onward, follow-ups incorporate previous outcomes to account for temporal dependencies within the regressive modeling framework. We divided the data into training and test sets throughout the follow-ups for model evaluation. We split the data into training and test sets at a 75%/25% ratio using the first follow-up samples. Data normalization helps smooth the fitting of the ML models. Hence, the feature variables are normalized using the training sample specific to each follow-up, and the minimum and maximum values are calculated for each feature across the training samples. For all ML models, the default hyperparameter values are used.

Examples

All machine learning algorithms are evaluated on the HRS dataset [36].

Accuracy of the Fitted ML Models for Training and Test Data for all Seven Follow-Ups

Table 4.3 presents the accuracy, sensitivity, specificity, and positive and negative predictive values for the training and test data across all seven time points. A 0.50 value as the probability threshold is used to calculate the model accuracy (proportion of correct classification for ADL). Training data accuracy ranges from 0.99 to 0.89 across different time points and models. Test accuracy varies from 0.92 to 0.88. We need to compare the training and test accuracies to conclude whether our fitted models are good enough to predict the risk for a new subject, that is, a subject that was not used to train our model. This will also show the generalizing ability of the fitted model(s). A comparison of training and test accuracy indicates overfitting for the RF and SVM models. Neither the Neural Network nor the Lasso showed any remarkable overfitting. However, our goal is to identify models that predict ADL-positive cases with reasonable accuracy. Additionally, it is important to select a model with good generalizability for risk prediction on unseen data points. Therefore, a model should also be free from both overfitting and underfitting.

Table 4.3 Accuracy and other statistics of the training and test data using the five models

	Training data							Test data						
	Follow-ups													
	1	2	3	4	5	6	7	1	2	3	4	5	6	7
Accuracy														
N. Net	0.91	0.91	0.91	0.91	0.91	0.89	0.89	0.89	0.91	0.90	0.90	0.89	0.89	0.89
R. F	0.99	0.98	0.98	0.98	0.97	0.97	0.96	0.89	0.91	0.90	0.89	0.88	0.88	0.89
D. Tree	0.92	0.92	0.92	0.92	0.91	0.91	0.91	0.88	0.91	0.89	0.88	0.88	0.88	0.88
SVM	0.95	0.96	0.97	0.97	0.97	0.98	0.97	0.88	0.89	0.88	0.87	0.86	0.86	0.86
Lasso	0.90	0.91	0.91	0.91	0.90	0.89	0.88	0.88	0.91	0.89	0.90	0.88	0.89	0.88
Sensitivity														
N. Net	0.41	0.50	0.56	0.55	0.56	0.54	0.61	0.38	0.56	0.55	0.55	0.53	0.56	0.63
R. F	0.90	0.84	0.82	0.83	0.79	0.78	0.76	0.29	0.44	0.42	0.41	0.42	0.44	0.54
D. Tree	0.46	0.44	0.56	0.54	0.51	0.54	0.65	0.38	0.46	0.47	0.42	0.43	0.49	0.63
SVM	0.58	0.67	0.76	0.79	0.81	0.85	0.82	0.22	0.31	0.37	0.34	0.42	0.42	0.49
Lasso	0.26	0.37	0.44	0.44	0.40	0.43	0.45	0.24	0.45	0.41	0.41	0.40	0.48	0.46
Specificity														
N. Net	0.98	0.97	0.97	0.97	0.97	0.96	0.95	0.97	0.97	0.96	0.96	0.96	0.96	0.95
R. F	1.00	1.00	1.00	1.00	1.00	1.00	1.00	0.98	0.98	0.98	0.98	0.98	0.98	0.97
D. Tree	0.97	0.98	0.98	0.98	0.98	0.97	0.97	0.96	0.97	0.96	0.96	0.97	0.97	0.95
SVM	1.00	1.00	1.00	1.00	1.00	1.00	1.00	0.98	0.97	0.97	0.96	0.96	0.96	0.95
Lasso	0.98	0.98	0.98	0.98	0.98	0.97	0.98	0.98	0.98	0.98	0.98	0.98	0.98	0.98
Positive predictive value														
N. Net	0.69	0.67	0.73	0.71	0.75	0.69	0.73	0.67	0.71	0.69	0.69	0.75	0.75	0.75
R. F	1.00	1.00	1.00	1.00	1.00	1.00	1.00	0.71	0.77	0.75	0.73	0.80	0.84	0.82
D. Tree	0.70	0.76	0.82	0.78	0.82	0.79	0.82	0.61	0.70	0.65	0.65	0.78	0.77	0.74
SVM	0.97	0.98	0.99	1.00	1.00	1.00	1.00	0.62	0.64	0.67	0.60	0.68	0.72	0.70
Lasso	0.65	0.71	0.78	0.75	0.81	0.75	0.83	0.65	0.74	0.74	0.74	0.81	0.85	0.86
Negative predictive value														
N. Net	0.93	0.93	0.93	0.93	0.93	0.92	0.92	0.91	0.94	0.93	0.93	0.90	0.91	0.91
R. F	0.99	0.98	0.97	0.97	0.96	0.96	0.95	0.90	0.92	0.91	0.91	0.89	0.89	0.90
D. Tree	0.93	0.93	0.93	0.93	0.92	0.92	0.93	0.91	0.93	0.91	0.91	0.89	0.89	0.91
SVM	0.95	0.96	0.96	0.97	0.97	0.97	0.96	0.89	0.91	0.90	0.90	0.89	0.88	0.88
Lasso	0.91	0.92	0.92	0.92	0.90	0.91	0.89	0.89	0.92	0.91	0.91	0.88	0.89	0.88

Variable Importance and Sparse Matrix

Variable importance (VI) in an ML model may help identify the features to include in the final model. VI values from the neural network and random forests are displayed in Table 4.4. The most significant (in a non-statistical sense) variables for the NN model are large muscle indices. In the RF model, large muscle index showed the highest importance across all seven time points, followed by income, BMI, CES-D, and age. The lasso sparse matrix is shown in Table 4.5. The large muscles showed the highest coefficient, followed by CESD, Ncond, and BMI. Lasso shrinks some coefficients to zero because they are not important predictors, thereby improving model performance. As noted earlier, not all ML models can estimate variable importance hierarchies, so we could not do so.

Table 4.4 The importance score of the feature variables using Neural Networks and Random Forests

	Neural network							Random forests						
	Follow-ups													
Features	1	2	3	4	5	6	7	1	2	3	4	5	6	7
Age	6.4	1.6	2.5	3.6	6.6	4.0	7.7	60.4	51.3	46.4	39.8	38.6	34.9	33.0
Mstat	6.9	0.8	2.1	1.0	1.5	0.2	0.0	15.5	12.2	11.9	11.1	10.6	8.3	9.0
Ncond	6.9	7.0	8.0	10.8	4.7	4.4	4.1	75.3	65.3	56.7	49.3	41.4	34.7	31.3
Drink	4.2	0.7	1.1	0.0	4.6	0.7	0.2	16.9	14.3	12.6	10.7	10.4	9.6	8.6
Gender	3.3	2.8	1.6	2.0	6.4	1.9	2.4	15.3	13.0	12.3	11.3	10.3	8.9	8.8
Race	5.4	0.9	1.9	1.1	6.8	1.3	0.5	15.6	13.5	12.6	9.3	9.6	9.0	7.1
Educ	8.9	3.9	2.2	0.6	2.4	5.3	3.1	63.8	48.5	48.1	39.6	37.3	31.8	29.8
Veteran	5.6	2.7	0.8	1.0	7.8	0.7	1.0	11.6	9.1	8.9	8.2	9.1	7.7	7.0
BMI	7.1	11.8	8.8	2.7	4.8	6.3	1.1	105.5	93.8	78.9	66.2	60.2	52.2	48.4
CESD	5.9	6.8	10.7	7.3	6.6	9.2	11.4	93.6	73.6	69.2	55.1	51.0	44.4	47.3
Lmuscle	16.5	16.1	19.8	20.3	15.5	20.0	22.2	171.1	113.3	100.4	78.7	92.0	69.5	78.8
Income	3.5	32.5	7.6	7.3	6.0	6.8	12.5	110.2	87.7	77.4	65.2	61.3	51.4	47.0
Memory	11.4	0.9	1.9	0.7	5.4	0.2	0.8	23.5	16.5	16.8	12.7	12.9	11.4	11.2
Wrecall	8.1	1.6	10.5	12.8	5.7	10.7	0.7	72.9	56.8	54.2	46.2	44.0	40.0	33.6
Y1		10.0	7.2	7.7	4.0	2.7	0.0		120.5	77.7	53.8	33.3	25.0	14.7
Y2			13.2	8.4	3.4	4.1	2.9			117.9	63.8	43.1	28.0	16.5
Y3				12.4	3.2	3.1	3.8				98.8	57.2	34.7	31.0
Y4					4.7	8.3	2.2					74.9	50.9	28.3
Y5						10.1	9.6						72.1	55.7
Y6							13.6							83.0

Table 4.5 The lasso sparse matrix for the seven-time points

	Follow-ups						
Variables	1	2	3	4	5	6	7
Intercept	0.00	0.00	0.00	0.00	0.00	0.00	0.00
Age	0.00	0.00	0.00	0.00	0.00	0.00	0.00
Mstat	0.00	0.00	0.00	0.00	0.00	0.00	0.00
Ncond	1.16	0.73	0.34	0.64	0.00	0.16	0.00
Drink	0.00	0.00	0.00	0.00	0.00	0.00	0.00
Gender	0.00	0.00	0.00	0.00	0.00	0.00	0.00
Race	0.00	0.00	0.00	0.00	0.00	0.00	0.00
Educ	0.00	0.00	0.00	0.00	0.00	0.00	0.00
Veteran	0.00	0.00	0.00	0.00	0.00	0.00	0.00
BMI	0.15	0.64	0.00	0.00	0.00	0.00	0.00
CESD	1.24	0.78	0.90	0.61	0.54	0.71	0.55
Lmuscle	3.30	2.51	2.13	2.04	2.16	2.42	2.02
Income	0.00	0.00	0.00	0.00	0.00	0.00	0.00
Memory	0.03	0.00	0.00	0.00	0.00	0.00	0.00
Wrecall	−0.53	0.00	0.09	−0.24	0.00	−0.31	0.00
Y1		1.63	0.78	0.69	0.03	0.22	0.00
Y2			1.63	0.71	0.35	0.15	0.00
Y3				1.41	0.74	0.25	0.11
Y4					1.13	0.98	0.01
Y5						1.32	0.91
Y6							1.25

Trajectory Risks for a Subject Using Five Machine Learning Models

To illustrate the usefulness of the predicted trajectory risks, we used a selected subject. For this specific subject, the predicted marginal, conditional, and joint probabilities for seven time points using NN, RF, DT, SVM, and Lasso models are shown in Table 4.6. This subject was included in the training dataset, with observed ADL problems at all seven time points. The estimated joint probabilities by all five models are shown in Fig. 4.3. The top line in the figure is using the RF model, followed by NN, DT, SVM, and Lasso, respectively. Because all seven time points for this subject were 1, we expect the joint probabilities to be close to 1. The RF model performs best for risk prediction. It may be noted that the joint probabilities decrease across the follow-ups. Because we are multiplying proportions, joint probabilities should be reduced. Also, joint probabilities pertain to the full sample, whereas conditional probabilities pertain to subgroups (partial samples).

Impact of Varying Covariate Values on the Trajectory Risk
Because the RF is the best-performing model, we compare the predicted marginal conditional risks for six subjects using the RF, as shown in Table 4.7. Subject 1 is the same subject from Table 4.6. All six subjects have ADL problems for all

Table 4.6 The calculation of marginal conditional and joint probabilities is shown in Fig. 4.3

Model	Marginal and conditional probabilities						
	Follow-ups						
	1	2	3	4	5	6	7
RF	0.84	0.86	0.95	0.92	0.92	0.94	0.92
NN	0.88	0.74	0.81	0.82	0.84	0.83	0.85
DT	0.74	0.83	0.85	0.78	0.87	0.81	0.87
SVM	0.69	0.68	0.77	0.74	0.77	0.79	0.77
Lasso	0.64	0.73	0.75	0.85	0.84	0.90	0.64
	Marginal and joint probabilities						
	Follow-ups						
	1	2	3	4	5	6	7
RF	0.84	0.73	0.69	0.69	0.59	0.55	0.51
NN	0.88	0.65	0.53	0.53	0.36	0.30	0.26
DT	0.74	0.62	0.52	0.52	0.36	0.29	0.25
SVM	0.69	0.47	0.36	0.36	0.20	0.16	0.12
Lasso	0.64	0.47	0.35	0.35	0.25	0.23	0.15

$1 =$ Column 1 under the Marginal probability $= \hat{p}(y_1|x)$, similarly, $2 = \hat{p}(y_2|;y_1|;x)$, $3 = \hat{p}(y_3|,;y_1|,;y_2|,;x)$ and so on are conditional probabilities. Similarly, the second part (Marginal and joint probabilities) column 1 = 1, 2 = 1 × 2, column 3 = 1 × 2 × 3, and so on

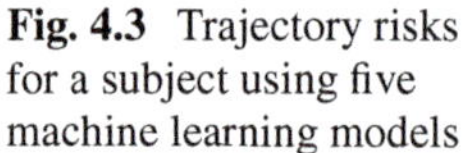

Fig. 4.3 Trajectory risks for a subject using five machine learning models

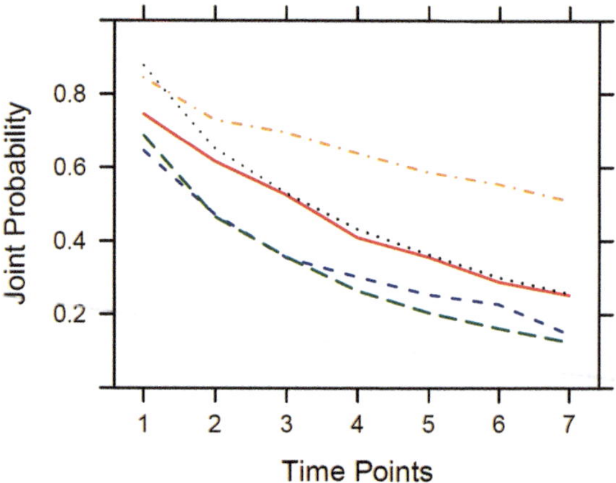

follow-ups. We are interested in finding how the varying covariate values of these six subjects affected the predicted trajectory risk. The subject's covariate values are different, as shown in Table 4.8. Trajectories for these six subjects are shown in Fig. 4.4. The joint probabilities decline gradually across the time points as expected. That is, trajectory risks have decreased and are below the threshold of 0.50. If the predicted risk is below 0.50, the subject will be considered free of ADL problems. However, because all six subjects had ADL present at all seven follow-ups, we expect their trajectories to be similar. To understand these, we should study the covariate impact on the trajectory. If we compare the first line from Fig. 4.4, which

Table 4.7 The calculation of marginal conditional and joint probabilities for six different subjects using the RF model

Subjects ID	Marginal and conditional probabilities						
	Follow-ups						
	1	2	3	4	5	6	7
1	0.84	0.86	0.95	0.92	0.92	0.94	0.92
2	0.57	0.79	0.91	0.89	0.94	0.95	0.91
3	0.68	0.76	0.83	0.89	0.90	0.89	0.96
4	0.75	0.82	0.90	0.95	0.98	0.91	0.99
5	0.59	0.75	0.83	0.85	0.90	0.86	0.92
6	0.70	0.83	0.91	0.90	0.91	0.88	0.94
	Marginal and joint probabilities						
	Follow-ups						
	1	2	3	4	5	6	7
1	0.84	0.73	0.69	0.64	0.59	0.55	0.51
2	0.57	0.45	0.41	0.37	0.35	0.33	0.30
3	0.68	0.52	0.43	0.38	0.34	0.31	0.29
4	0.75	0.61	0.55	0.52	0.51	0.46	0.46
5	0.59	0.44	0.37	0.31	0.28	0.24	0.22
6	0.70	0.58	0.53	0.48	0.44	0.39	0.36

Table 4.8 Features values for six different subjects are shown in Figs. 4.3 and 4.4

ID	X1	X2	X3	X4	X5	X6	X7	X8	X9	X10	X11	X12	X13	X14	Follow-ups
1	69	0	2	0	2	0	8	0	21.1	7	4	9768.00	1	6	1
1	71	0	2	0	2	0	8	0	26.3	6	4	7500.00	1	2	2
1	73	0	3	0	2	0	8	0	27.1	5	3	8100.00	1	5	3
1	75	0	3	0	2	0	8	0	26.6	4	4	8572.00	1	4	4
1	78	0	3	0	2	0	8	0	23.0	7	4	10800.00	1	7	5
1	79	0	3	0	2	0	8	0	23.0	4	4	11376.00	1	3	6
1	81	0	4	0	2	0	8	0	23.5	4	2	9660.00	1	2	7
2	68	0	2	0	2	1	12	0	39.5	1	3	16926.98	0	12	1
2	69	0	2	0	2	1	12	0	38.0	3	4	25408.00	0	10	2
2	71	0	2	0	2	1	12	0	43.4	2	4	4773.00	0	7	3
2	74	0	2	0	2	1	12	0	42.8	3	4	15802.00	0	9	4
2	76	0	2	0	2	1	12	0	40.4	1	4	17592.00	0	13	5
2	78	0	3	0	2	1	12	0	42.0	1	3	12634.19	0	13	6
2	80	0	3	0	2	1	12	0	35.5	1	4	15389.56	0	9	7
3	64	0	0	0	1	0	10	0	19.9	0	3	8088.00	0	11	1
3	65	0	0	0	1	0	10	0	17.8	1	3	6348.00	0	8	2
3	68	0	0	0	1	0	10	0	19.0	2	3	7236.00	0	10	3
3	69	0	0	0	1	0	10	0	19.2	0	3	10367.45	0	11	4
3	71	0	0	0	1	0	10	0	19.6	3	2	11368.27	1	10	5
3	74	0	0	0	1	0	10	0	17.9	3	3	8376.00	1	8	6

(continued)

Table 4.8 (continued)

ID	X1	X2	X3	X4	X5	X6	X7	X8	X9	X10	X11	X12	X13	X14	Follow-ups
3	75	0	1	0	1	0	10	0	20.5	2	4	17136.00	1	10	7
4	64	0	5	0	2	1	11	0	25.6	6	4	6864.00	0	10	1
4	66	0	5	0	2	1	11	0	27.8	8	4	15504.00	1	11	2
4	68	0	5	0	2	1	11	0	30.2	6	4	8796.00	0	12	3
4	70	0	5	0	2	1	11	0	30.5	1	4	7944.00	0	7	4
4	73	0	6	0	2	1	11	0	30.3	7	4	13056.00	1	6	5
4	74	0	6	0	2	1	11	0	31.7	7	3	8350.00	1	5	6
4	76	0	6	0	2	1	11	0	30.3	5	4	16872.00	1	5	7
5	64	0	1	0	1	0	14	1	28.6	0	3	9552.00	0	6	1
5	67	0	1	0	1	0	14	1	28.6	0	4	22176.00	1	6	2
5	69	0	1	0	1	0	14	1	26.7	0	3	14688.00	0	8	3
5	71	0	1	0	1	0	14	1	28.5	0	2	11700.00	0	6	4
5	73	1	1	0	1	0	14	1	28.6	0	4	24480.00	1	4	5
5	75	0	1	0	1	0	14	1	27.0	1	2	12000.00	0	2	6
5	76	0	1	0	1	0	14	1	24.7	0	4	13212.00	0	5	7
6	69	0	5	0	2	1	11	0	23.6	6	4	28884.00	1	10	1
6	71	0	6	0	2	1	11	0	24.1	6	3	24348.00	1	8	2
6	73	0	6	0	2	1	11	0	24.9	3	4	26856.00	1	10	3
6	75	0	6	0	2	1	11	0	21.7	3	4	28368.00	1	8	4
6	77	0	6	0	2	1	11	0	19.5	7	3	28800.00	1	3	5
6	79	0	6	1	2	1	11	0	28.7	5	3	35700.00	1	6	6
6	81	0	6	0	2	1	11	0	28.9	7	3	33600.00	1	7	7

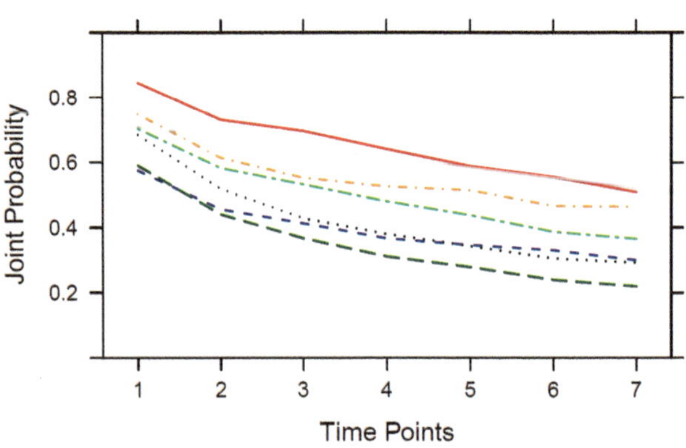

Fig. 4.4 Trajectory risks for six subjects using random forest models

is the Subject with ID 1 (Table 4.8), to that of the last line in Fig. 4.4, which is the Subject with ID 5 from Table 4.8. We observe a noticeable reduction in CESD (X10) feature values across time points, and a larger muscle index for the 5th subject than for the 1st. Such findings would be highly useful for patient education. Additionally, we can predict risks for a new subject by varying feature values to demonstrate the disease risk reduction and communicate these results to patients to support adherence to their physicians' recommendations.

Discussion

The elderly population is growing rapidly worldwide and more rapidly in developed countries. This elderly population experiences various types of adverse health conditions and frequent chronic problems. Digital healthcare, including recent advancements in wearable devices and related technologies, has made it possible to continuously collect health data from people via the internet. These wearable devices are useful for monitoring and collecting data from older adults and young adults. These data are highly valuable for evaluating the potential predictive relationships between various adverse health conditions and risk factors. Many companies sell these devices that collect real-time data and store it in their databases. These types of data constitute a rich repository of longitudinal and time-series data, and big data is a valuable resource that can be generated through proper analysis and modeling. Because these data are longitudinal, they offer opportunities to address a range of useful questions. For example, we can study the disease course (trajectory) by predicting the trajectory risk. To do this, we used ML models for the classification of ADL categories (0 = No ADL problem and 1 = ADL problem). Also, identifying significant, controllable predictors of ADLs could help manage the condition. Existing chronic ADL problems are a precursor of Instrumental Activities of Daily Living (IADL) problems among the elderly [37]. Other studies also found ADL as a significant predictor of IADL [38, 39]. So, it is important to understand how ADL and its trajectory risk change over time.

To predict trajectory risk, we need to fit joint probabilities for a subject across time points, which requires a joint model for categorical outcomes, which is rarely available. We employed a Markov chain to predict trajectory risk, enabling us to derive the joint probability of the trajectory by combining marginal and conditional probabilities. The main advantage of this approach is that the conditional probability can be estimated using conditional models in the univariate case; hence, a multivariate (joint) model is not required. Using various machine learning algorithms for trajectory risk prediction, we demonstrated approaches to analyzing such longitudinal datasets and how predictive results can be used to provide feedback to patients to improve their health outcomes.

Conclusions

Longitudinal data exhibit inherent temporal dependence that must be accounted for during model fitting, necessitating a multivariate model. Unfortunately, such a multivariate logistic regression model is not available. Therefore, it is a significant challenge to analyze such data in real time to identify risks, trends, and patterns and to provide informed, online, automated, and predictive feedback to the user so that they can improve their adverse health conditions. We proposed a framework for trajectory risk prediction and illustrated it using various ML models and real-life datasets for the elderly from the USA. The predictions of ADL categories are very high for all five ML models (N. Net, R.F, D. Tree, SVM, and Lasso). The prediction accuracies range from 0.88 to 0.98 for the training data and from 0.88 to 0.91 for the test data. The predictors, large muscle index, total income, BMI, depression score (CESD), and age emerged as the significant predictors of ADL problems, and some of these are controllable. The proposed predictive modeling framework for trajectory risk prediction proved highly useful, with the added advantage of reducing a multivariate problem to a univariate one. This framework can be applied to many longitudinal datasets from other disciplines.

Acknowledgments The authors acknowledge the National Institute on Aging of the University of Michigan for sharing the US Health and Retirement Study data.

Appendix

R Code Example to Fit the Neural Network Model

```
library(foreach)
 library(doParallel)
 library(data.table)
 library(dplyr)
 library(MASS)
 library(caret)
 library(glmnet) ## Lasso
 library(randomForest)
 library(tree)
 library(e1071)

 setwd("C:\\paper")
 source("userFunction.R")
  set.seed(34567)

 load("allTrnor.RData")  # Training data set same structure
as in Table 2
 load("allNor.RData")  # Both training and test data set
the same structure as in Table 2

 # Features name
 indvars <- c("Age", "Mstat", "Ncond", "Drink", "Gender",
"Race", "Educ",
              "Veteran", "BMI", "CESD", "Lmuscle", "Income",
"Memory", "Wrecall")

 idvar   <- "hhidpn"   # Subject ID feature
 depvar <- "Adla"     # Output
 b        <- 15            # Total number of features
plus output
 totfol  <- 7              # Total time points

 ##########################################################
###################
## Model fitting NN (Neural Network)

 registerDoParallel(7)
  system.time(
   Bo2 <- foreach(i = 1:totfol, .
```

```
packages=c('MASS','caret')) %dopar% {

          trainDatN <- as.data.frame(allTrnor[Wave==i,])
          trainDatN$Adla <- factor(trainDatN$Adla)

          if(i>1){indvars<-c(indvars,paste("Y",(i-1),sep=""))}
          mymodel <- paste(depvar, paste(indvars, collapse=" +
"), sep=" ~ ")
          ttDat   <- trainDatN[,1:(i+b)]

          binmod  <- train(Adla~., data=ttDat[,2:dim(ttDat)[2]],
method='nnet',
                    trControl=trainControl(method='cv'), number =
10, repeats = 5)

          newdat <- allNor[allNor$Wave==i,] #[,1:(i+b)]
          prob   <- predict(binmod, newdat ,type='prob')
          prob   <- prob[,2]
          Yh     <- ifelse(prob > 0.50, 1, 0)
          prob   <- as.data.frame(cbind(hhidpn = newdat$hhidpn, Y
= newdat$Adla,
                                             Yh = Yh, prob = prob,
Type = newdat$Type))
          mls    <- list(binmod,prob)
         })
      stopImplicitCluster()

        cpBo2 <- cpjp(totfol, Bo2)    # Creating data file
including conditional and joint probabilities


     # Computing accuracy and other statistics
        accNn <- accuMat(totfol,Bo2) #First 7 columns is for
Train and next seven for Test
        round(accNn,3)
```

Similar structures of codes are used for the other four machine-learning models.

References

1. United Nations Department of Economic and Social Affairs, Population Division. World population ageing 2023: challenges and opportunities of population aging in the least developed countries. UN DESA/POP/2023/TR/NO.5; 2023.
2. Tandel V, Kumari A, Tanwar S, Singh A, Sharma R, Yamsani N. Intelligent wearable-assisted digital healthcare industry 5.0. Artif Intell Med. 2024;157:103000.
3. Ranganathan I, Poongodi T, Suresh P, Balamurugan B. The growing role of internet of things in healthcare wearables. In: Emergence of pharmaceutical industry growth with industrial IoT approach. Academic Press; 2020. p. 163–94.
4. Beck RW, Riddlesworth T, Ruedy K, et al. Effect of continuous glucose monitoring on glycemic control in adults with type 1 diabetes using insulin injections: the DIAMOND randomized clinical trial. JAMA. 2017;317:371–8.
5. Jafleh EA, Alnaqbi FA, Almaeeni HA, Faqeeh S, Alzaabi MA, Al Zaman K. The role of wearable devices in chronic disease monitoring and patient care: a comprehensive review. Cureus. 2024;16(9):e68921.
6. Bent B, Goldstein BA, Kibbe WA, Dunn JP. Investigating sources of inaccuracy in wearable optical heart rate sensors. NPJ Digit Med. 2020;3:18. https://doi.org/10.1038/s41746-020-0226-6.
7. Gungormus DB, Garcia-Moreno FM, Bermudez-Edo M, Sánchez-Bermejo L, Garrido JL, Rodríguez-Fórtiz MJ, Pérez-Mármol JM. A semi-automatic mHealth system using wearable devices for identifying pain-related parameters in elderly individuals. Int J Med Inform. 2024;184:105371.
8. Cai L, Zhu Y. The challenges of data quality and data quality assessment in the big data era. CODATA. 2015;14:2.
9. Silva BM, Rodrigues JJ, de la Torre Díez I, López-Coronado M, Saleem KJ. Mobile-health: a review of current state in 2015. J Biomed Inform. 2015;56:265–72.
10. Ozcan M, Peker S. A classification and regression tree algorithm for heart disease modeling and prediction. Healthcare Anal. 2023;3:100130.
11. Chang V, Bhavani VR, Xu AQ, Hossain MA. An artificial intelligence model for heart disease detection using machine learning algorithms. Healthcare Anal. 2022;2:100016.
12. Islam MM, Hassan S, Akter S, Jibon FA, Sahidullah M. A comprehensive review of predictive analytics models for mental illness using machine learning algorithms. Healthcare Anal. 2024;6:100350.
13. Mahmoud A, Takaoka E. An enhanced machine learning approach with stacking ensemble learner for accurate liver cancer diagnosis using feature selection and gene expression data. Healthcare Anal. 2025;7:100373.
14. Han Y, Wang S. Disability risk prediction model based on machine learning among Chinese healthy older adults: results from the China Health and Retirement Longitudinal Study. Front Public Health. 2023;11:1271595.
15. Zhang H, Zhou W, He J, Liu X, Shen J. Machine learning insights on activities of daily living disorders in Chinese older adults. Exp Gerontol. 2024;198:112641.
16. Chen J, Ren Y, Ding J, et al. Construction of disability risk prediction model for the elderly based on machine learning. Sci Rep. 2025;15:16247.
17. Jafari-Koulaee A, Mohammadi E, Fox MT, et al. Predictors of basic and instrumental activities of daily living among older adults with multiple chronic conditions. BMC Geriatr. 2024;24:383.
18. Islam MA, Chowdhury RI. Prediction of disease status: a regressive model approach for repeated measures. Stat Methodol. 2010;7:520–40.
19. Singer JD, Willett JB. Applied longitudinal data analysis: modeling change and event occurrence. Oxford University Press; 2003.
20. Twisk JWR. Applied longitudinal data analysis for epidemiology. Cambridge University Press; 2013.
21. Tripepi G, Heinze G, Jager KJ, Stel VS, Dekker FW, Zoccali C. Risk prediction models. Nephrol Dial Transplant. 2013;28(8):1975–80.

22. Chowdhury RI, Islam MA. Regressive models for risk prediction for repeated multinomial outcomes: an illustration using health and retirement study (HRS) data. Biom J. 2020:1–18.
23. Islam, M.A., Chowdhury, R.: Analysis of repeated measures data. Singapore: Springer Nature. https://doi.org/10.1007/978-981-10-3794-8. (2017).
24. McCulloch WS, Pitts W. A logical calculus of the ideas immanent in nervous activity. Bull Math Biophys. 1943;5:115–33.
25. Hoff JR, Edward M. Learning phenomena in networks of adaptive switching circuits. Stanford University; 1962.
26. Rosenblatt F. Principles of neurodynamics. Perceptrons and the theory of brain mechanisms. Buffalo: Cornell Aeronautical Lab Inc; 1961.
27. Kutner MH, Nachtsheim CJ, Neter J, Li W. Applied linear statistical models. 5th ed. New York: McGraw-Hill, Irwin; 2005.
28. Ripley BD. Pattern recognition and neural networks. Cambridge University Press; 2007.
29. Breiman L. Random forests. Mach Learn. 2001;45:5–32.
30. Tibshirani RJ, Efron B. An introduction to the bootstrap. Monogr Statist Appl Probab. 1993;57(1):1–436.
31. Breiman L. Classification and regression trees. Routledge; 2017.
32. Boser BE, Guyon IM, Vapnik VN. A training algorithm for optimal margin classifiers. In: Proceedings of the fifth annual workshop on computational learning theory; 1992.
33. Cortes C, Vapnik V. Support-vector networks. Mach Learn. 1995;20:273.
34. Tibshirani R. Regression shrinkage and selection via the lasso. J R Stat Soc Ser B Methodol. 1996;58(1):267–88.
35. Lee S-I, Lee H, Abbeel P, Andrew YN. Efficient l~ 1 regularized logistic regression. Aaai. 2006;6:401–8.
36. HRS. Public-use dataset: health and retirement study. Ann Arbor: University of Michigan; 2019.
37. Chowdhury R, Bari W, Hasan MT, Hossain Z, Rahman M. Artificial intelligence-based models for predicting disease course risk using patient data. Computers. 2026;15:113.
38. Rice K, Chen J, Kakara R, Haddad YK. Risk of diminished activities of daily living (ADLs) and instrumental activities of daily living (IADLs) after an older adult fall, medicare current beneficiary survey, 2015–2020. Am J Lifestyle Med. 2025:15598276251368863. Online ahead of print.
39. Guo HJ, Sapra A. Instrumental activity of daily living. [Updated 2022 Nov 14]. In StatPearls [Internet]. StatPearls Publishing: Treasure Island; 2025. Available online at: https://www.ncbi.nlm.nih.gov/books/NBK553126/.

Chapter 5
Empowering Healthcare: Harnessing the Potential of the Medical Internet of Things for Advanced Patient Care

S. Delsi Robinsha and B. Amutha

Introduction

Overview

Technical advancements, as well as clinical practices, have been presented with a blend of innovation that has transformed the way patients are treated in modern healthcare facilities. This progress is largely attributed to the development and implementation of the *Medical Internet of Things (MIoT)*, a relatively young and rapidly evolving discipline that involves the use of digital platforms, sensors, and interconnected devices to optimize the delivery of medical care. The integration of the IoT paradigm enables the real-time collection, processing, and transmission of data related to various aspects of medical treatment and patient management. In this chapter, emphasis will be placed on examining the major trends in the application of the Internet of Things (IoT) in healthcare, in order to highlight its potential to improve treatment quality, enhance healthcare delivery, and shape the overall development of the healthcare sector. This chapter aims to provide readers with a clear understanding of the revolutionary capabilities of IoT by exploring its historical evolution, its current functions, and possible future directions. At its core, the Internet of Things (IoT) represents the convergence of connectivity, data analytics, and healthcare knowledge. IoT holds the potential to support a wide range of applications, including remote patient monitoring, personalized approaches to medical care, and many others. It assists stakeholders by providing healthcare practitioners with actionable information that can enable early interventions before a patient's condition deteriorates. Furthermore, IoT facilitates the integration of various

S. Delsi Robinsha (✉) · B. Amutha
Department of Computing Technologies, School of Computing, Faculty of Engineering and Technology, SRM Institute of Science and Technology, Kattankulathur, Tamil Nadu, India
e-mail: ds8912@srmist.edu.in; amuthab@srmist.edu.in

P. Eappen et al. (eds.), *Advancing Healthcare with the Medical Internet of Things*, Health Informatics, https://doi.org/10.1007/978-3-032-23933-4_5

systems and devices throughout a patient's care journey, supporting better self-management and continuity of care [1].

At the same time, it is important to recognize that alongside its benefits, IoT presents several challenges that must be addressed to ensure its safe and effective use. Risks related to data security, privacy, cross-platform compatibility, legal regulations, and ethical considerations remain significant concerns. Coherent and coordinated actions are necessary to mitigate these risks and fully realize the potential of the Internet of Things. Nevertheless, it would be misleading to overlook the transformative potential of IoT in healthcare. By embracing IoT technologies and processes, healthcare stakeholders can enhance patient outcomes, manage resources more efficiently, and drive innovation within the sector. Ultimately, IoT is fostering the development of patient-centric healthcare models that prioritize personalized treatment and proactive prevention over reactive care.

IoT in healthcare, as demonstrated in Fig. 5.1, provides the opportunity to make timely decisions, and in relation to reporting and monitoring, it allows doing it in real-time, whereas the end-to-end connectivity increases communication between devices and healthcare providers.

It is crucial to begin our journey into the sphere of the Internet of Things (IoT) within the healthcare sector by stating two things: first, the promise of this technology is enormous; and second, the challenges arising from the introduction of IoT cannot be dismissed as insignificant [2]. In the next decade, with the help of IoT, a new level of patient care and healthcare industry evolution is possible only if all these risks will be overcome with adequate attention, ideas, and focus on patients.

- The chapter "Empowering Healthcare": The paper Making Sense of the Medical Internet of Things: Opportunities and Challenges which this chapter explores contains several central ideas focused on the explication of the role of the Medical Internet of Things in patient centered care.

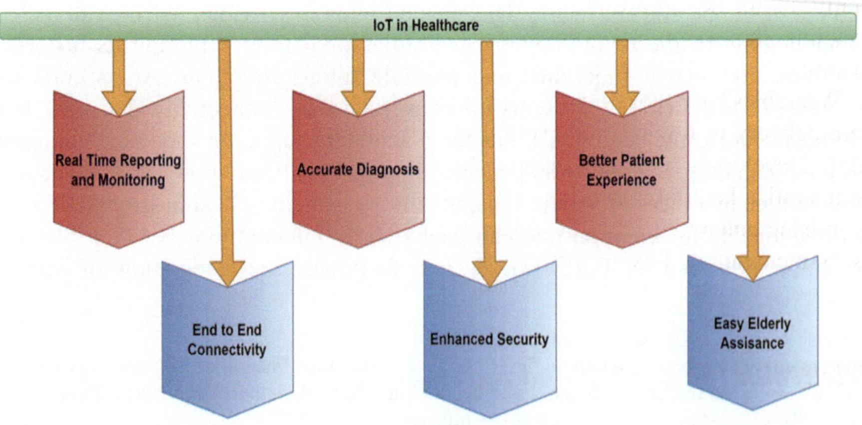

Fig. 5.1 Internet of things in healthcare

- First, it put a lot of weight on the interconnectivity of devices, sensors, and applications, which allow for real-time data processing and collection to improve patient status. Thus, MIoT helps in the individualized and preventive approach to health promotion while adapting resources in healthcare facilities with their help of technologies like artificial intelligence, cloud storage, and wearable devices.
- Second, the chapter discusses the topic of development in the course of MIoT, which brought improvements in wearable health monitoring, sensors, and telemedicine. This documents how these innovations support self-management of patient's health while helping care givers target disease therapies according to the received information.
- Also, as part of the MIoT research, this chapter also discusses some of the significant issues pertaining to the MIoT among them being security, integration, and standardization, and compliance questions. Due to these findings, it emphasizes the importance of having adequate security measures and compliance with best practices that would allow for the secure utilization of MIoT technologies in healthcare.

Lastly, the chapter calls for the integration of MIoT into patient care by increasing the level of cooperation between healthcare practitioners, technologists, and policy makers to fully unleash MIoT capabilities and foster evolution to patient-centered care domain. In highlighting these aspects in the chapter, the work establishes the importance of MIoT in transforming healthcare and patients' well-being.

Evolution of the Medical Internet of Things

The MIoT has significantly transformed the healthcare system by acting as an enabler of fresh models in delivering healthcare services such as telemedicine, smart-connected medical devices, wearable health solutions besides remote patient monitoring. These changes reflect improvements over the standard healthcare models, maintaining high and actually enhancing patients' satisfaction as well as optimization of processes in delivering healthcare. MIoT has one significant advantage: it allows watching data and their further analysis in real-time. The MIoT marks a transformative first stage in the evolution of modern healthcare by introducing new models of care delivery that extend far beyond traditional, facility-based systems. Early applications of MIoT have focused on integrating technologies such as telemedicine, smart-connected FDA cleared medical devices, wearable technologies and monitoring, and remote patient monitoring. These innovations allow healthcare services to reach patients in real-time, regardless of location, while enhancing patient satisfaction, improving treatment outcomes, and optimizing operational processes. A defining advantage of MIoT is its capacity real-time data collection and analysis, for which empowers healthcare professionals to continuously monitor patient health and intervene promptly when necessary. This proactive approach has been shown to significantly reduce hospital readmissions, particularly for chronic disease management. In contrast, conventional healthcare relies on periodic physical examinations and delayed diagnostic processes, which can postpone critical treatment decisions. Additionally, MIoT has streamlined healthcare workflows by automating the gathering and analysis of patient data, reducing reliance on manual processes that are often time-consuming and prone to human error. This first stage of MIoT evolution has not only redefined how care is delivered but also laid the foundation for a more connected, efficient, and patient-centered healthcare system.

The advancement and complexity of connected devices, sensors, and digital platform in the healthcare sector is the progression of the medical internet of things (MIoT) as observed in [3]. MIoT technologies have also increased patient satisfaction as a result of digitized communication technologies. Patients state that the elements such as monitoring from the distance and the variety of telemedicine options provide them with more engagement and help to simplify their lives. Due [4] to the long hours spent waiting and limited access to their wanted providers, people can literally get unhappy in conventional care contexts. The Internet of Things (IoT) resolves these issues by providing additional control over the demand for healthcare and allowing people to discuss with their doctors from home. Still, there are certain issues relating to the application of MIoT in healthcare even with these developments made. To get the best out of MIoT, issues ranging from security and privacy of data, compatibility issues and the need to obey existing rules have to be resolved.

(i) *Research Gaps*

Research Gaps of Medical Internet of Things (MIoT) in healthcare include several significant aspects that must be researched. First, there is a clear requirement for enhanced protection of data since the patients provide some very sensitive information about their health. Second, devices of MIoT in healthcare integrate with other systems, and still there is a need for research in setting standards and protocols for proper integration. Moreover, the awareness of the related regulation of MIoT technologies varies depending on the region; thus, the proper approach should be determined. Factors in user experience and adoption also need research in order to improve the usability of MIoT systems, both for the healthcare providers and the patients. Last but not the least, the process of evaluating the clinical outcomes linked to MIoT implementations is still continuing to evaluate the efficiency of the embedded solutions for enhancing care to patients as well as the delivery of healthcare services.

Data Quality, Reliability, and Accuracy: Many MIoT devices generate large amounts of real-time data, but the accuracy, consistency, and clinical validity of this data can vary. False alarms, sensor drift, and inconsistent measurements limit clinical decision-making. Research is needed on data validation methods, machine learning filters, and AI models that can distinguish between clinically relevant signals and noise.

Clinical Integration and Decision Support: There is limited research on how MIoT data can be effectively integrated into existing Electronic Health Records

(EHRs) and clinical workflows. Research is required to design decision support systems that help clinicians translate MIoT data into actionable, evidence-based interventions.

Usability and Human Factors Many devices are not designed with end-user (patients and clinicians) needs in mind, leading to poor adoption, compliance, or understanding. Research into user-centered design, human-machine interaction, and behavioral acceptance of MIoT devices is lacking.

Scalability and Cost-Effectiveness: Most MIoT applications are still limited to pilot studies or specialized settings. Research is needed to assess large-scale deployment, economic sustainability, and cost-benefit analysis across diverse healthcare systems.

Ethical and Legal Considerations: Issues related to informed consent, data ownership, algorithmic bias, and patient autonomy are underexplored in the context of MIoT. Legal frameworks governing cross-border data sharing and the use of AI-driven decisions in healthcare are not well defined.

Environmental and Energy Sustainability: Many MIoT devices are battery-dependent or resource-intensive, raising concerns about energy consumption and electronic waste. Research on energy-efficient MIoT systems, green IoT, and biodegradable devices is still in its infancy.

Outcome Evaluation and Long-Term Impact: While MIoT shows promise in improving patient monitoring and outcomes, there is a lack of longitudinal studies demonstrating sustained clinical benefit, cost savings, or population health improvement over time.

Personalization and Predictive Analytics: More research is needed to harness MIoT data for personalized medicine and predictive risk modeling using advanced AI, especially for chronic disease management and preventive care.

Multiple critical phases characterize the development of MIoT

A New Era in Wearable Health Monitoring

Smart garments like belts, watches, and bracelets are some of the products that were brought in the first phase during the conception of the IoT. These devices included sensors for capturing biometrics of the user; for example, pulse rates, level of mobility, and sleep. Apart from regular clinical environment, these gadgets opened the possibility for transitioning to personal health management [4].

Technological Progress in Sensors

Integrated devices, biosensors, accelerometers, and even environmental sensors for the purpose of IoT are attributable to innovative enhancements in sensor technology. Thus, these small sensors that are inexpensive must be incorporated into several medical devices and wearable because it is able to continuously monitor the physiological parameters, as well as the environmental factors [5].

Interoperability and Connectivity

Interoperability and flow from one system to another was becoming even more pronounced as more devices were connected to the IoT. "Identifying patients" care requirements, co-ordination, and data exchange have benefitted from improved communication channels including Bluetooth, Wi-Fi, and cellular networks. These protocols have simplified a method through which; devices, healthcare institutions, and EHRs can exchange health information.

A common IoT healthcare system consists of multiple layers, the first being perception layer that contains multiple sensors and the second being the application layer that allows decision-making and analysis. This stratified design guarantees data capture, safe communication, data storage, and integration to provide efficient healthcare delivery (see Fig. 5.2).

Utilization of Analytics Data

Data analytics and machine learning algorithms embedded in computer systems linked to IoT have made it possible for the healthcare providers to derive high value from large amounts of health data generated by IoT devices. Doctors may know patients' status, anticipate health outcomes, and look for anomalies, which helps to propose individualized approaches.

Growth in the Field of Telemedicine and Online Health

Integration with telemedicine and virtual care has also occurred with the advancement of the Internet of Things (IoT) where COVID-19 has caused specific advancement. Teleconferencing, home monitoring, and digital care applications are now central to the Internet of Things (IoT), thus assisting in delivering healthcare services without much physical contact [6].

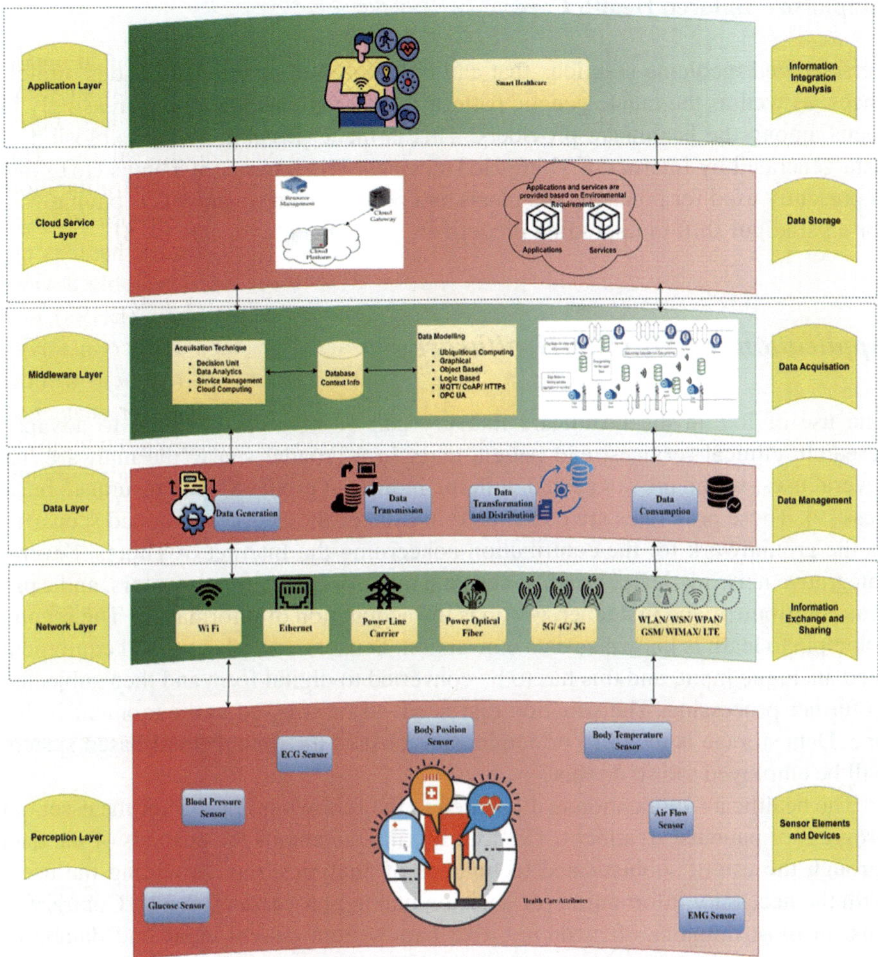

Fig. 5.2 Evolution of the medical IoT

Application of AI

The IoT solutions have been slowly implementing AI technologies like Natural Language Processing, Computer vision, and Predictive analytics to increase the existing automation level, improve the diagnosing ability, and improve the patients' experience in correspondingly sequences. Diagnostic algorithms, prediction models, and virtual health assistants that incorporate artificial intelligence in their functions are altering the face and functional capabilities of the health care sector making it more efficient and effective in the process.

Emphasize Tailored Health Care

Personalized medicine solutions that can be tailored to the characteristics, preferences, as well as the innate genetic patterns of the patients are now increasingly in focus among the healthcare providers. This is made possible by the explosion of data generated by Internet of Things IoT devices. The Internet of Things (IoT) that is presently used for precision diagnosis and personalized treatments is paving way for a paradigm shift in upgrading proactively patient centered care [7, 8].

Applications of MIoT in Healthcare

The use of IoT in the healthcare industry can be of great potential to advance research, clinical services, and patient care. In a broader sense, the malware has several uses, which are connected with the industrial processes and insurance business [9]. These principles are considered in each of the above-mentioned scenarios as the groundwork for the contribution concerning the Internet of Things. Several integrative network devices such as sensors, monitors, detectors, equators, and cameras contribute to the first tenet, which is the acquisition of information. The second principle to learn is known as data conversion. Sensors and other related equipment feed analogue input, and this has to be converted to digital form and then subjected to further processing. The situation that needs to be stressed at the moment is this one. Data storage is the third principle, and most of the time a cloud-based system will be employed too so do this.

The healthcare application is illustrated in the following Fig. 5.3 for the essential progress of patients' treatment. The fourth principle entails the analysis of the data through the use of sophisticated techniques of analytics, thus providing the users with the necessary information for decision making processes [10, 11]. Contrary to this, in most domains of medicine, like handwritten patient chart and databases interconnected in laboratories, the norms that were introduced previously are already implemented. One of the major risks is that data is always persistent, and the outline of things informed by the IoT can have an influence at any successive moment. This is what makes the different from other Internet of Thing's systems. Below are some of the applications in the MIoT.

Remote Patient Monitoring System

To effectively deliver long-distance healthcare and to give the patients a chance to be monitored from a distance, tele healthcare is utilized. Tele healthcare to a certain extent has closed up part of the gap that developed between patients and their healthcare provider(s). The main advantages of tele healthcare are that patients will not visit frequent to the hospital therefore; it has the potential of cutting costs greatly. It avails health care services and consultancy to the patients irrespective of

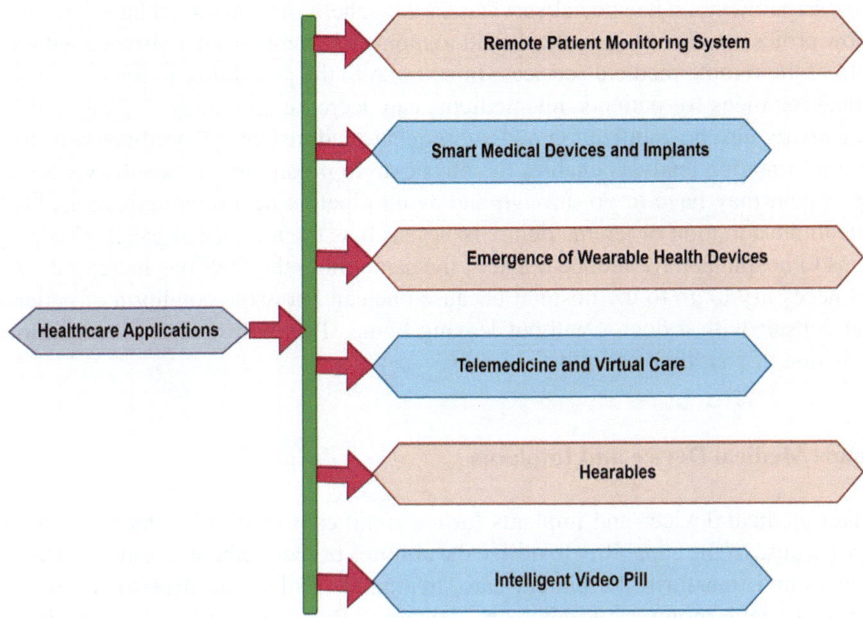

Fig. 5.3 Applications of MIoT

the place they are in through the use of mobile technology, computers, and telecommunication. Recently the transmission of data over networks has been involving several ways.

On the other hand, a number of specialists have identified an algorithm for path finding in networks purposely for the telesurgery. Thus, with the help of medical applications like health monitors with telesurgery options, they were able to do it. This optimization of Medical Quality of Service (m-QoS) is especially important in the era of epidemic, where most of the civilized world's population cannot leave without medical help. In [12], the writers developed a system, which is dependable and trustworthy to help in the facilitation of interaction between clinicians and patients. This was done to make the probability of carrying out the surgery while at distant areas. With this, a successful surgery could be carried out from greater distance. Moreover, the provided mechanism will be employed to observe these connections because it makes it possible to receive data in real-time. The over-arching research question for the study is therefore how can the study increase buffer space as this can be effectively used to minimize the time taken by data from source to destination. Smart Route control algorithm, referred to as the S-RCA, is a new algorithm designed for the first time in this chapter. By means of its help, data can be transmitted much easier with establishing the smart routes between two points in the virtual world. This concern-oriented reliable connectivity will help surgical treatments because it ensures that all the instructions will be delivered on time. Thus, this method improves the M-QoS in remote surgery through utilizing the more reliable pathways. The special services in the sphere of medical technologies will allow professionals of the medical field to monitor patients from a distance with the help of the remote medical services. In addition to the possibility to prescribe individual regimens for patients, telemedicine can decrease the number of cases when patients require hospitalization and subsequent readmissions. Coordinated healthcare information analysis enables the physician to predict major health events that the patient may have to go through and avoid pipeline health complications [13]. Due to the adoption of telemedicine, issues such as the number of patients' admissions to hospitals have reduced, and at the same time, the QoS has increased. It is not necessary to go to the hospital because one can know the condition of patients and consult with a doctor without leaving home. This will lead to a tremendous reduction of wait time as follows.

Smart Medical Device and Implants

Smart medical devices and implants form a significant shift in healthcare technology because of the capability to utilize the abilities of the Medical Internet of Things (MioT) and transform the patient care, treatment results, and disease control. In terms of health monitoring indicators, delivering treatment, and exchanging information with the doctors, these devices use Internet of Things, sensors, and connection elements. Some examples of such devices are continuous glucose monitors (CGMs), which give the patient's doctors and the patient real-time glucose levels; implantable cardiac devices such as pacemakers or implantable cardioverter-defibrillators that diagnose the disturbances in the regular heartbeat and apply the proper electric shock or pacing to restore the standard rhythm of the heart; and smart inhalers that contain sensors and connectivity capabilities to deal with asthma more efficiently by monitoring the usage. Some of the positive aspects that come with smart MDs include real time screen; individual patient interactions; tele monitoring; increased patient involvement; better health outcomes; and cost reduction resulting from the elimination of unnecessary hospitalization; or emergency room visits; or costly consequences of uncontrolled long-term conditions. Smart medical device delivery of healthcare is improving the healthcare of citizens globally and also enriching the patients perceptive. These devices function in the manner that involves patients in matters concerning their own treatment, provide real-time data, and help in the quick response to any ailments.

Emergence of Wearable Health Device

They are not as intrusive, make it possible to speak without a hold anything, and come packed with several ways of communication. They are portable displays worn on the hand, bodycams, and augmented reality headsets. "Phones" and "apps" go together with wearable devices. According to Antonelli, applications on computers and other portable devices are wearables' interfaces [14]. Consequently, cellphones perform and/or store individuals' device information in the cloud or fog. Mobile tech and wearable tech are related [15]. On the other hand, smarter and stronger wearables may 1 day work without computers. The fact that people can readily use services with wearables; Similar to lighting, the use of voice can be used as a replacement to typing or even moving around. Smart watches and spectacles are special forms of active wearables that can do so. They can used to command devices near or far. The other kind of gear that is worn is not as noisy as the foregoing examples of armory and harness. Wearable-tech IoT healthcare system: Fitness Trackers, Step Counters, Heart Rate Monitors, and Blood Pressure Monitors are some of the wearable medical devices. These gadgets can instantly monitor the patients' heart rate, blood pressure, as well as glucose levels. Since these measures are not prescriptive, they do not have to be memorized or written down by patients. One can practice self-care in the confines of his or her home as long as they have medical wearables. Specifically, early warnings and monitoring of medical vital signs are made to the patients. Analytics allows execution of doctors to be traced by patients' treatment. This benefit assists patients with mental disorders or chronic diseases. Clinical staff may also be told of patient mishaps in or outside the health institution. If the examined outpatient with heart failure is not making enough steps per day, something is wrong with him and he should be checked out. If a child has diabetes and is given blood glucose monitor alarms that suggest that the glucose level is high, teach the parents of the child the benefits of appropriate diets. Using analyses and the use of big data, the use of wearable technology enhances doctor-patient relationships. Better prevention may result. It reveals to the patients their reverse behaviors or challenges merely by looking at their blood oxygen level, pulse, or blood sugar levels. This makes the patients more involved in their health status and the processes that are meeting out their treatment. Wearable equipment assists in tracking the patients' status without the need for a doctor. Integrated circuits (system on chips), biosensors, advanced energy technologies like energy harvesting, wireless charging, nanotechnology and materials science, IPv6 over LoWPAN, and ultra-low power device to device networking enable this. Among the issues are the compatibility issues between the devices, incorrect or inconsistent data stored in them, the invasion of privacy, the security flaws, low battery capacity, and affectation of the signals for communication.

Telemedicine and Virtual Care

Telemedicine may also be referred to as E-Health or M-Health, E-Visits, or telemedicine if the m symbolizes mobile. It is the provision of healthcare services with the use Information Communication Technology. The implication of this is that is health care that doctors provide you over the wires and not the typical clinic room. On the whole, though, telemedicine is in some ways novel. This is due to the spread of video conferencing, which makes the occurrence quite common. The truth, however, is that telemedicine is not a relatively new concept, and it has been around for more than a couple of decades. In the past, doctors were allowed to do consultations through phone calls. Next, facsimile made it possible for people to converse with their physicians. Synchronous video consulting is generally occurring more often, but patients can still phone or email their GP. Essentials of telemedicine show that not everybody is too busy to be served through these noble practices. Initially, such a form of patient treatment was great news for those people who live in unfavorable conditions or in the countryside. It was safer to receive medical treatment in this manner during the COVID-19 pandemic. It is becoming quite valuable for those people who simply do not have time to go to the doctor and then sit in a waiting room for hours.

Hearables

Hearables of the current epoch have dramatically altered the modalities of using hearing aids by individuals with hearing impairment with regard to interacting with the surrounding world. Currently, electronic hearing aids have been fitted with Bluetooth; this enables you to connect through your smartphone. With the help of this piece of software, real-world sounds can be filtered, equalized, and overlaid with additional characteristics. The vest example leading to this understanding is Doppler Labs.

Intelligent Video Pills

For efficient diagnosis, a smart pill is ingested and allows doctors to see a live image of the patient's internal condition. It thereby can share those images to a wearable device that synchronizes with applications specific for medical use.

Case Studies

MIoT has also improved ways of deliverance in the health sector through enabling real-time tracking of patients, better results on the cases treated, and sharing of information that is real time. The following are the different case studies that show how MIoT works in real life healthcare systems and the advantages accrued.

A. *Telemonitoring in the Management of Chronic Illness*

Case Study: Diabetes Management
An AP of a healthcare facility in the United States adopted the use of RPM to cater for patients suffering from diabetes. Clients were provided with CGM, which sends out the ongoing glucose values to the healthcare givers. This made it possible to make appropriate revisions on the management and treatment recommendations depending on the information that was received.

Outcomes

Reduction in Hospital Readmissions: The use of the tool in the implementation process resulted in the reduction of readmission rates among patients that were monitored to 30%.

Improved Patient Engagement: Respondents affirmed that they became more engaged in their condition's management since they could see glucose levels and address food impacts.

Cost Savings: Due to the healthcare provider's assistance, specific costs linked to intervention measures and sudden hospitalization were reduced.

Thus, MIoT helps in the proper management of chronic diseases as it offers consistent monitoring and preventive medical interventions.

B. *Smart medical device and implants*

Case Study: Cardiac Monitoring with Smart Pacemakers

A hospital in Europe adopted use of smart pacemakers that are associated with the MIoT. These devices track the heart rate and may even report abnormalities to the concerned medical practitioners.

Outcomes:

Real-Time Data Transmission: These pacemakers ensured that the physicians received constant information on the health of the patients' heart causing them to respond in case of an emergent occurrence.

Reduction in Emergency Visits: Admitted they had smart pacemakers, their use added that emergency room visit was reduced by 40% since their conditions were well managed.

Enhanced Quality of Life: The patients also expressed enhanced self-efficacy in their overall health since there was check-up of their cardiac health all the time.

The real-life case brought out that MIoT can assist to offer current health information, which can promote timely action and better quality of life among the patients.

C. *Telemedicine Integration*

Case Study: Telehealth Services During COVID-19 a Qualitative Study Performed at Taif University, KSA

During the COVID-19 outbreak, a healthcare facility incorporated telemedicine together with technologies within the MIoT context whereby patients could speak to their healthcare practitioners online from the comfort of their homes. Patients engaged in remote video consultations and passed their physical stats to the doctors.

Outcomes:

Increased Access to Care: Such patients included those in remote areas or those who had some form of difficulty in physically moving from one place to another, could get healthcare, without having to physically attend the heath facilities.

Higher Patient Satisfaction: Patients and doctors reported a 25% increase in the perception of received care since the remote consultations did not pose any risks to the patients' health.

Continuity of Care: They also made sure patients would be able to receive the necessary care during lock down through integration.

This case also depicts a scene where MIoT enhances the support of telemedicine solutions to patients and ensures the continuity of the patients' management.

D. *Wearable health devices are used for identifying potential health risks and disease in consumers before they become major problems.*

Case Study: Sports Wearables in Health Monitoring

A wellness program implemented in the corporate environment provided wearable health devices to track employees' movement, heart rate, and sleep. Quantitative data was collected from the patients, and recommendations given based on that data to help the patients lead healthy lives.

Outcomes:

Improved Employee Health: Most of the participants stated that their activity level increased and that they had improved sleep patterns, which proactively enhanced their health status.

Reduced Healthcare Costs: The company reported less cases of healthcare claims especially those concerning lifestyle diseases, which would have enormous implications on the firm's financial status.

Enhanced Engagement: The human resource management enabled the members of the workforce to be in charge of the kind of health that the organization promoted, enhancing the company's wellness culture.

This case also shows all the possibilities of MIoT wearables for the prevention of diseases and employee's health maintenance.

Regulatory Landscape Governing MIoT

Currently, the legal framework of MIoT is quite dissimilar across the different regions in the world, all of which are striving to overcome problems and implement measures for efficient compliance.

(i) *United States*

The Food and Drug Administration (FDA) in the United States has spelt out policies on the distinction of IoT gadgets used in medical devices. The FDA aims at providing protection of these devices in aspect of safety and effectiveness accompanied by paramount importance of secure protection of patients' records.

(ii) *European Union*

In Europe, there is a law known as General Data Protection Regulation (GDPR) that provides high-sensitivity requirements to MIoT devices. The GDPR helps to protect patient's information by ensuring that it is well protected and guarantee whoever's information it is, they have full control. Also, the EU is working in its regulatory agenda for the connective technologies of digital health including questions like compatibility, data quality, and clinical testing

(iii) *Asia-Pacific*

Implementing nations, like Japan and Singapore of the Asia-Pacific, are stimulating MIoT through policies and financing for healthcare innovations. However, these nations are also solving the issue of data security and problem of interoperability to make safe the usage of MIoT.

Best Practices for Compliance

To make compliance worldwide smoother in the view of MIoT, few safer directions can be followed: Firstly, the issue of standardization is significant; appearances of standard MIoT devices can contribute to the issue of compatibility and the governing policies' harmonization. Such a claim ensures that devices are able to exchange information within and between health systems, hence promoting and effective integrated system.

Second, most activities involve stakeholder collaboration. Therefore, continual dialogue with the key stakeholders involving the healthcare providers, technology developers, and regulators can lead to solving such problems more efficiently. Such relations enhance a deep understanding of the requirements and the general perspectives of all the sides so that the requirements and regulations would be more realistic and useful.

Another identifies the implementation of appropriate data security controls as another strategic best practice. Effective measures such as message encryption or access restrictions for specific categories of information as well as the preparation of reaction on incidents can also reduce the risks of adverse effects on confidentiality of patients' data. Since the MIoT devices are concerned with collecting data pertaining to the user's health, concerns with data security cannot be overemphasized.

Transparency as well as the consent of the patient is also another consideration. Overcoming the patient's misunderstanding of data collection, usage, and sharing enables healthcare organizations and developers of MIoT technologies to promote ethical practices. One of the critical components of the relationship between patients and the providers is evaluating their understanding of how their data is used and getting their consent.

Finally, the constant assessment of MIoT devices is needed to cope with innovative technologies in this field. Periodic review of the effectiveness and safety of these devices, as well as revising aspects of regulation depending on the newly available information and consumers' experiences, guarantees that the rules and regulations are still useful and efficient. Thus, applying these best practices, the stakeholders can improve compliance and promote the further deployment of MIoT technologies in healthcare safely and efficiently.

Challenges and Consideration

Data Security and Privacy

IoT faced some key challenges that include data security and privacy which is among the biggest headaches of IoT. Smart gadgets for the Internet of Things deliver real-time data acquisition ability; however, it is significant to note that most of them are not compliant with data protocols and standards. In the big pool of information, it is quite difficult to define ownership and regulation of the data content. Internet protocol device data storage results in theft and easy access to the fraudsters, who obtain the heath information of patients. Two examples of how the collected data from the Internet of Things devices is misused are forging documents like identification cards for the purchase and sales of the drugs and counterfeiting claims to health facilities. Figure 5.4 looks at some of the challenges that are likely to be faced in the integration of medical IoT.

Integration: Multiple Devices and Protocols

The Internet of Things can only be useful in the healthcare sector if several different kinds of devices are integrated. This problem originated from the industry's inability to agree on the protocols and standards used by the manufacturers of these devices. This will give rise to various ecosystems of the Internet of Things devices from various manufacturers, which prevented products from companies in the same industry from being compatible. This indicates that there is no synchronous protocol that can be utilized as the method of data aggregation in this case. Due to this, the procedure is a little on the complicated side, and hence, the ability of IoT in the healthcare field may not be as wide as has been anticipated.

Data Overload and Accuracy

Perhaps the toughest task is that of aggregating information when it is required for integrated views and further research due to no homogeneity of the conversation protocols and information. IoT currently gathers information in large volumes, and in an effort to analyze data effectively, the information has to be sliced into data portions that possess given exactness while avoiding too much strain on the system.

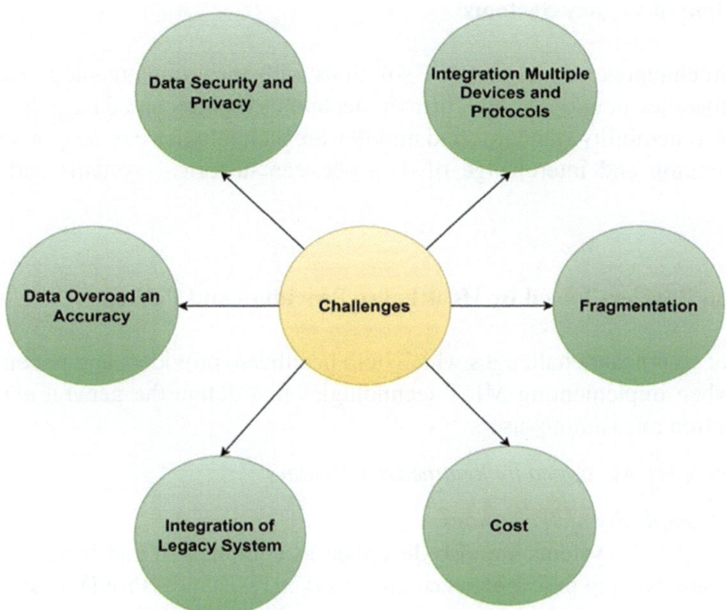

Fig. 5.4 Challenges in MIoT

At the same time, a large amount of information can, in the long run, affect the decision-making process within the field of hospitality.

Cost

One of the major challenges for considering mobile healthcare solutions in Systems through creating IoT apps is finding the financial link. Therefore, if the Internet of Things implementation solves a pain point accurately, the costs are justified. Of course, the creation of the IoT application will take considerable time and effort, but this investment will be compensated when your company implements better and more efficient processes, saves money and time, generates additional income, and discovers new opportunities for its development.

Fragmentation

The healthcare domain is highly dispersed, and individual's systems, old technologies, and diverse data models constitute the healthcare industry. There is a need for conscious endeavors toward integrating standards and simplifying the means of generally adopting them in the middle of such complexity.

Integration of Legacy Systems

The main challenge of merging IoT solutions with early implemented legacy systems is that they employ wholly different technology stacks and data exchange formats. Interoperability standards and middleware technologies can help in achieving the integration and interchange of data between historical systems and today's systems.

Adoption Barriers Faced by Healthcare Providers and Patients

There are significant challenges which both healthcare providers and patients experience when implementing MIoT technologies that define the general experience and adoption rates among users.

(i) *Solving issues capped by healthcare providers*

   (a) *Complexity of Technology*:
   MIoT systems are also described as complicated and hard to integrate into existing practice, hence the observed resistance. Providers should also have the technical know—how in handling these new technologies, but often this may not be the case due to high learning curve involved in handling the new technologies.

   (b) *Data Integration*:
   The challenge of integrating data from various MIoT devices into EHR systems can be a deciding issue. Sometimes, two systems are incompatible, and there is always a requirement to normalize data, which can lead to the emergence of obstacles that impede efficient data work.

   (c) *Regulatory Compliance*:
   The rules and regulations in countries like USA regarding privacy and security of data are stringent, and following the guidelines like the Health Insurance Portability and Accountability Act (HIPAA) is very challenging and consumes considerable time for the healthcare professionals. Another challenge for MIoT technologies' adoption is stakeholders' fear of not following various rules and legal restrictions that may arise in addition to legal problems.

(ii) *Challenges Faced by Patients*

   (a) *Technological Literacy*:
   Like any other application or devices, some patients especially those who are less computer literate or those who are old may have some challenges in handling MIoT devices and applications. For this reason, [personal communication] could fail or lead to the development of frustration and avoidance of these technologies.

   (b) *Data Privacy Concerns*:Perceived health data insecurity is a major concern from the patients, which may lead to reluctance in the adoption of MIoT devices. The concerns people have about their data being stolen and accessed by unauthorized persons can be a major concern to the adoption of such technologies.

(c) *Cost of Devices*:

MIoT devices may be costly for the patients, where they require purchasing cost and frequent replacement in the event of damage, especially for the less- to moderate-income earner. These expenses make it costly for patients to afford these technologies, hence may not adopt them.

(d) *Lack of Trust*:

It means that if the patient does not trust the healthcare provider or the technology and devices used in it, they will not agree to use MIoT technologies. Thus, to entice patients, it is necessary to build trust and to enhance the clarity of data use and protection.

Ethical Consideration

The concept of the Medical Internet of Things has helped improve healthcare delivery by bringing changes like remote patient care, smart medical gadgets, wearable health enhancing gadgets, and tele-care systems. These have made patients experience better health than those in the traditional health care systems, increased operation efficiency, and ultimate patient satisfaction. A critical advantage that MIoT brings to healthcare is the constant monitoring and real-time monitoring pared with conventional care that enables healthcare providers to manage health conditions In this case, there are better patient outcomes. Another factor is that of efficiency; the connectivity of devices and the automation of data flow significantly increase organizational efficiency and decrease the volume of paperwork and administrative tasks. It has also been found that patient satisfaction has increased with the help of MIoT technologies as features such as remote monitoring, and telemedicine options were made available to the patients. However, there are still some issues that can be observed in application of MIoT in healthcare. Challenges like security, privacy, data compatibility, and adherence to standards and regulations have to be met to achieve the true benefits of MIoT. These challenges need to be tackled by involving as many players across the care continuum as possible to invest in the proper infrastructure and to take comprehensive measures to protect the patients' privacy and sensitive data.

Future Directions and Opportunities in the MIoT

Significant trends and opportunities concerning the healthcare delivery and patient care are emerging and being influenced by the changing dynamics of Medical Internet of Things (MIoT). These future trends include shifting of practices in healthcare, new technologies, and developing applications. Chances and trends connected with implementation of medical IoT are presented in Table 5.1.

Potential future hotspots and areas of concentration for MIoT include the following:

The Integration of IoMT Ecosystems

The integration of IoT devices and systems into a broader IoMT structure would enable integration among healthcare institutions, research establishments, and technological companies through sharing of information. The next 5 years will enable the creation of harmonized solutions for healthcare that are patient-centric if open standards, the interoperability framework, and data sharing efforts are promoted.

Transformation of Healthcare Delivery

IoT application will further intensify bespoke healthcare delivery models, increasing patient-centered treatment, and reliance on technology. IoT will benefit patients, improve healthcare providers' organization in communicating care instructions, and streamline the numerous procedures in an extensively broad health spectrum. This will be achieved by developing concepts in home monitoring, point of care, and health management.

Digital Health Applications

Telemedicine, self-management of chronic diseases, other services that use IoT to facilitate personalized care plans, and other services are examples of digital health applications. These applications are designed for interacting with patients and increasing their compliance with the suggested treatment schedules.

Table 5.1 Future trends and opportunities in MIoT

Future trends and opportunities	Description
AI-driven healthcare	Incorporation of AI into diagnostics, treatment planning, and analytics for the future
Connected healthcare ecosystem	Harmonization of healthcare records from various sources
Next-generation wearables	Mobile gadgets that can be worn and have better sensors and features
Remote surgery	Executing surgical operations with unmanned aerial vehicles
Precision health monitoring	Ensuring precise and accurate monitoring of health parameters

Automated Drug Delivery Systems

IoT-enabled drug delivery systems that can automatically adjust drug dosages based on patient needs and biometric data, improving treatment outcomes and reducing side effects.

Connected Inhalers

Internet of Things (IoT) inhalers that can track how patients use them and give them immediate feedback on how to use them correctly to increase the effectiveness and adherence to their prescription.

Health Monitoring Wearables

Wearable health monitors—Internet of Things (IoT) devices that can track vital signs including heart rate, blood pressure, and the quality of a person's sleep, giving doctors and patients more information to use in treatment and prevention.

Conceiving of a Delicate and Power-Efficient Fixture

Anticipation of energy consumption and the lack of developed solution for optimizing resources in smart healthcare systems are also important concerns. Thus, there is a need to develop a new, lightweight, and energy-efficient ML-based data aggregation technique as most of the current solutions do not possess these properties. It also requires the emergence of new schemes for the delegation of work to the various parts of the IoT that are yet to be discovered. Such schemes require something beyond solving the problem of restrictive resources in these networks.

Apply Algorithms That Make Data More Private

Health records are especially susceptible to such threats due to the content of records; accordingly, security and privacy are required to be highly protective. Thus, it brings to the necessity of building stronger, low overhead, and energy efficient processes for managing aggregation of data in ML. The solutions have to safeguard the data and not permit privacy breaches with the use of conventional data privacy protection strategies. Two emerging techniques in the protection of personal information are differential privacy and Blockchain. This would also enhance the security of data since data from other/private networks and identities would be well protected. In other words, there is the need for further development of better access control to enhance the security of the network. Again, there is the physical security aspect whereby the devices should not be so easily messed with or physically affected.

Making the Right Devices

One of the biggest issues that healthcare industry is facing is the issue of the authenticity of the data that is being gathered through wearable gadgets. In subsequent development, projects must take the aspect of adaptable movement in projects especially in movement detection and all systems that requires sensors to be able to accept individual gait data. Regarding these challenges, it is necessary to address the exploration of the contact-based and contactless schemes to develop DL models for the identification of real and fake values.

Guaranteeing the Interoperability of Semantic

For interoperability concerns to be well addressed, it is very imperative to put up a standard and protocol that is well recognized internationally. Thus, one of the approaches that might be performed in the future is Semantic Interoperability of maintaining Healthcare Information. To achieve this, it is essential to ensure that wherever one system of healthcare or one device passes information to another, they are both able to understand the stuff as safely as possible regarding the meaning of the messages and their context.

Based on the findings, the following recommendations for implementing secure and easy-to-use MIoT should be considered: First, the interface must be natural; submenus should not be very deep, and buttons and menus must be easily recognizable in order to facilitate a healthcare provider's work or a patient. More important, it can also help smooth the buy-in process by providing extensive training and support for users so that they are ready to take advantage of the tools being offered to them.

Technological infrastructure and security procedures should also be strong to meet people's expectations concerning privacy. Amelioration of risks pertaining to data breaches can be done by enhancing available measures such as encryption, access control, and data storage security measures. Further, creating awareness and ensuring that patient's consent in the use of their data will help develop trust and match ethical standards of conducting the research.

Achieving compatibility of the MIoT devices with other healthcare systems is very important in promoting adoptions. Stating more common standards we can simplify the exchange of data and improve users' experience. Finally, there should be an accumulation of the constant feedback from the users to update those MIoT systems to be fit for the everyday use. Thus, awareness of these areas will allow healthcare organizations to increase the utilization of MIoT technologies and optimize the quality of patient service.

The MIoT has revolutionized the healthcare management systems in practice through inventions such as Remote Patient Monitoring, Smart Medical Devices, Wearable Health Technologies, and Telemedicine. Such developments have resulted in the better quality of patients' health, effectiveness of services offered, and levels of satisfaction in patients than the traditional modes of healthcare delivery. MIoT can help in constantly tracking patients' conditions or obtaining real-time data to manage health conditions and leading to improved patient outcomes. Another advantage of MIoT is optimum importance since connected gadgets as well as emphasis on the automatic acquisition of information limit service time and make it possible to cut down on clerical work. The patient satisfaction level has also increased with MIoT technologies because of the features like remote monitoring or using telemedicine. Nevertheless, some issues will persist in the MIoT adoption in the healthcare system. Thus, the challenges that need to be solved for MIoT include data protection, privacy, integration with other systems and legal requirements. These issues can only be addressed through cooperation and joint effort of all stakeholders, proper infrastructural support, and all the measures to protect patient's right to privacy and his or her files and records.

Conclusion

The Internet of Things (IoT) is leading to influencing solutions, enhancing opportunities for patients to get a treatment, and the overall autonomy of patient's health. This is done through wearable health devices, technologies in remote patient monitoring, an improved way of data analysis, and various precision medicine approaches. Technology advancements, information exchange, and smart personal health care still remain the promising ways to enhance the results of treatment, minimize the expensed of healthcare, and improve the population health. Such shifts are envisaged to happen as the IoT advances. The IoT stands for the Interconnect of Things. For the Internet of Things to bring about the desired change in the future of the healthcare industry though, challenges like data safety, privacy issues, and legal issues would have to be addresses. As this chapter also showed, the ecosystem of conjoined technology can work to produce a system of healthcare that is improved, patient-centric, and effective for all the stakeholders if only the healthcare organizations would act in acceptance of the IoT and engage in strategic partnerships.

References

1. Kaur C, Al Ansari MS, Dwivedi VK, Suganthi D. An intelligent IoT-based healthcare system using fuzzy neural networks. In: Advances in fuzzy-based internet of medical things (IoMT); 2024. p. 121–33. https://doi.org/10.1002/9781394242252.
2. Hosary AG, Emran A, El-Saghir B. Design of service oriented architecture for an IoT healthcare management system. Indones J Electr Eng Inform. 2024;12(1):87–100. https://doi.org/10.52549/ijeei.v12i1.5191.

3. Arul R, Alroobaea R, Tariq U, Almulihi AH, Alharithi FS, Shoaib U. IoT-enabled healthcare systems using block chain-dependent adaptable services. Pers Ubiquit Comput. 2024;28(1):43–57. https://doi.org/10.1007/s00779-021-01584-7.
4. Nachiappan N, Sreevijnya M, Thanigaivel G. Time and accuracy optimized IoT based elderly healthcare system. In: 2024 2nd international conference on intelligent data communication technologies and internet of things (IDCIoT). IEEE; 2024. p. 25–30. https://doi.org/10.1109/IDCIoT59759.2024.10467831.
5. Divya NJ, Kanniga Devi R, Muthukannan M. Privacy-aware IoT-based multi-disease diagnosis model for healthcare system. In: Computer vision and AI-integrated IoT technologies in the medical ecosystem; 2024. p. 376–406. https://doi.org/10.1201/9781003429609.
6. Srinivasan A, Rampur V, Rao MMS, Singh R. Implementation of IoT in healthcare barriers and future challenges. In: Advances in fuzzy-based internet of medical things (IoMT); 2024. p. 271–86. https://doi.org/10.1002/9781394242252.ch18.
7. Ala A, Simic V, Pamucar D, Bacanin N. Enhancing patient information performance in internet of things-based smart healthcare system: hybrid artificial intelligence and optimization approaches. Eng Appl Artif Intell. 2024;131:107889. https://doi.org/10.1016/j.engappai.2024.107889.
8. Robinsha SD, Amutha B. IoT architecture for energy management in smart cities. Int J Serv Oper Inform. 2023;12(4):325–43. https://doi.org/10.1504/IJSOI.2023.137474.
9. Jabeen T, Jabeen I, Humaira Ashraf NZ, Jhanjhi AY, Shamim Hossain M. An intelligent healthcare system using IoT in wireless sensor network. Sensors. 2023;23(11):5055. https://doi.org/10.3390/s23115055.
10. Kumar P, Kumar R, Gupta GP, Tripathi R, Jolfaei A, Najmul Islam AKM. A blockchain-orchestrated deep learning approach for secure data transmission in IoT-enabled healthcare system. J Parallel Distrib Comput. 2023;172:69–83. https://doi.org/10.1016/j.jpdc.2022.10.002.
11. Sardar A, Umer S, Rout RK, Wang S-H, Tanveer M. A secure face recognition for IoT-enabled healthcare system. ACM Trans Sens Netw. 2023;19(3):1–23. https://doi.org/10.1145/3534122.
12. Subhan F, Mirza A, Su'ud MBM, Alam MM, Nisar S, Habib U, Iqbal MZ. AI-enabled wearable medical internet of things in healthcare system: a survey. Appl Sci. 2023;13(3):1394. https://doi.org/10.3390/app13031394.
13. Nahid AM, Haleem A, Javaid M. Scope of health care system in rural areas under Medical 4.0 environment. Intell Pharm. 2023;1(4):217–23. https://doi.org/10.1016/j.ipha.2023.07.003.
14. Izhar M, Naqvi SAA, Ahmed A, Abdullah S, Alturki N, Jamel L. Enhancing healthcare efficacy through IoT-edge fusion: a novel approach for smart health monitoring and diagnosis. IEEE Access. 2023;11:136456–67. https://doi.org/10.1109/ACCESS.2023.3337092.
15. Kumar D, Sood SK, Rawat KS. Empowering elderly care with intelligent IoT-driven smart toilets for home-based infectious health monitoring. Artif Intell Med. 2023;144:102666. https://doi.org/10.1016/j.artmed.2023.102666.

Chapter 6
Integrating Genomic and Imaging Data: Advancing Radiogenomics in Modern Radiology

Mohd. Arfat and Taiba

Introduction

Radiogenome is made up of two words, "radio" and "genome." It comes from the word "Radio," which means "Radiation," and "genome" refers to all of a living thing's genes or genetic material. To sum up, radiogenomics is the study of how radiation affects genetic material (Fig. 6.1). Following the genomic revolution in the early 1990s, scientists have been driven to investigate the genetic causes of human diseases and to develop precise cancer treatments tailored to the specific genetic makeup of a tumour. To match the new therapeutic ideas developed in the age of precision medicine, diagnostic tests must also be accurate, multi-layered, and high-tech to find the relevant genetic mutations that make cancers treatable. A new approach to medical research has emerged due to significant advancements in training, medical imaging methods, image analysis, and the development of high-throughput technologies that enable the extraction and integration of numerous imaging parameters with genomic data. Radiogenomics is the name of this new method. Radiogenomics tries to connect the way tumours look (the imaging appearance) with gene expression patterns, gene mutations, and other genome-related traits to learn more about how tumours work and how they are different from one another. The main goal of radiogenomics is to make imaging biomarkers that can predict outcomes based on both genotypic and phenotypic measures. Radiogenomics is a new field that is growing quickly, and early results look good. This is because

M. Arfat (✉)
Medical Radiology and Imaging Technology, Paramedical College, Faculty of Medicine, Aligarh Muslim University (AMU), Aligarh, India
e-mail: marfat.pmc@amu.ac.in

Taiba
Medical Imaging Technology, Allied Healthcare & Sciences, SAHSR-Jamia Hmadard, New Delhi, India

P. Eappen et al. (eds.), *Advancing Healthcare with the Medical Internet of Things*, Health Informatics, https://doi.org/10.1007/978-3-032-23933-4_6

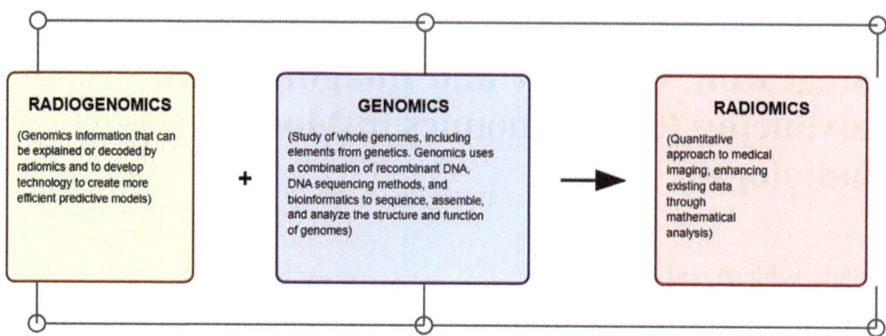

Fig. 6.1 Work flow for radiogenomic study

medical imaging is safe and widely used in clinical practice. Radiogenomics combines big data imaging with genetic profiling to create non-invasive biomarkers that show the molecular landscape of diseases, mostly cancer [1]. Radiomics is an important part of this field because it takes medical images and turns them into high-dimensional datasets using standard methods that pull out features like texture, shape, intensity, and wavelet-based features [2]. These traits often show modest phenotypic signs of the underlying biology of the tumour, like necrosis, angiogenesis, or cellular heterogeneity, that cannot be seen with the naked eye [3]. A strict workflow begins with acquiring images consistently, using the same scanner settings and resolution factors to minimise differences to a minimum. After preprocessing steps like normalisation and bias-field correction, tumours are divided into clinically important subregions, such as the enhancing core, the non-enhancing tumour, and the infiltrative margins. This can be done by hand or with the help of AI-assisted tools. Segmentation accuracy is critical because the quality of feature extraction later on rests on accurately delineating the tumour. Reproducibility is improved when semi-automated or standard tools are used [4]. Following the rules set by the Image Biomarker Standardisation Initiative (IBSI), the next step is feature extraction. This creates a library of quantitative descriptors that include first-order statistics (like entropy and skewness), second-order textures (like GLCM and GLRLM), and higher-level morphological and filter-derived features [2, 5]. These traits stand in for physically important traits like tumour size, sharpness of the margins, and internal heterogeneity [2]. Advanced statistical selection methods, such as LASSO regression, principal components analysis, and mutual information filtering, are used to handle the large set of features. These methods decrease the number of dimensions and find the most predictive variables [6]. This is where machine learning (like random forests and SVM) or deep learning models (like convolutional neural networks) come in. They are taught to predict genomic ends like IDH mutation or MGMT methylation [7]. Cross-validation methods are used to test how well the model works, and then it is validated by an outside group of people from multiple centres. This is very important for showing that the model is reliable in the real world [8]. In the case of glioblastoma, radiogenomic models using MRI-based texture and enhancement metrics have successfully predicted IDH mutation status, MGMT promoter methylation, and even EGFRvIII mutations, with AUC values often topping 0.85 [7, 9]. It is important to note that tumour radiomics have been compared with pathway-level data, like angiogenesis and DNA repair mechanisms, using transcriptomics datasets. This makes imaging-genotype associations more biologically plausible [9]. In the same way, dynamic contrast-enhanced MRI features in breast cancer, such as wash-in and wash-out kinetics and shape descriptors, have been linked to molecular subtypes (e.g., Luminal A, HER2-enriched, triple-negative) and risk stratification scores like Oncotype DX, which helps doctors make decisions about non-invasive treatments [10]. Despite these positive steps, there are still problems to solve. Variability depending on the scanner, problems with preprocessing, and feature issues in different software versions all make it harder to reproduce [4, 6]. Most of the results from radiogenomic studies are from single-centre, historical studies. This shows how important it is to do large-scale, prospective, multi-institutional trials [8]. Also, deep learning models are still hard to understand, so we need AI systems that can be explained to make things clear and build trust among clinicians [9]. Multi-omics, which includes radiogenomics, transcriptomics, proteomics, and pathomics, will help us learn more about disease biology from the picture level to the molecule level in the future. Radiogenomic tools will be easier to understand and use in clinical processes with explainable models, and shared repositories like TCGA/TCIA will make it easier for multi-centre projects to be validated and approved by regulators [8]. By connecting imaging signatures with molecular behaviour, radiogenomics helps doctors figure out how different types of tumours respond to and fight treatment. In the case of non-small cell lung cancer, EGFR and KRAS mutation status have been strongly linked to CT-based radiomic traits like edge sharpness and texture heterogeneity. A study with more than 400 patients found that a random forest model trained on these features had AUCs above 0.80 for predicting outcomes, which meant it could point patients quickly and without harm to them to specific therapies. Additionally, AI-enhanced radiogenomic models have successfully forecast PD-L1 expression levels, which helps doctors decide if immunotherapy is right for a patient without having to take more tissue samples. It can also be used in neuro-oncology to track the effects of treatment and distinguish between changes caused by treatment, such as pseudoprogression or radiation necrosis, and changes caused by tumour growth. Radiomic features, especially texture and dynamic perfusion parameters, were found to be related to underlying molecular markers in glioblastoma patients receiving chemoradiation. This helped in evaluating the early treatment response. Based on these results, radiogenomics might help lower the need for complicated or invasive testing methods by providing a real-time, image-based alternative. In addition, multi-modal interaction is making radiogenomics more useful. Recent studies have successfully combined PET radiomic traits (like metabolic heterogeneity from FDG uptake) with MRI texture to identify different types of tumours better and predict survival in people with head-and-neck cancer. By combining metabolic, structural, and molecular data sets, this multi-parametric approach makes imaging biomarkers easier to understand from a biological point of view. Some radiogenomic processes now have automatic image processing, quality control, and clinical decision-support layers to make sure that the results are used in the right way in the clinic. A breast cancer prospective trial used a cloud-based tool with automated segmentation, batch-standardised feature extraction, and AI-based Oncotype DX score prediction, showing that it could be used in real-life clinical settings. The results showed that radiogenomic estimates were accurate for about 85% of cases, which is a good step towards cost-effective, image-guided treatment planning [9]. Even with these improvements, providing radiogenomics on a large scale means dealing with several problems. One significant challenge is that AI models are difficult to interpret, as deep learning architectures like convolutional neural networks can operate in a manner akin to "black boxes." Explainable AI (XAI) methods, like attention mapping and feature attribution, are being studied to find out which parts of an image affect predictions. Another issue to think about is the rules about data sharing and privacy. To test how to train radiogenomic models across institutions without having to centralise private data, shared learning systems are being used. Overall, radiogenomics has the power to completely change cancer and other fields by allowing non-invasive, comprehensive molecular profiling. But for this promise to come true, the field needs to keep working on standardised processes, strong multi-centre validation, AI interpretability, and moral frameworks. As these infrastructure parts improve, radiogenomic tools are expected to significantly impact how diagnoses are made significantly, treatments are chosen, and patient care is provided [10].

Clinical and Research Significance

Radiogenomics has enormous practical value because it gives us non-invasive biomarkers that show how tumours are made at the molecular level. These biomarkers help with diagnosis, planning treatment, and figuring out how likely a tumour is to come back [11]. In the case of glioblastoma, MRI-derived radiomic features can predict IDH mutation and MGMT promoter methylation status, which are very important for deciding how to treat the cancer and its outcome [12]. In the same way, radiogenomic models have shown links between imaging features on dynamic contrast-enhanced MRI and molecular groups like Luminal A/B, HER2, and triple-negative breast cancers [13]. In lung cancer, CT radiogenomic models have been used to guess the EGFR mutation status and the level of PD-L1 expression, which helps with planning treatment [14]. Radiogenomics is being used for more than just cancer research. It is also being used to study brain diseases and liver fibrosis [15]. Radiogenomics helps researchers learn more about how different tumours change over time by combining genetic and spatial data across whole tumour volumes, which is something that biopsies alone cannot do [16]. It can also be used to sort patients into groups for clinical trials, make prediction models, and find new imaging biomarkers that are linked to better treatment results [4]. This area pushes for a move towards data-driven precision medicine, which uses AI, imaging, and genetic analytics to provide better care that is tailored to each patient [17].

Scope and Object of the Chapter: Structure Overview

The first part of this chapter talks about how genomes and radiology have changed over time, laying the groundwork for how they will work together in the field of radiogenomics. Then it talks about the main ideas of radiogenomics, such as radiomics, feature extraction, genomic annotation, and association analysis. The parts that follow talk about how it can be used in clinical settings to treat different types of cancer, mainly brain, breast, and lung cancer, as well as how it can be used in translational research. The chapter also discusses the current technological, moral, and methodological challenges that hinder the widespread adoption of radiogenomics in everyday clinical practice. Finally, the chapter ends with some thoughts on the future and suggestions for how to make radiogenomic integration in personalised medicine even better.

Genomic Concept: Biological Foundation

DNA

DNA is made up of nucleotides that are grouped in a straight line. Genetic information is stored in DNA. Two strands of nucleotides are complementary to each other and hold DNA molecules together. Hydrogen bonds hold these strands together between base pairs that are G-C and A-T. To make a copy of the genetic material, one strand of DNA is used as a model to make a second strand that is the same. Genome duplication is the name for this process. There are directions for all the proteins that an organism will ever make stored in its DNA. This information will stay with the organism for its whole life. [18].

DNA Repair and Replication

Each daughter cell needs the same DNA when the parent cell splits. The DNA copies itself to do this. During the S phase of the cell cycle, which comes before mitosis or meiosis, DNA replication takes place. The double helix shape gave us a hint about DNA replication. Adenine always pairs with thymine, and cytosine pairs with guanine. This means that the strands go well together. One strand of DNA has the nucleotide code AGTCATGA, and the other has TCAGTACT. Since the two lines work well together, one may copy the other. In this replication theory, the two strands of the double helix split during replication and use each other as models to make copies of the other strand. Each double-helix strand of DNA is used as a model to make copies of different strands. The "old" or maternal strand will go well with the new one. There is one father strand and one daughter strand in each new double strand. This is known as semiconservative duplication. Two copies of DNA with the same nucleotide bases are split into two daughter cells [19].

Gene

A gene is a genetic unit on a chromosome. Genes work by influencing protein synthesis.

Chemical Structure of Gene

- Promoter Region: DNA that starts gene transcription.
- Introns and Exons: Exons are coding regions appearing in the final RNA product.
- Non-coding introns are deleted during RNA processing.

Most genes are formed of DNA, but some viruses use RNA, a related material. DNA has two nucleotide chains. These chains are rope-like. Sugar and phosphates form the ladder's sides, and nitrogenous bases join to form the rungs. A, G, C, and T are these bases. A–T ladder rungs are made by connecting A and T chains.

Gene Mutation

Changes in base order or number can cause mutations in a gene (Fig. 6.2). When nucleotides are deleted, copied, changed, or swapped, they have different effects. Mutations don't have much of an impact on living things, but they can kill or spread them. Until they become popular, populations will accept mutations that are good for them. Changes in genes affect people and other species.

The primary categories of genes involved in cancer are:

(1) Ongensgenes (2) Tumour suppressor genes (3) Genes relevant to DNA repair [20].

Radiomic

Radiomics analyses tumour features using quantitative feature extraction from medical pictures. This method emphasises ROI segmentation, picture acquisition, and descriptive feature estimation [21] (Figs. 6.3 and 6.4).

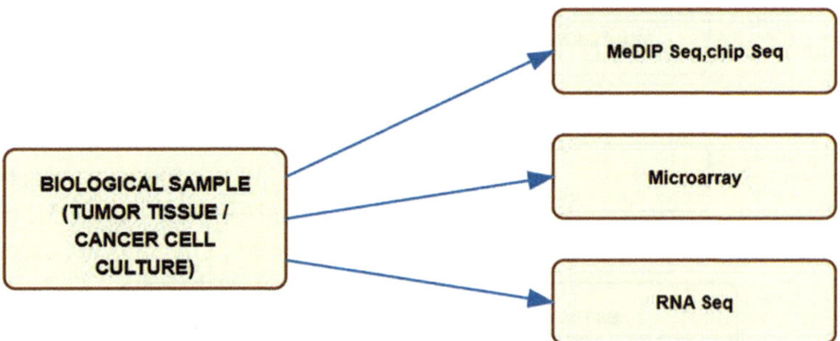

Fig. 6.2 The flow chart shows the steps involved in studying tumour tissue or cancer cell cultures using three techniques. First, a biological sample is collected. Then, RNA is extracted for *RNA-Seq* to measure gene activity. Next, *MeDIP-Seq* is used to study DNA methylation changes, which can affect gene function. Finally, *ChIP-Seq* is used to analyse protein-DNA interactions, helping to understand how genes are regulated in cancer cells

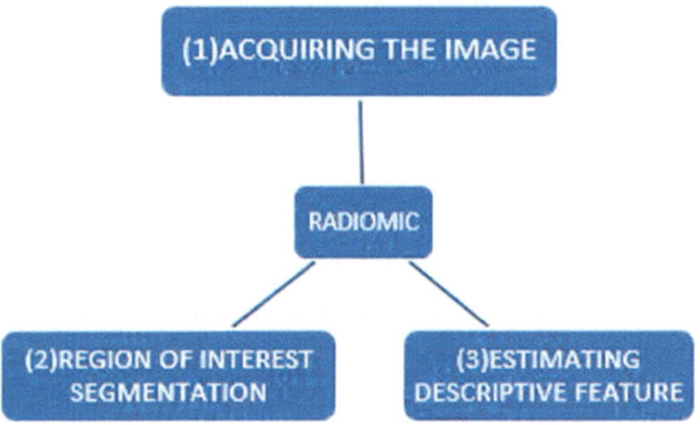

Fig. 6.3 The radiomics workflow begins with acquiring high-quality medical images using imaging modalities such as CT, MRI, or PET, ensuring optimal parameters for precise and accurate representation. The next step involves segmenting the region of interest (ROI) to isolate the relevant tissue or lesion for detailed analysis. Finally, descriptive features, including texture, shape, and intensity, are extracted from the segmented ROI, offering valuable insights into the tissue's characteristics, which aid in clinical diagnosis, prognosis, and treatment planning

Genetic Variation

Genetic variation refers to differences in DNA sequences among individuals, which contribute to phenotypic diversity, disease susceptibility, and population evolution. The most common type is the single-nucleotide polymorphism (SNP), a variation in a single base pair that can influence disease risk, drug response, and gene expression regulation through effects on coding and non-coding regions [22]. Copy number variations (CNVs)—which involve duplications or deletions of large segments of DNA—also play a crucial role in human diseases such as autism, schizophrenia, and cancer, by altering gene dosage. Studies have shown that CNVs affect more nucleotides than SNPs and are often linked to gene expression change. Other types

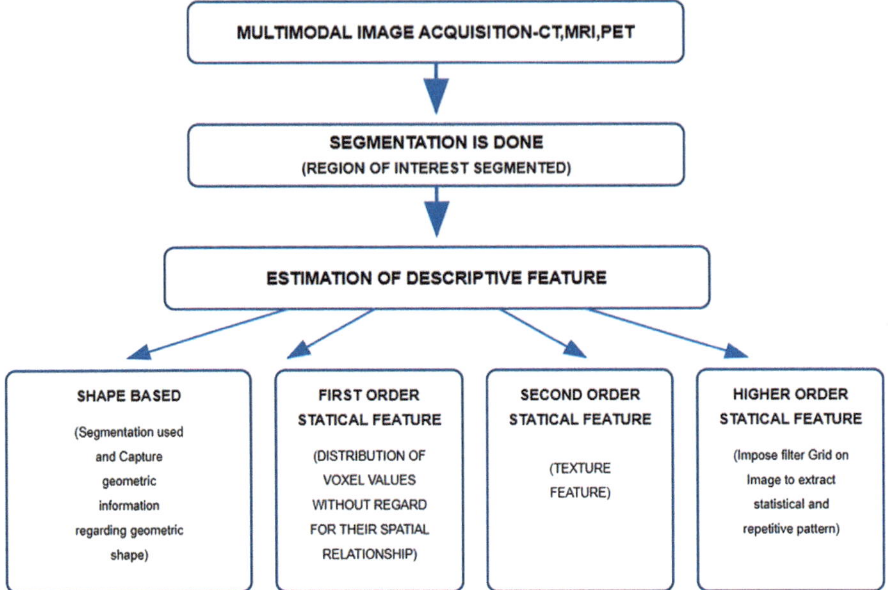

Fig. 6.4 Flow chart showing radiogenomic

include insertions/deletions (indels) and significant structural variants like inversions and translocations, which can disrupt gene function or regulatory elements. Large-scale genome projects like the 1000 Genomes Project revealed that an average human genome contains over 3 million SNPs and thousands of CNVs and indels, underlining the complexity of the human genome [20]. These variations are central to genome-wide association studies (GWAS), which identify genetic markers linked to common diseases and traits. As research advances, tools like GEMINI and VEP (Variant Effect Predictor) help scientists interpret genetic variation data by connecting them with known phenotypes and biological pathways [23]. Understanding these variations is crucial for developing personalised medicine, predicting disease risk, and exploring human evolutionary patterns.

Genetic differences mainly cause different responses to radiation treatment and side effects. Up to 80% of these differences can be traced back to genetic factors. A single-nucleotide polymorphism (SNP) is the most basic type of individual variation in DNA. These straightforward alterations can be either transitional or transversional in nature, and they happen roughly once every 1000 base pairs across the genome [24]. In sequencing projects, SNPs are distinguished from DNA mutations based on their frequency in the population: "Single Nucleotide Polymorphisms" (SNPs) and DNA mutations are defined as DNA variants detectable in >1% or <1% of the population, respectively [20]. Both coding and non-coding parts of the genome may have these differences, which could affect how a gene functions, how susceptible a person is to disease, and how well a treatment works [25]. Single nucleotide polymorphisms (SNPs), which are passed down in haplotypes, have a significant effect on radiosensitivity, primarily through DNA repair genes like ATM. This can cause diseases like ataxia telangiectasia. These uncommon genetic diseases show how genetics can have a significant impact on how radiation works, both right away and over time. This shows how vital personalised radiation treatments are. On the other hand, most people do not have such severe side effects. Early research on candidate genes like ATM and BRCA1 mostly looked at genes whose roles were already known, not taking into account the fact that many genes cause radiosensitivity. As a result, many studies failed to establish strong links between genetic differences and radiation-related harm due to insufficient sample sizes, unresolved issues from multiple tests, or over-reliance on known candidate genes. It helps us better understand how genes affect radiation therapy and create more personalised treatment plans [26].

Candidate Gene Studies

Candidate gene studies are a hypothesis-driven way to look into how genetic differences are linked to specific traits or illnesses. Researchers use this method to choose one or more genes, called candidate genes, based on what they already know about biology or evidence that points to their part in the disease pathway1. Then, genetic variants, usually single-nucleotide polymorphisms (SNPs), are looked for in these genes to see if there is a statistically significant difference in allele rates between people who have the disease (cases) and people who don't have it (controls) [27].

The choice of candidate genes is generally based on how biologically related they are to the condition being studied. For instance, the APOE gene is extensively researched in Alzheimer's disease as it is known to play a part in the breakdown of lipids and the repair of neurons33. Similarly, TP53 and BRCA1/2 are popular candidate genes in cancer research due to their critical role in DNA repair and tumour suppression [28]. When a researcher has a reasonable hypothesis, candidate gene studies are helpful and do not cost much. However, they are often limited by small sample numbers, publication bias, and the chance of false-positive results because of how the population is divided [29]. Also, this method might miss meaningful connections in genes that were not thought to be involved in the disease process before.

Even with these problems, candidate gene studies have helped us learn more about how different diseases are caused genetically and set the stage for bigger studies like Genome-Wide Association Studies (GWAS), which do not use assumptions and instead look at the whole genome. Early radiogenomics studies identified ATM, BRCA1, and TGF-β1 genes as potential contributors to radiation-induced damage. However, TGF-β1 studies did not reliably link common SNPs to higher radiosensitivity. Small sample numbers, reliance on known gene functions, and lack of control for multiple testing may explain inconsistent results. This highlights the need for more rigorous genomic techniques to investigate radiosensitivity's complicated genetic components. The 2009 World Radiogenomics Consortium (RGC), with 219 partners from 32 nations and 129 institutions, promoted large-scale investigations to address these issues. GWAS, which evaluate genetic variations without preconceptions, have advanced radiogenomics. These studies use linkage disequilibrium to identify 300,000–1000,000 tag SNPs. Different genetic linkages for radiation damage in prostate and breast cancer patients have been found in larger investigations like the UK RAPPER group. The TANC1 gene was linked to late-onset urinary and rectal damage, highlighting tissue-specific radiation responses. Long-term effects of radiation, including second cancers, have been studied, and frequent genetic variants can affect radiation exposure, particularly in Hodgkin's lymphoma and childhood cancer survivors [30].

Applications

Radiogenomic Study of Breast Cancer

Radiogenomic analysis of breast cancer was studied by looking at the link between MRI image features and gene expression patterns in breast cancer. The researchers used a small group of 10 patients from a bigger group of 353 patients to connect 26 imaging features and gene expression data. The study found a strong link between the type of interferon and breast cancer and different enhancement patterns. It achieved this by identifying 21 image features that were associated with 71% of the genes examined. Also, 11 imaging traits were linked with gene sets that help predict prognosis and 12 were connected with gene sets that are important for breast cancer. The study shows how crucial radiogenomic analysis is as a cutting-edge way to understand how breast cancer starts at the molecular level. Putting together genetic and imaging data in this way could lead to better patient outcomes and more personalised treatment choices [31] (Table 6.1).

Radiogenomic Study for Lung Cancer

Conventional imaging tests for lung cancer mostly look at morphological factors, such as the density, borders, and size of the lesions. Radiomics improves this method by using higher-order statistics to look at imaging traits. This gives us a better understanding of how different things are inside lesions (Fig. 6.5). This difference might have something to do with the genetic and protein information inside the tumour. The goal of this study is to shed light on the radiogenomics of lung cancer by highlighting cutting-edge machine learning (ML) and artificial intelligence (AI) methods and exploring their practical applications. Radiogenomic analysis of non-small cell lung cancer (NSCLC) can be used to find out about the cancer's molecular properties without having to cut the tumour out. This is possible because it finds

Table 6.1 Showing radiogenomic workflow in breast cancer

Steps	Process	Description	Tools/technologies used
1	Patient selection and data collection	Selection of breast cancer patients with available imaging and genomic data	Clinical criteria, consent, and HER
2	Imaging acquisition	High-resolution imaging of breast tissue	Clinical criteria, consent, and HER
3	Image preprocessing and annotation	Standardisation and segmentation of tumours in images	AI tools, radiomics software (e.g., pyradiomics)
4	Radiomic feature extraction	Quantification of imaging biomarkers (e.g., shape, texture, intensity)	Radiomic pipelines, machine learning
5	Genomic data collection	Extraction of DNA/RNA from biopsy samples for molecular analysis	NGS (Next-Gen Sequencing), microarrays
6	Bioinformatics analysis	Processing genomic data to identify gene expression, mutations, etc.	Tools like GATK, DESeq2, and Bioconductor
7	Data integration	Correlating radiomic features with genomic alterations	Statistical modelling, deep learning, data fusion platforms
8	Model development and validation	Build predictive models for diagnosis, prognosis, and treatment response	Machine learning (e.g., Random Forest, CNNs)
9	Clinical interpretation and decision support	Translate findings into actionable clinical insights	CDSS, tumour boards, genomic-radiologic maps
10	Outcome monitoring and feedback	Longitudinal tracking of treatment response and outcomes	Imaging follow-up, genomic reassessment

many links between semantic picture elements and metagenes that follow normal molecular pathways [32] (Table 6.2).

Radiogenomics Analysis for Predicting Prognosis in Gastric Cancer

Radiogenomics analysis for gastric cancer (GC) prognosis combines genomic data with imaging biomarkers from contrast-enhanced CT (CECT) to tailor patient management. Genetic variables and imaging markers that reflect tumour heterogeneity help comprehend a patient's tumour biology. A GC study included CECT pictures from 46 patients and RNA sequencing data from 407 GC patients from The Cancer Genome Atlas (TCGA) and The Cancer Imaging Archive. Additional CECT photos from 392 Nanfang Hospital patients were added. They found radiation damage and tumour progression-linked gene modules using weighted gene co-expression network analysis (WGCNA). These modules were linked to imaging features, revealing

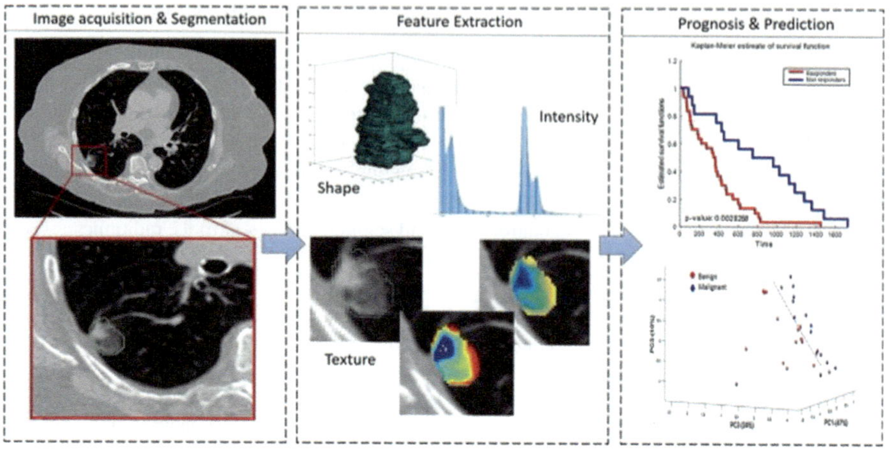

Fig. 6.5 Overview of a typical Radiomic workflow. CT image acquisition is followed by automatic or manual expert segmentation. Radiomic features (such as texture, shape) are extracted quantitatively to build machine learning based models. The output of the machine learning models can be predictive or prognostic in nature, depending on the clinical question

three imaging biomarkers with high survival relationships. Then, they built a nomogram that incorporated radiomics scores and clinicopathological factors to predict overall survival better than TNM staging (AUC = 0.838 vs. 0.765, $P = 0.011$). The nomogram increased clinical utility, calibration, and discrimination in both training and validation groups, suggesting clinical application. This radiogenomics approach can help physicians make better judgments, improving tailored treatments and precision theranostics. To improve gastric cancer radiogenomics accuracy and clinical usefulness, future research should increase patient cohorts, integrate more omics data, and build more advanced machine learning models [33] (Table 6.3).

Radiogenomic Analysis of Papillary Thyroid Carcinoma for Prediction of Cervical Lymph Node Metastasis

Papillary thyroid carcinoma (PTC) is frequently identified by the presence of metastases to cervical lymph nodes (CLNs), which has a substantial impact on the surgical strategy for patients who are affected. The purpose of this study was to create a radiomic signature for predicting CLN status using preoperative thyroid ultrasound and to investigate the association between radiomic features and PTC tumour molecular characteristics. The prospective study included a total of 270 patients. Radiomic characteristics were retrieved using recognised procedures, and a radiomic signature was created and confirmed in distinct cohorts. The radiomic signature performed well, with an AUC of 0.873 in the training group and 0.831 in the validation cohort. To study the molecular basis, proteins from tumour samples were evaluated using

Table 6.2 Radiogenomic workflow in lung cancer

Steps	Process	Description	Tools/technologies used
1	Patient enrolment and clinical data collection	Selection of lung cancer patients: record demographics, history, and tumour stage	EHR, clinical protocols, consent forms
2	Imaging acquisition	Capture tumour images to assess morphology and spread	Chest CT, PET/CT, MRI (optional)
3	Image preprocessing and segmentation	Standardise and segment tumour regions for analysis	DICOM tools, AI-based segmentation, radiology software
4	Radiomic feature extraction	Extract quantitative features (e.g., shape, texture, intensity) from images.	Pyradiomics, MATLAB, radiomics toolkits
5	Tumour biopsy and genomic profiling	Obtain tumour tissue and analyse genomic alterations	NGS, PCR, FISH, RNA-Seq
6	Bioinformatics and genomic analysis	Process raw data to identify mutations and biomarkers	GATK, Bioconductor, cBioPortal, Ensembl VEP
7	Imaging-genomic data integration	Correlate radiomic features with genomic signatures	Machine learning, multivariate statistical models
8	Model development and validation	Predict molecular profiles, therapy response, or prognosis	AI/ML algorithms (Random Forest, SVM, CNN), cross-validation
9	Clinical interpretation and decision support	Translate findings to guide treatment decisions	Clinical decision support systems (CDSS), tumour boards
10	Longitudinal monitoring and feedback	Track therapy response, recurrence, and update data	Follow-up CT/PET imaging, repeat biopsy if needed

liquid chromatography/mass spectrometry (LC/MS) and isobaric tags for relative and absolute quantitation (iTRAQ) technology. Clustering was used to identify gene modules associated with metastasis, which were then evaluated using a radiogenomic map created using the Spearman correlation matrix. This mapping found strong relationships between radiomic characteristics and biological pathways. MEmeganta, which is connected with telomere maintenance and cell-cell adhesion, and MEblue, which captures cell-cell adhesion and glycolysis, were the two most prominent gene modules. These modules were associated with specific radiomic parameters such as tumour margin, internal echogenicity, and minimum calcification area, all of which represent tumour characteristics detectable on imaging. The study also discovered hub genes inside these modules using protein-protein interaction (PPI) networks. Immunohistochemistry indicated that LAMC1 and THBS1 expression levels differed significantly between metastatic and non-metastatic tissues. LAMC1 was substantially associated with tumour margin and echogenicity characteristics, whereas THBS1 was linked to calcification. Finally, the study shows that a radiomic signature can noninvasively predict CLN status in PTC patients, offering valuable preoperative insights. Furthermore, by combining imaging phenotypes and

Table 6.3 Showing workflow in gastric cancer

Steps	Process	Description	Tools/technologies used
1	Patient selection and data collection	Selection of gastric cancer patients and collection of clinical records, including histological type, stage, and comorbidities	Electronic health records (EHR), biobank consent
2	Imaging acquisition	Perform imaging to assess tumour location, invasion, and metastasis	Contrast-enhanced CT, MRI, endoscopic ultrasound (EUS), PET/CT
3	Image preprocessing and tumour segmentation	Standardise image formats and segment the primary tumour and lymph nodes	DICOM software, semi-automated or AI segmentation tools
4	Radiomic feature extraction	Derive features describing tumour shape, size, density, and texture	Radiomics software (e.g., PyRadiomics, ITK-SNAP)
5	Biopsy and genomic profiling	Obtain gastric tumour tissues via endoscopy or surgery for molecular analysis	Next-generation sequencing (NGS), whole exome sequencing (WES), PCR
6	Bioinformatics analysis	Analyse genomic data to identify mutations and signatures	Tools: GATK, Bioconductor, TCGA, Ensembl, OncoKB
7	Data integration	Correlate radiomic features with genomic alterations (e.g., MSI status, TP53 mutation, HER2 amplification)	Multivariate models, statistical analysis, ML algorithms
8	Predictive modelling	Develop models for predicting tumour subtype, prognosis, and therapy response	Machine learning/deep learning (e.g., SVM, RF, CNN)
9	Clinical decision support	Use integrated radiogenomic data to assist in treatment planning and personalised therapy (e.g., immunotherapy, HER2-targeted)	CDSS, tumour board integration, NCCN/ESMO guidelines
10	Monitoring and re-evaluation	Track patient outcomes and adapt treatment through follow-up imaging and potential re-biopsy	Serial CT/MRI, genomic reassessment, EHR feedback loop

genomic data, the study demonstrates the ability to correlate molecular aspects of PTC tumours to radiomic traits. This technique could help with clinical decision-making and tailored management strategies for PTC patients [34] (Table 6.4).

Conclusion

Radiogenomics has advanced our understanding of how genetic variants affect radiation therapy toxicity and long-term effects. In early investigations, genes including ATM, BRCA1, and TGF-β1 were identified, but small sample numbers and limited

Table 6.4 Showing work workflow in papillary thyroid

Steps	Process	Description	Tools/ technologies used
1	Patient selection and clinical evaluation	Inclusion of PTC patients with preoperative imaging and biopsy data; documentation of tumour size, thyroid function, and cervical lymphadenopathy	Electronic health records (EHR), ultrasound reports
2	Imaging acquisition	Perform high-resolution imaging of the thyroid and neck to evaluate tumour characteristics and lymph nodes	Neck ultrasound (US), contrast-enhanced CT, sometimes MRI
3	Tumour and lymph node segmentation	Delineate the primary thyroid tumour and suspicious lymph nodes on imaging	AI/manual segmentation using software like ITK-SNAP, 3D slicer
4	Radiomic feature extraction	Extract quantitative features such as margin, echogenicity, vascularity, shape, and calcification patterns	Radiomics software, MATLAB, PyRadiomics
5	Fine-needle aspiration and genomic profiling	Obtain a biopsy and perform molecular testing to identify key genetic mutations	BRAF V600E, TERT promoter, RAS mutations via PCR/NGS
6	Bioinformatics and mutation analysis	Analyse and annotate mutations; evaluate mutation burden and correlation with aggressiveness	Bioconductor, cBioPortal, Ensembl VEP
7	Data integration	Combine imaging phenotypes (e.g., hypoechogenicity, microcalcifications) with mutation profiles to find predictive associations	Correlation matrix, logistic regression, AI fusion models
8	Predictive modelling for lymph node metastasis	Build and train ML models to predict the likelihood of cervical lymph node involvement	Random Forest, XGBoost, deep learning, validation on test datasets
9	Clinical translation and decision support	Use prediction to assist in surgical planning (e.g., prophylactic neck dissection vs. conservative approach)	Clinical decision support systems (CDSS), multidisciplinary teams
10	Postoperative monitoring and feedback	Monitor outcomes and validate model predictions with surgical pathology and imaging follow-up	Post-op ultrasound, serum thyroglobulin, histopathology

methodologies caused inconsistent findings. Modern genome-wide association studies (GWAS) have discovered intricate genetic linkages, such as the TANC1 gene's significance in late radiation damage. Identifying genetic characteristics that can lead to individualised radiation therapies, increasing patient outcomes and reducing hazards requires ongoing research and collaboration, particularly through the World Radiogenomics Consortium. Radiogenomics is changing clinical radiology by making it possible to understand tumour biology through regular images without cutting the tumour open. By taking quantitative features from MRI and CT scans, like texture, shape, and contrast enhancement, and connecting them with genetic data, doctors can figure out molecular characteristics that were previously only possible through invasive biopsies [2]. Extensive studies with more than 800 patients have shown that machine-learning models using common MRI traits (like

T1, T2, and FLAIR) can predict how well someone with IDH wild-type glioblastoma will do in the future. RNA sequencing proved that these models were correct in a biological sense, showing connections with pathways that control cell growth, the reaction to DNA damage, and the activation of the immune system.

In the same way, contrast-enhanced T1-weighted MRI features can accurately predict MGMT promoter methylation status, which is a key biomarker for chemotherapy response, and be both sensitive and specific in both exploratory and validation groups [35]. A prospective study of 95 women with breast cancer using MRI radiogenomics found a link between image features (such as the shape of the mass and the different types of lesions) and changes in gene expression (such as CCL3L1, MIR421) that are unique to oestrogen receptor-positive and other subtypes [36]. Also, several new studies have shown that radiomic features from dynamic contrast-enhanced MRI and diffusion-weighted imaging can predict Oncotype DX repeat scores. This provides a non-invasive way to determine who should receive treatment and plan surgery.

These studies show a few of the most essential benefits of radiogenomics:

Whole-tumour evaluation: Imaging shows differences in shape and size across the whole tumour, while biopsy samples can only be taken from small areas [3]. Non-invasive monitoring: MRI-based radiogenomic signatures allow multiple readings over time without the need for extra procedures, which makes it possible to track how the tumour changes over time. Predictive imaging biomarkers can help doctors make treatment decisions. For example, they can find patients who are likely to react to temozolomide or who need aggressive treatments right away. Despite this, radiogenomics has many problems. Significant differences in imaging protocols, scanners, and feature-extraction software can make it hard to replicate results across centres. This shows how important it is to standardise and follow reporting standards. Also, retrospective and single-institution studies are helpful, but prospective multicentre trials are needed to test prediction models thoroughly and show they are useful in the real world [3, 37].

Radiogenomics is set to become an essential part of precision medicine, even with these problems. The adoption of artificial intelligence in radiology is increasing at a faster pace due to advancements in analytics, the availability of larger, multi-modal datasets, and growing interest among doctors. In the end, radiogenomics offers personalised care that is safer, faster, and cheaper by using everyday imaging to find deep biological insights. This will lead to better patient outcomes and less reliance on invasive diagnostic procedures.

Future Recommendation

Future investigations in radiogenomics should focus on larger, more heterogeneous cohorts and the integration of multi-omics data to enhance understanding of the genetic determinants that affect radiosensitivity. Advanced machine learning methodologies and longitudinal research will be crucial for discovering novel biomarkers and optimising individualised radiation therapy to improve patient outcomes.

Use of Artificial Intelligence and Machine Learning in Radiogenomics

For the future of radiogenomics to succeed, it is essential to combine artificial intelligence (AI), especially machine learning (ML), and deep learning methods. High-dimensional imaging and genomic datasets can be managed with these tools to find subtle trends that people might miss. Examples of how AI can improve model accuracy include predicting genetic mutations, treatment results, and disease progression in glioblastoma and lung cancer [38]. Future work should focus on creating AI models that can be explained so that clinical choices can be understood and trusted. Using multi-modal AI platforms that combine genomics, imaging, and clinical data will help make diagnosis and treatment plans even more accurate [39].

Development of Standardised, Multi-institutional Datasets

Different imaging protocols and small sample sizes are currently holding back radiogenomics studies. Large, standardised databases with linked imaging, genomics, and clinical outcome data need to be established as soon as possible across multiple centres.

The Cancer Imaging Archive (TCIA) and The Cancer Genome Atlas (TCGA) are two projects that have started the process. However, more data that is consistent across all types of imaging, platforms, and groups is required. It will be easier for institutions to validate models and make copies of them if image acquisition, radiomic feature extraction (e.g. by following IBSI guidelines), and annotation methods are all standardised [40].

Integration with Transcriptomics and Pathomics

To fully understand how tumours work, radiogenomics needs to grow into a multi-omics paradigm. Using imaging data along with transcriptomics (gene expression profiles) and pathomics (digital pathology features) can help us learn more about tumours at the molecular level. Such integration will make it easier to find biomarkers, create models for prognosis, and predict how a treatment will work. In recent studies [3], for example, using both radiomic features and RNA-seq data together has made risk classification better in IDH wild-type glioblastoma and ER+ breast cancer. For more useful clinical insights, future studies should focus on collecting data simultaneously and identifying connections between different types of genes.

Ethical and Regulatory Considerations

As radiogenomics grows, it brings up important moral and legal issues. Some of these are data privacy, getting informed permission for genomic profiling, holding AI models accountable, and the possibility of algorithmic bias.

To protect patient rights, regulatory groups need to come up with rules for how AI can be used in healthcare, how predictive models can be checked, and how data can be shared. Governance models should also look at how radiogenomic predictions affect patient autonomy, especially when results are unclear or not expected [8].

Educational and Training Needs for Future Practitioners

As radiogenomics grows, it brings up important moral and legal issues. Some of these are data privacy, getting informed permission for genomic profiling, holding AI models accountable, and the possibility of algorithmic bias.

To protect patient rights, regulatory groups need to come up with rules for how AI can be used in healthcare, how predictive models can be checked, and how data can be shared. Governance models should also look at how radiogenomic predictions affect patient autonomy, especially when results are unclear or not expected [18]. To get the next crop of radiologists and clinicians ready to use radiogenomics in their daily work, we need workshops, certifications, and integrated medical education programs. It will be better for translational studies and clinical deployment if clinical and computational experts collaborate to learn.

References

1. Pinker K, Shitano F, Sala E, Do RK, Young RJ, Wibmer AG, et al. Background, current role, and potential applications of radiogenomics. J Magn Reson Imaging. 2018;47(2):604–20. https://doi.org/10.1002/jmri.25875.
2. Gillies RJ, Kinahan PE, Hricak H. Radiomics: images are more than pictures, they are data. Radiology. 2016;278(2):563–77. https://doi.org/10.1148/radiol.2015151169.
3. Zwanenburg A, Leger S, Vallières M, Löck S. Image biomarker standardisation initiative. Radiother Oncol. 2020;146:35–40. https://doi.org/10.1016/j.radonc.2020.01.001.
4. Aerts HJWL, Velazquez ER, Leijenaar RTH, et al. Decoding tumour phenotype by noninvasive imaging using a quantitative radiomics approach. Nat Commun. 2014;5:4006. https://doi.org/10.1038/ncomms5006.

5. Li S, Zhou B. Radiogenomics in oncology: framework and standardization need. Med Phys. 2019;46(8):3636–44. https://doi.org/10.1002/mp.13607.
6. Kickingereder P, Bonekamp D, Nowosielski M, et al. Radiogenomics of glioblastoma: machine learning–based classification of molecular characteristics by multi-parametric MRI features. Radiology. 2016;281(3):907–18. https://doi.org/10.1148/radiol.2016160775.
7. Bakas S, Akbari H, Sotiras A, et al. RSNA–MICCAI brain tumor radiogenomic classification: 2021 challenge outcomes. Med Image Anal. 2022;76:102303. https://doi.org/10.1016/j.media.2021.102303.
8. Park AY, Han MR, Seo BK, et al. MRI-based breast cancer radiogenomics using RNA profiling: prospective study. Breast Cancer Res. 2023;25(1):79. https://doi.org/10.1186/s13058-023-01653-7.
9. Li H, Zhu Y, Burnside ES, et al. MR imaging radiomics signatures for predicting the risk of breast cancer recurrence. Radiology. 2016;281(2):382–91. https://doi.org/10.1148/radiol.2016152112.
10. Zanfardino M, Franzese M, Pane K, et al. Integrated radiogenomics, pathomics, and transcriptomics in cancer: future directions. J Clin Med. 2022;11(7):1986. https://doi.org/10.3390/jcm11071986.
11. Liu X, Zhang H, Li Z, et al. MRI based radiomics model for predicting MGMT promoter methylation in glioblastoma. Sci Rep. 2023;13:13501. https://doi.org/10.1038/s41598-023-40632-0.
12. Gao L, Li H, Luo Z, et al. Radiomics signature for IDH mutation detection in high grade gliomas. Neuro-Oncology. 2023;25(4):657–68. https://doi.org/10.1093/neuonc/noac253.
13. Wu J, Yang X, Xie C, et al. Association of DCE MRI radiomic features with PAM50 subtypes in breast cancer. Cancer Imaging. 2022;22:67. https://doi.org/10.1186/s40644-022-00513-3.
14. Li Y, Zhao W, Yang W, et al. CT radiomics predicts EGFR mutation and PD L1 expression in NSCLC. Front Immunol. 2022;13:813072. https://doi.org/10.3389/fimmu.2022.813072.
15. Chen M, Tang Z, Lin L, et al. Radiomics in liver fibrosis staging: a systematic review. Eur Radiol. 2024;34:1567–79. https://doi.org/10.1007/s00330-023-09600-2.
16. Zhang P, Li X, Wang X, et al. Radiomics for early detection of neurological disorders. NeuroImage. 2023;278:119505. https://doi.org/10.1016/j.neuroimage.2023.119505.
17. Mello J, Bessho H, Watanabe M, et al. Federated learning in radiogenomics. NPJ Digit Med. 2024;7(1):112. https://doi.org/10.1038/s41746-024-01038-z.
18. Alberts B, Johnson A, Lewis J, Raff M, Roberts K, Walter P. Molecular biology of the cell. 6th ed. New York: Garland Science; 2014.
19. Karki R, Pandya D, Elston RC, et al. Defining “mutation” and “polymorphism” in the era of personal genomics. BMC Med Genet. 2015;8:37. https://doi.org/10.1186/s12920-015-0115-z.
20. OpenStax: DNA replication. In: Human biology. University of Minnesota. https://open.lib.umn.edu/humanbiology/chapter/6-3-dna-replication/. Last accessed 25 June 2024.
21. Visscher PM, Brown MA, McCarthy MI, Yang J. Five years of GWAS discovery. Am J Hum Genet. 2012;90(1):7–24. https://doi.org/10.1016/j.ajhg.2011.11.029.
22. 1000 Genomes Project Consortium, Auton A, Brooks LD, Durbin RM, et al. A global reference for human genetic variation. Nature. 2015;526(7571):68–74. https://doi.org/10.1038/nature15393.
23. Paila U, Chapman BA, Kirchner R, Quinlan AR. GEMINI: integrative exploration of genetic variation and genome annotations. PLoS Comput Biol. 2013;9(7):e1003153. https://doi.org/10.1371/journal.pcbi.1003153.
24. Shastry BS. SNPs: impact on gene function and phenotype. Methods Mol Biol. 2009;578:3–22. https://doi.org/10.1007/978-1-60327-411-1_1.
25. Aiello M, Infante T, Cavaliere C. Radiogenomic analysis of oncological data: a technical survey. Future Oncol. 2021;17(8):981–93. https://doi.org/10.2217/fon-2020-0899.
26. Corder EH, Saunders AM, Strittmatter WJ, et al. Gene dose of apolipoprotein E type 4 allele and the risk of Alzheimer’s disease. Science. 1993;261(5123):921–3. https://doi.org/10.1126/science.8346443.

27. Ioannidis JP, Ntzani EE, Trikalinos TA, Contopoulos-Ioannidis DG. Replication validity of genetic association studies. Nat Genet. 2001;29(3):306–9. https://doi.org/10.1038/ng749.
28. Hirschhorn JN, Daly MJ. Genome-wide association studies for common diseases and complex traits. Nat Rev Genet. 2005;6(2):95–108. https://doi.org/10.1038/nrg1521.
29. Brothwell MRS, West CM, Dunning AM, Burnet NG, Barnett GC. Radiogenomics in the era of advanced radiotherapy. Clin Oncol (R Coll Radiol). 2019;31(5):319–25. https://doi.org/10.1016/j.clon.2019.02.006.
30. Yamamoto S, Maki DD, Korn RL, Kuo MD. Radiogenomic analysis of breast cancer using MRI: a preliminary study to define the landscape. AJR Am J Roentgenol. 2012;199(3):654–63. https://doi.org/10.2214/AJR.11.7824.
31. Liu H, Wang Y, Liu Y, et al. Contrast-enhanced computed tomography–based radiogenomics analysis for predicting prognosis in gastric cancer. J Gastrointest Oncol. 2022;13(3):1250–61. https://doi.org/10.21037/jgo-22-20
32. Ferro M, de Cobelli O, Vartolomei MD, et al. Prostate cancer radiogenomics—from imaging to molecular characterization. Int J Mol Sci. 2021;22(18):9971. https://doi.org/10.3390/ijms22189971.
33. Tong Y, Sun P, Yong J, et al. Radiogenomic analysis of papillary thyroid carcinoma for prediction of cervical lymph node metastasis: a preliminary study. Front Oncol. 2021;11:682998. https://doi.org/10.3389/fonc.2021.682998.
34. Bibault JE, Giraud P, Burgun A. Big data and machine learning in radiation oncology: state of the art and future prospects. Cancer Lett. 2016;382(1):110–7. https://doi.org/10.1016/j.canlet.2016.01.037.
35. Chang K, Bai HX, Zhou H, et al. Residual convolutional neural network for predicting MGMT methylation status in glioblastoma. Clin Cancer Res. 2018;24(5):1073–81. https://doi.org/10.1158/1078-0432.CCR-17-1257.
36. Bakas S, Akbari H, Sotiras A, et al. Advancing the cancer genome atlas glioma MRI collections with expert segmentation labels and radiomic features. Sci Data. 2017;4:170117. https://doi.org/10.1038/sdata.2017.117.
37. Gerke S, Minssen T, Cohen G. Ethical and legal challenges of artificial intelligence-driven healthcare. Artif Intell Med. 2020;109:101964. https://doi.org/10.1016/j.artmed.2020.101964.
38. Hosny A, Parmar C, Quackenbush J, Schwartz LH, Aerts HJWL. Artificial intelligence in radiology. Nat Rev Cancer. 2018;18(8):500–10. https://doi.org/10.1038/s41568-018-0016-5.
39. Guan F, Wang Z, Qiu Y, et al. Biological underpinnings of radiomic MRI phenotypes for risk stratification in IDH wild-type glioblastoma: large-cohort study. J Transl Med. 2023;21:841. https://doi.org/10.1186/s12967-023-04483-0.
40. Mahajan A, Ghosh R, Singh R, et al. Prediction of MGMT promoter methylation status in glioblastoma by conventional contrast-enhanced T1 weighted MRI qualitative features. Neurooncol Adv. 2024;6(1):vdae016. https://doi.org/10.1093/noajnl/vdae016.

Chapter 7
Neuroscience, Technology, and Solutions for the Public Health Mental Health Crisis

Ryan Brown, Justin Kennedy, Marlene Gonzalez, and Amin Sanaia

Introduction

As societies worldwide confront an escalating mental health crisis, the integration of technology into public health strategies has become increasingly vital. Mental health issues, once relegated to the background of public health priorities, are now recognized as a leading cause of disability and morbidity, affecting millions globally. This crisis is not only a health issue but a societal one that influences productivity, social stability, and overall quality of life.

The current landscape of mental health care is primarily reactive, often addressing mental illness only after it has reached a critical stage. This approach has significant drawbacks, including delayed treatment, increased healthcare costs, and suboptimal outcomes for individuals. However, the advent of wearable technology offers a paradigm shift toward a more proactive and preventive strategy. Wearables, equipped with sensors to monitor various physiological and neurophysiological data, provide continuous insights into an individual's mental and emotional state, allowing for early detection and intervention of mental health issues.

Incorporating the principles of neuroscience and neuroplasticity, wearables can play a pivotal role in understanding and enhancing the brain's ability to reorganize itself by forming new neural connections in response to learning or experience.

R. Brown (✉)
Dalhousie University, Halifax, NS, Canada
e-mail: ryan.brown@dal.ca

J. Kennedy · M. Gonzalez
Monarch Business School, Walchwil Zug, Switzerland
e-mail: jj@profkennedy.com; marlene.gonzalez@lcgnow.com

A. Sanaia
SAN Consulting, West Palm Beach, FL, USA
e-mail: dramin@sanconsultingenterprise.net

P. Eappen et al. (eds.), *Advancing Healthcare with the Medical Internet of Things*, Health Informatics, https://doi.org/10.1007/978-3-032-23933-4_7

This adaptability of the brain is central to resilience and recovery in mental health, making wearables a key tool in personalized medicine approaches that cater to the dynamic nature of individual neurological and cognitive function.

By continuously monitoring indicators such as heart rate variability, sleep patterns, and activity levels, wearables offer a unique window into the wearer's daily health status, potentially identifying early signs of stress, depression, or anxiety. These devices not only collect data but can also deliver neuroplasticity-promoting interventions, such as biofeedback and stress management exercises, tailored to the user's specific neurological patterns and needs.

Moreover, the role of wearables extends beyond individual monitoring to contribute valuable data for public health research. By aggregating data from a large population of users, researchers can gain insights into broader mental health trends, evaluate the impact of public health interventions, and improve strategies for mental health management on a community or national level.

This chapter explores the intersection of wearable technology, neuroscience, and public health in the realm of mental health, emphasizing how these devices are transforming the landscape from one of reactive intervention to proactive, personalized care. It delves into the technical capabilities of current wearable devices, discusses the challenges and ethical considerations of their use, and examines case studies where wearables have successfully contributed to mental health strategies. The aim is to provide a comprehensive overview of how wearable technology can be harnessed to address the public health mental health crisis, fostering a future where technology and healthcare converge to enhance the well-being of populations worldwide.

The Public Health Mental Health Crisis: Mental Health, Mental Illness, and Resilience

The mental health crisis represents one of the most pressing public health challenges of our time. While often thought of in terms of infectious disease and hygiene, public health is concerned with any aspect of human health impacted at the population level. This spans communicable disease, chronic disease and mental health. Mental health is extraordinarily complex, and issues with mental health and mental illness are at epidemic proportions in society today. Its complexity stems from the interplay between individual, societal, and environmental factors. Often misunderstood, the terms "mental health" and "mental illness" are used interchangeably; however, they represent distinct, though interconnected, aspects of human psychology and physiology. Mental health encompasses overall well-being, resilience, and the capacity to cope with life's challenges, while mental illness refers to specific conditions that disrupt these capacities. By unpacking these distinctions and highlighting resilience and loneliness as critical concepts, we can better understand and address the mental health crisis.

Mental health is a state of well-being in which individuals can realize their potential, cope with normal stressors, work productively, and contribute to their community. It is not merely the absence of mental illness but a positive state of emotional, psychological, and social well-being. Central to mental health is the concept of resilience—the ability to adapt to adversity and bounce back from challenges.

In contrast, mental illness refers to a range of diagnosable conditions that affect mood, thinking, and behavior. These include depression, anxiety disorders, bipolar disorder, schizophrenia, and more. Mental illnesses often impair daily functioning and require clinical intervention. While mental health is a universal concept applicable to all, mental illness pertains to those experiencing specific symptoms that meet diagnostic criteria.

This distinction is critical for framing the public health crisis. Addressing mental health involves promoting well-being for all individuals, while addressing mental illness requires targeted interventions for those diagnosed with specific conditions. The Canadian Mental Health Association estimates that 1 in 5 individuals will experience issues with mental health or mental illness in any given year and that, by the age of 40, 50% of the population will have, or will have had, a mental illness [1, 2].

Societal and Environmental Impacts on Mental Health

Mental health does not exist in isolation; it is profoundly influenced by societal and environmental factors. Social determinants of health, including income, education, employment, and access to healthcare, play a pivotal role in shaping mental well-being. For instance, individuals living in poverty often face chronic stress, which can erode mental health over time as can those who are employed in situations that are not psychologically safe. Similarly, systemic inequities, such as racism and discrimination, contribute to disparities in mental health outcomes.

Environmental factors also exert significant influence. Natural disasters, climate change, and urbanization create stressors that challenge individual and community resilience. The COVID-19 pandemic further highlighted how isolation and loneliness, compounded by uncertainty and fear, can have a profound impact on mental health. During the pandemic, lockdowns and social distancing measures, while necessary for physical health, intensified feelings of loneliness for many, leading to a surge in mental health challenges.

Resilience as a Critical Concept

Resilience is the ability to adapt positively in the face of adversity, trauma, or significant stress. It serves as a protective factor that mitigates the impact of negative experiences on mental health. While some individuals appear naturally resilient, resilience is not an innate trait but a skill that can be developed.

Factors contributing to resilience include strong social connections, a sense of purpose, and adaptive coping mechanisms. For example, community support networks can provide a buffer against stress, while mindfulness practices can enhance an individual's capacity to manage emotional challenges. Notably, addressing loneliness is critical for fostering resilience. Creating opportunities for meaningful social interactions can strengthen resilience, providing individuals with the support and resources needed to navigate life's challenges.

Efforts to build resilience must also account for structural barriers. For example, individuals in underserved communities may lack access to mental health resources or supportive social networks, making it harder to develop resilience. Public health initiatives must therefore aim to reduce these disparities and create environments that support mental well-being.

The Complexity of Mental Health and Mental Illness

The relationship between mental health and mental illness is not binary but exists on a continuum. An individual can experience poor mental health without having a diagnosable mental illness and vice versa. For example, someone may feel overwhelmed or stressed due to life circumstances yet not meet the criteria for a mental illness. Conversely, individuals with chronic mental illnesses can achieve good mental health by effectively managing their symptoms and building resilience.

This complexity highlights the need for a nuanced approach to addressing the mental health crisis. Public health initiatives must focus on promoting mental health for all while providing targeted support for those with mental illnesses. This dual approach ensures that mental well-being is prioritized at both individual and societal levels.

The Role of Loneliness in the Mental Health Crisis

Loneliness is increasingly recognized as a significant contributor to the public health mental health crisis and can be considered a public health crisis in its own right. Defined as the subjective feeling of being socially isolated or lacking meaningful connections, loneliness affects mental health by heightening stress and emotional distress. While loneliness is often associated with older adults, it is pervasive across all age groups, with studies showing a sharp increase in loneliness among young adults, particularly in the wake of the COVID-19 pandemic. It should, however, be noted that this crisis existed prior to COVID, and, while an exacerbating factor, many new uses of existing and novel technologies have come out of the COVID-19 pandemic that mitigate loneliness [3].

Loneliness can undermine mental health in profound ways. Prolonged loneliness is associated with increased risks of depression, anxiety, and suicidal ideation. It activates the body's stress response, leading to elevated cortisol levels, which, over time, can impair physical health and cognitive functioning. Moreover, loneliness reduces the perception of social support, a critical buffer against life's challenges, thereby exacerbating feelings of vulnerability and helplessness.

The societal shifts that contribute to loneliness—such as the erosion of community ties, increased reliance on digital interactions, and urbanization—underscore the urgent need to address this issue. Loneliness is not merely a personal experience but a public health concern that requires systemic solutions [4].

Loneliness significantly impacts mental health and must be a priority in public health strategies. Effective approaches include fostering social connections through community-based programs like volunteering, group activities, and mentorship initiatives. Inclusive urban planning can promote interaction by creating spaces such as parks and community centers [3]. Technology, when used wisely, can bridge social gaps through virtual support groups, online counseling, and community-building apps. Public education campaigns can raise awareness about the mental health implications of loneliness and encourage individuals to seek meaningful connections. Additionally, workplaces can play a critical role by fostering inclusive cultures, organizing team-building activities, and providing resources to enhance employee connections and support.

Strategies to Address the Public Health Mental Health Crisis

Addressing the mental health crisis requires a multifaceted approach that includes prevention, early intervention, and treatment. Key strategies include:

1. Promoting Mental Health Education: Increasing awareness about mental health and mental illness can reduce stigma and encourage individuals to seek help. Educational programs in schools, workplaces, and communities can foster understanding and support.
2. Strengthening Social Support Systems: Strong social connections are critical for mental health. Initiatives to build community resilience, such as peer support groups and mental health hotlines, can provide essential resources.
3. Improving Access to Mental Health Services: Barriers to mental healthcare, including cost, availability, and stigma, must be addressed. Expanding access to affordable, culturally sensitive mental health services is vital.
4. Integrating Mental Health into Primary Care: By embedding mental health services within primary care settings, individuals can receive timely interventions, reducing the burden of untreated mental illness.
5. Addressing Societal Inequities: Tackling systemic issues such as poverty, discrimination, and unequal access to healthcare can create an environment conducive to better mental health outcomes.

6. Leveraging Technology for Mental Health: Technology offers innovative solutions to expand access to mental health support. Digital mental health tools, such as apps for mindfulness, cognitive behavioral therapy, and stress management, empower individuals to manage their mental well-being independently. Telehealth platforms enable remote therapy sessions, breaking geographical and accessibility barriers, particularly for underserved populations. Online support groups and community-building apps can foster social connections, reducing feelings of loneliness and isolation. Wearable technologies, such as smartwatches and fitness trackers, add another dimension by monitoring physical and emotional health indicators like heart rate variability, sleep patterns, and activity levels, which can provide insights into mental health status. These devices often integrate with mental health apps to offer personalized feedback and real-time interventions, encouraging users to make healthier lifestyle choices and recognize early signs of mental distress. However, it is critical to ensure that all these tools, including wearables, are evidence-based, secure, and user-friendly to maximize their effectiveness in addressing the mental health crisis.

The public health mental health crisis is a multifaceted challenge that demands a comprehensive and nuanced response. By distinguishing between mental health and mental illness and addressing loneliness as a critical determinant, we can better understand the scope of the crisis and identify targeted solutions. Promoting mental well-being, building resilience, and addressing societal and environmental determinants are key strategies for creating a healthier and more equitable society.

Resilience and social connection are critical concepts, bridging the gap between mental health promotion and mental illness prevention. Addressing loneliness, fostering meaningful relationships, and creating supportive environments are essential to building resilient individuals and communities. Ultimately, tackling the mental health crisis requires collective action, with a focus on reducing loneliness, promoting resilience, and enabling all individuals to thrive.

The application of wearable technology in the context of mental health and resilience will be explored in depth as this chapter progresses. The leveraging of these technologies will be looked at through the lens of theoretical organizational neuroscience as well as applied neuroscience and neuroplasticity.

The Neuroscience Behind Resilience and Recovery: Application of Neuroplasticity

Introduction to Neuroplasticity and Resilience

The intersection of neuroscience and behavior change offers transformative potential for fostering resilience and recovery, particularly through the lens of neuroplasticity. This section explores how neuroplasticity enhances well-being, addresses mental health challenges, and builds resilience. It introduces the concept of the

Neuroplastician, a non-clinical coach skilled in leveraging neuroplasticity to guide clients in behavior change and achieving health-related goals. Grounded in the work of Dr. Selma Kalkavan and Dr. Justin James Kennedy [5], the protocol demonstrates how neuroplasticity-based tools can reshape behavior, improve cognitive function, and promote mental health.

Advancements in Neuroscience and Mental Health

The exploration of themes such as attachment, trauma, sensory processing, and creativity has been instrumental in advancing mental health neuroscience. Zhang [6] highlighted ten influential articles published in Brain Sciences that exemplify multidisciplinary efforts to understand cognition and emotion. These include Fonagy et al.'s [7] exploration of attachment and trauma, Deste et al.'s [8] review of exercise and cognitive remediation for schizophrenia, and Yan et al.'s [9] study on olfactory bulb morphology and dysfunction. Together, they underscore the significance of neurotransmitters like dopamine and serotonin in sensory and emotional regulation [6, 10].

Emerging studies increasingly integrate computational models to unravel mechanisms underlying empathy, theory of mind, and social learning. This interdisciplinary approach highlights the complex interplay between neurotransmitters such as acetylcholine and norepinephrine in modulating cognition and emotion [11]. These advancements pave the way for therapeutic breakthroughs to enhance individual neuroplasticity, social and general well-being.

Mental Health, Mental Illness, and the Role of Neuroplasticity

Viewing mental health and mental illness as points on a continuum, rather than binary states, reveals the complexity of human functioning. Effective management strategies can enable individuals with mental illnesses to achieve high levels of mental health, while others without diagnosable conditions may struggle with poor mental health. This continuum-based perspective is critical for shaping public health interventions to universally promote mental well-being and target support for those with mental illnesses [12].

The Neuroscience of Resilience

Resilience, the ability to adapt positively to adversity, is a cornerstone of mental health. Neuroscientific research has revealed that resilience relies on brain plasticity, stress regulation mechanisms, and social connectivity. Neurotransmitters like endorphins play a key role in moderating stress and enhancing positive emotions [13]. Resilient individuals exhibit robust functioning in the prefrontal cortex, amygdala, and hippocampus, which are critical for decision-making, emotional regulation, and memory.

Functional magnetic resonance imaging (fMRI) studies show heightened prefrontal cortex activity during stress in resilient individuals, facilitating better emotional regulation [14]. Conversely, chronic stress and emotional dysregulation in non-resilient individuals are associated with amygdala overactivation. Balanced levels of neurotransmitters, such as norepinephrine and acetylcholine, further enhance adaptive responses to adversity [15].

Building Resilience: Factors and Interventions

Resilience is not a fixed trait but a dynamic capacity that can be cultivated through intentional practices and interventions. Key factors include:

- Social Support: Strong relationships activate brain regions associated with reward and stress buffering, mitigating the effects of adversity.
- Cognitive Flexibility: Reframing challenges as opportunities promotes adaptive emotional responses.
- Mindfulness Practices: Techniques like meditation enhance neural connectivity between the prefrontal cortex and other brain regions, reducing stress reactivity.
- Sense of Purpose: Engaging with meaningful life goals activates the brain's reward pathways, fostering resilience even under difficult circumstances.

These factors underscore the interplay between psychological strategies and neuroplasticity, enabling the brain to adapt and reorganize in response to challenges [14].

Neuroplasticity: The Foundation of Change

Neuroplasticity, the brain's ability to reorganize by forming new neural connections, underpins resilience and recovery. It involves three primary mechanisms:

1. Synaptic Plasticity: Strengthening or weakening synaptic connections based on activity
2. Neurogenesis: Creation of new neurons, particularly in the hippocampus, supporting learning and emotional regulation
3. Structural Remodeling: Altering white matter pathways to enhance communication between brain regions [15]

Both internal factors (e.g., genetics and hormones) and external factors (e.g., environment and learning experiences) shape neuroplasticity. Understanding these mechanisms is crucial for leveraging neuroplasticity to address mental health challenges.

Neuroplasticity in Mental Health Interventions

Neuroplasticity provides a framework for innovative mental health interventions. For instance:

- Depression: Reduced hippocampal volume in depression can be mitigated through interventions like antidepressants, physical exercise, and cognitive-behavioral therapy (CBT), which promote neurogenesis and strengthen synaptic connections.
- Anxiety Disorders: Maladaptive neural circuits between the amygdala and prefrontal cortex can be rewired through exposure therapy and mindfulness, improving emotional regulation and stress responses [16].

The Neuroplastician: Bridging Science and Practice

The Neuroplastician, as conceptualized by Kalkavan and Kennedy [5], integrates neuroplasticity-based tools to guide clients toward sustainable well-being. These practitioners employ strategies like:

- Cognitive Restructuring: Identifying and reframing negative thought patterns to reshape maladaptive neural pathways
- Mindfulness-Based Interventions: Strengthening prefrontal cortex connectivity to enhance emotional regulation
- Lifestyle Modifications: Encouraging activities like physical exercise and learning new skills to promote neural health

Functional imaging studies confirm that these interventions strengthen neural connections, reducing symptoms of anxiety and depression.

Technology and Neuroplasticity

Technology-driven interventions further harness neuroplasticity's potential. Digital therapeutic apps like Calm and Headspace enhance prefrontal cortex activation and reduce amygdala hyperactivity. Virtual reality therapies provide immersive environments for addressing anxiety-provoking stimuli, desensitizing maladaptive fear responses. Non-invasive brain stimulation techniques, such as transcranial magnetic stimulation (TMS), modulate neural activity to improve mood and cognitive function [17].

Cognitive Restructuring and Neural Rewiring

Cognitive restructuring is a cornerstone of neuroplasticity-based interventions. By identifying habitual negative thought patterns, challenging their validity, and reframing them into constructive beliefs, individuals can rewire neural pathways.

This process underscores how repeated use of adaptive cognitive patterns strengthens neural connections, fostering resilience and mental health.

Interventions and Neuroplasticity

Everyday activities significantly impact neuroplasticity:

- Physical Exercise: Increases brain-derived neurotrophic factor (BDNF), essential for neural health and plasticity
- Skill Learning: Enhances synaptic plasticity and cognitive reserve
- Quality Sleep: Consolidates learning and emotional processing, supporting neuroplasticity [13]

The importance of neuroplasticity in maintaining cognitive function later in life is well-documented [18]. These findings highlight the relevance of lifestyle interventions in promoting lifelong resilience and mental health.

Public Health Implications

The mental health crisis demands scalable neuroplasticity-based solutions. Public health campaigns can raise awareness of the brain's adaptability and encourage practices like mindfulness, exercise, and social connection. Integrating neuroplasticity-based approaches into primary care, including screenings and referrals for CBT or digital therapeutics, can enhance early intervention strategies [16].

The neuroscience of mental health and neuroplasticity provides profound insights into addressing the global mental health crisis. By distinguishing mental health from mental illness, emphasizing resilience, and leveraging neuroplasticity-based tools, a comprehensive framework for enhancing mental well-being emerges. Continued collaboration among neuroscientists, clinicians, and public health experts is essential to effectively implement these solutions, reaching diverse populations and fostering a resilient society.

The Application of Wearables in Resilience and Mental Health Monitoring

The integration of wearable technology into mental health and resilience monitoring is revolutionizing the way psychological well-being is understood, predicted, and managed. Historically, mental health assessments have depended on clinical evaluations, often intervening only after symptoms have become severe. However, neuroscience-backed wearables now enable proactive mental health strategies by providing continuous, real-time data on neural activity and emotional states. These tools are reshaping the field, addressing the mental health crisis, building resilience, and fostering recovery. Platforms like Immersion Neuroscience empower individuals, clinicians, and researchers to monitor emotional fitness, predict mental health challenges, and implement timely interventions [11, 18].

The global mental health crisis highlights the urgency of innovative solutions. In the United States alone, one in five individuals will face clinical depression during their lifetime, with millions more experiencing anxiety disorders annually. The economic and social costs—stemming from suicide rates, productivity losses, and healthcare expenses—underscore the need to shift from reactive to proactive mental health strategies. Wearable technology offers a path forward, addressing these concerns through continuous and objective monitoring [7].

Traditional mental health tools, such as self-reported surveys and clinical assessments, are limited by reliance on subjective inputs. These methods often suffer from inaccuracies, recency bias, and survey fatigue. In contrast, wearables equipped with sensors capture real-time physiological and neurophysiological markers, such as heart rate variability, movement, and neurochemical signals. These devices create a comprehensive, data-driven picture of an individual's mental and emotional states [19]. For instance, the Immersion Neuroscience platform quantifies neurochemical activity linked to dopamine and oxytocin—key regulators of emotional regulation and social bonding.

Using photoplethysmography (PPG) sensors, the platform computes a composite measure, "Immersion," representing neural value derived from experiences. Peaks and troughs in Immersion data correlate strongly with emotional fitness and mood variability, enabling the identification of pre-depressive symptoms and the promotion of resilience [5].

Practical Applications of Wearable Technology

Wearable technology has significant practical applications in mental health contexts as mood variability is a characteristic feature of mental health conditions like depression, anxiety, and wearables with neurophysiological monitoring detect patterns of mood variability by tracking Immersion peaks and troughs offer insights that help clinicians anticipate emotional lows and capitalize on positive experiences, for example, a study using Immersion Neuroscience monitored participants for 8–10 h daily over 3 weeks and predicted mood states with 90% accuracy as observed by Merritt and Zak [20]. Furthermore, emotional fitness, defined as the ability to regulate emotions, build resilience, and thrive, can be actively cultivated using wearables with physiological data signaling wellbeing and thriving or highlighting the need for health improvement intervention.

By analyzing this data, targeted strategies—such as engaging in mindfulness practices, physical activities, or social interactions—can be implemented to enhance well-being [5]. Wearables bridge the gap between episodic clinical visits and daily life by providing clinicians with detailed, objective data on emotional and physiological states. For instance, Immersion data can reveal prolonged troughs, prompting health coaches and clinicians to explore contributing factors and develop tailored treatment plans [11].

Resilience Building Through Wearable Technology

Resilience, the capacity to adapt positively to adversity, is essential for mental health. Wearables contribute to resilience-building by identifying stress triggers, promoting positive behaviors, and supporting mindfulness practices. Continuous data collection detects patterns in stress responses, enabling individuals to recognize and address triggers proactively. Additionally, wearables integrate with apps that guide reflective practices and track their impact on emotional states, fostering resilience through actionable insights [7].

Despite their potential, challenges must be addressed to maximize the effectiveness of wearables, and the collection of sensitive physiological data raises concerns about privacy. Ensuring robust encryption, adherence to health data regulations, and transparent practices is essential to building user trust [6]. Wearables must be accessible to diverse populations, including underserved communities. Affordability, cultural sensitivity, and technological literacy are crucial to prevent widening health disparities [18]. For widespread adoption, wearable data must seamlessly integrate with existing healthcare systems. Interoperability between wearable platforms and electronic health records (EHRs) streamlines data sharing and enhances clinical workflows as per Dinh-Le et al. [21].

Emerging Trends and Future Directions

Wearables represent a transformative solution to the global mental health crisis. By addressing accessibility, privacy, and integration challenges, they empower individuals and clinicians to enhance emotional fitness and resilience. Platforms like Immersion Neuroscience demonstrate how neuroscience and technology converge to support well-being, predict mood variability, and foster recovery. As the field advances, wearables will play an increasingly central role in creating a proactive, data-driven approach to wellness as observed by Merritt and Zak [20]. The evolution of wearables from monitoring tools to active agents of change presents exciting possibilities. Wearables can provide real-time feedback and personalized interventions, such as guiding users through breathing exercises during stress or recommending mood-enhancing activities. AI-powered analytics enhance the predictive accuracy of wearables, uncovering complex patterns in neurophysiological data. Extended monitoring periods enable researchers to track mood and resilience trends over time, offering deeper insights into the long-term impact of interventions observed [22].

Petrowski et al. [23] describe the revised Short Screening Version of the Profile of Mood States (POMS). POMS is the default psychological assessment tool designed to measure mood and emotional states across six dimensions, including tension, depression, anger, vigor, fatigue, and confusion. Psychologists use it to evaluate temporary mood fluctuations and emotional responses, often in clinical or research settings, by administering a questionnaire where individuals rate their feelings on a standardized scale. POMS-16 is a valid and reliable measure of mood states with minimal losses compared to the 35-item version, and where a brief assessment is needed, the POMS-16 should be considered. According to Penner and Stoddard [24], affective neuroscience emphasizes the study of the neural mechanisms underlying emotions and affective states. It is relevant as it bridges psychology and neuroscience, offering insights into how brain activity influences emotions, which is crucial for understanding mental health and developing targeted interventions for emotional disorders.

Understanding neurotransmission is vital to advancing research in affective neuroscience, where questions about the neural basis of emotions like valence (pleasure-displeasure) and arousal remain unresolved. Early models focused on identifying specific brain regions responsible for these dimensions, but research has not consistently uncovered reliable or unique neural circuits for affective experiences [25–27]. This gap has led to a shift toward predictive processing models, which propose that the brain generates affect through predictions and prediction errors rather than fixed neural signatures. These challenge traditional views by emphasizing variability across individuals and contexts. Lee, Ferreira-Santos, and Satpute [28] critique current neuroimaging practices in affective neuroscience, highlighting how rigid assumptions about uniform brain activation patterns slow progress. Predictive models suggest that instead of searching for static "on/off" neural circuits, researchers should explore how predictions dynamically shape subjective experiences [29, 30]. This approach calls for changes in experimental design, data analysis, and theoretical frameworks, emphasizing ecological and external validity.

By integrating predictive processing into affective neuroscience, the field can move beyond outdated feature detector models. This perspective not only advances our understanding of emotions but also reshapes how researchers study the intricate relationship between neural activity and subjective experience by offering real-time data. Merritt and Zak [20] addressed this challenge by leveraging neurophysiologic immersion—a state defined by sustained attention and emotional resonance—as a reliable metric for understanding mood fluctuations in relation to neurotransmission. This study highlights the integration of wearable sensors and artificial intelligence to track neurophysiologic signals, offering a non-invasive approach to mood monitoring. Recent advances in wearable technology and neurophysiological data have enabled researchers to explore the potential of real-time mood prediction.

Case Study 1: The Impact of Wearable Technology on Engagement and Resilience in High-Pressure Industries

Wearable technology has significantly transformed training practices and human resources practices across high-pressure industries, providing real-time insights into engagement, psychological safety, and physiological responses. The experience in the sports sector demonstrates how tools such as biosensors and heart rate monitors can enhance learning environments by offering actionable data to trainers. Although expertise is found outside healthcare, the parallels between these industries suggest that similar technologies could benefit executives who face equally demanding and high-pressure scenarios, not to mention clinicians. By applying these tools, organizations can support leadership development and resilience in ways that address the unique challenges of their fields.

Insights from the Sports Executive Pilot

This pilot program demonstrated how wearable technology could optimize training by providing real-time physiological data. Participants wore devices capable of tracking metrics like heart rate variability and electrodermal activity, which correlate with stress and emotional engagement. Insights derived from this data allowed trainers to identify peak engagement moments and adjust pacing and content delivery in real time, ensuring participants remained focused. These dynamic interventions created a more responsive and impactful training environment. Additionally, a significant percentage of participants reported a strong sense of security during the program, fostering deeper engagement and retention of material. These findings suggest that training programs in various sectors could also benefit from integrating wearable technology to monitor and enhance participants' emotional and cognitive states [31].

Integrating wearable technology into training offers an opportunity to address the unique demands of various industries through data-driven strategies. Tools like heart rate monitors and biosensors can provide real-time feedback, enabling trainers to make immediate adjustments that improve engagement and retention. Wearables can detect stress spikes during simulations, prompting trainers to pause or adjust the difficulty to ensure participants remain focused and productive. Building emotional resilience is another area where wearables can play a critical role in training by tracking stress levels and emotional responses in real time. This approach not only helps executives develop resilience but also equips them to manage stress effectively in real-world scenarios.

In emergency response simulations, wearable devices can track physiological responses, helping trainers assess participants' reactions under pressure. Improving communication skills is another vital application, as wearables monitor emotional responses during role-playing exercises, providing feedback on moments where participants may struggle with empathy or clarity. Team-based training can also benefit from wearable insights, particularly in revealing how group dynamics impact individual performance.

Psychological safety, a team's shared belief that it is safe to take interpersonal risks, is foundational for effective team dynamics, particularly in critical care settings where rapid decision-making and vulnerability are commonplace. Wearable technology, through its real-time monitoring capabilities, plays a pivotal role in fostering this environment. Devices that measure physiological responses such as heart rate variability and stress levels can provide immediate feedback to team leaders and trainers, highlighting moments when team members might be feeling overwhelmed or anxious.

This data enables leaders to create targeted interventions to support team members, such as initiating debriefs, adjusting workloads, or providing immediate emotional support. For example, if a team member's stress markers rise during a simulation of a high-stakes procedure, trainers can intervene to offer guidance and reassurance, helping to normalize the acceptance of support and reducing the stigma around expressing vulnerability. This not only aids in maintaining focus during critical tasks but also reinforces a culture where team members feel valued and supported, enhancing overall team cohesion and psychological safety.

Building Resilience Through Data-Driven Insights

Resilience in critical care teams is essential not just for the wellbeing of the healthcare professionals but also for the quality of care they provide. Wearables can detect subtle physiological changes that precede visible signs of stress and burnout, allowing for preemptive action to bolster resilience. By analyzing this data, trainers and leaders can identify patterns that may indicate resilience or vulnerability to stress, tailoring training programs to reinforce coping mechanisms and stress management strategies.

Training sessions enhanced with wearable technology can simulate stressful scenarios that are common in critical care settings, providing a safe space for team members to engage with these stressors. The insights gathered from wearables during these simulations enable trainers to offer personalized feedback and develop individualized resilience-building plans. For instance, if a team member consistently shows elevated stress levels during pediatric emergencies, additional training can be provided in this area, alongside techniques to manage emotional responses effectively.

Impact on Critical Care Outcomes

The long-term impact of integrating wearable technology into critical care training is profound. Enhanced psychological safety leads to more open communication, reduced errors, and a more supportive workplace culture. As team members feel safer and more supported, their ability to handle stress improves, which is critical in environments where the margin for error is slim.

Moreover, resilient teams are better equipped to handle the emotional and physical demands of critical care. This not only improves their personal health outcomes, reducing the incidence of burnout and turnover, but also enhances patient care quality. Wearable technology provides the data needed to continuously refine training processes and team dynamics, ensuring that the critical care teams are prepared to meet challenges head-on. By providing real-time, actionable insights into physiological and emotional states, wearables help create safer, more supportive, and resilient healthcare environments. This technology not only impacts the individuals within these teams but also the very nature of patient care delivery, ultimately leading to better health outcomes and more efficient healthcare systems.

This pilot program demonstrated how wearable technology can transform training by providing real-time insights into engagement, stress, and psychological safety. These findings suggest that similar tools could revolutionize training for executives, where effective leadership development is critical for managing the complexities of modern industries. By integrating wearable devices into training programs, organizations can create adaptive learning environments that foster resilience, improve decision-making, and enhance team dynamics.

Case Study 2: Continuous Remote Monitoring of Neurophysiologic Data to Accurately Predict Affect and General Mood in a Residential Living Facility

Neurological health assessments traditionally rely on subjective self-reports and infrequent clinical evaluations, creating a reactive approach to mental health care. This paradigm limits early identification and intervention for conditions like depression and anxiety. Recent advancements in wearable technology and neurophysiological data analysis offer promising solutions by enabling continuous, proactive monitoring of mental well-being. By analyzing neurochemical activities, particularly the release of oxytocin and dopamine, critical roles in human connection, attention, memory, behavior, and overall well-being can be observed [32]. These advancements enable the measurement of neurochemical releases through subtle changes in cardiac rhythms, detectable via wearable devices like smartwatches and fitness trackers. Sophisticated algorithms applied to this data provide real-time insights into the brain's valuation processes, predicting behaviors and informing strategies in areas such as mental health and emotional well-being.

A pioneering study by Merritt and Zak [20], published in Frontiers in Digital Health, explored the potential of continuously monitoring neurophysiological data to predict mood states. The study utilized the Immersion Neuroscience platform, a commercial technology quantifying the neural value of social-emotional experiences via real-time monitoring of associated dopamine and oxytocin levels.

The study involved 24 participants who wore the Immersion Neuroscience device for 8–10 h daily over 3 weeks. Continuous neurophysiological data were collected at a 1 Hz sampling rate. Concurrently, participants provided self-reported measures of their mood and energy levels, serving as the ground truth for validating the predictive algorithms. The researchers analyzed the data using machine learning models trained to correlate immersion levels with self-reported mood scores. The longitudinal design enabled capturing a wide range of mood states over time. Contextual data, such as time of day and activity type, were also incorporated to enhance predictive accuracy.

The study yielded several significant findings. Identification of "Troughs" and "Peaks": Researchers identified distinct neurophysiological patterns characterized as "troughs" (periods of low neural value) and "peaks" (periods of high neural value). These patterns closely corresponded to fluctuations in participants' mood states.

Predictive Accuracy: Utilizing regression and machine learning models, the study achieved a predictive accuracy of 90% for daily mood based on the frequency and characteristics of these events was employed. The predictive model demonstrated high sensitivity (87%) and specificity (85%), outperforming traditional mood tracking methods like self-reporting.

Individual Variability: Participants with higher baseline heart rate variability (HRV) exhibited more stable mood predictions compared to those with lower HRV, underscoring the need for personalized models to account for individual physiological and behavioral differences.

Gender Differences: Women showed a higher propensity for low mood compared to men, revealing potential gender-specific patterns in mood variability. A particularly striking finding was the model's ability to detect subtle mood changes up to 30 minutes before participants consciously recognized them. This capability suggests immense potential for early intervention in mood-related disorders.

Implications

The implications of this research are profound for mental health and human performance optimization. Continuous, passive, and objective mood monitoring could transform how clinicians diagnose and manage conditions like depression and anxiety. Early identification of mood disturbances allows timely interventions, potentially improving treatment outcomes and reducing symptom severity. Personalized healthcare is another promising avenue. By analyzing individual patterns of "troughs" and "peaks," clinicians can tailor interventions, such as recommending mindfulness exercises during periods of low neural value or incorporating activities that consistently elicit "peaks" into daily routines to enhance well-being.

The study also advances the field of digital phenotyping by demonstrating how wearable technologies and machine learning algorithms can analyze complex behavioral and physiological data. Digital phenotyping holds the promise of identifying individual-level patterns and trajectories of mental health conditions, leading to more precise diagnoses and targeted interventions. While the findings are promising, several ethical considerations must be addressed to ensure responsible use of this technology. Continuous collection of sensitive neurophysiological data raises concerns regarding data privacy, informed consent, and potential misuse. Robust ethical frameworks and stringent data security measures are essential to mitigate these risks and build public trust. Despite its promising results, the study had limitations that warrant further investigation:

Sample Size: The study's small sample size ($N = 24$) limits the generalizability of the findings. Future research with larger, more diverse populations is crucial.

Diverse Populations: The study primarily focused on a specific demographic. Future studies should explore findings across clinical populations with varying mental health conditions, ages, and cultural backgrounds.

Technology Replicability: The study relied on a single commercial neuroscience platform. Future research should investigate whether similar findings can be replicated using different technologies.

Long-Term Predictions: The study focused on short-term mood predictions. Further research is needed to evaluate the long-term predictive validity of this approach.

Significance of Findings

Merritt and Zak's [20] study represents a significant milestone in leveraging digital phenotyping for mental health. By demonstrating the predictive power of continuous neurophysiological monitoring, the researchers opened new avenues for proactive mood assessment and personalized mental health interventions. The findings emphasize the transformative potential of wearable technologies to enhance resilience, improve emotional fitness, and support mental well-being. Continuous, passive monitoring provides a groundbreaking tool for designing personalized healthcare strategies. Organizations could use this technology to enhance employee well-being and productivity by identifying stressors and creating responsive environments.

Participants experienced an average of 2.25 neurophysiologic troughs per day (SD = 3.70, Min = 0, Max = 25) and 3.28 peaks per day (SD = 3.97, Min = 0, Max = 25). These metrics predicted daily mood with 90% accuracy, underscoring the reliability of immersion as a mood proxy. This protocol highlights the potential to proactively assess mood and energy, providing valuable insights into vulnerabilities and indicators of thriving.

Future research should focus on refining predictive algorithms, addressing ethical challenges, and exploring applications across diverse populations. Continuous remote monitoring of neurophysiologic immersion could revolutionize mental health management, offering a proactive, data-driven approach to well-being. Capturing unconscious value during interactions provides actionable insights into emotional engagement and the effectiveness of resilience-building interventions.

Ultimately, Merritt and Zak's [20] work underscores the importance of integrating objective, data-driven methods into mental healthcare. The ability to continuously and passively measure value using wearable technology offers a transformative tool for designing personalized healthcare and resilience-building strategies that promote long-term well-being. As this technology evolves, it promises to enhance quality of life worldwide. This case study serves as a foundational reference for scholars and practitioners interested in wearable digital phenotyping, mental health, and emotional fitness.

Conclusion

The integration of wearable technology into the landscape of mental health represents a pivotal shift toward a more proactive and personalized approach to healthcare. As demonstrated throughout this chapter, wearables offer a unique capacity to monitor and manage mental health in real-time, transforming our understanding and intervention strategies from reactive to predictive.

Wearable devices, equipped with advanced sensors, provide continuous data on various physiological and neurophysiological parameters, such as heart rate variability, sleep patterns, and stress levels. This data is not only vital for individual health monitoring but also enriches our broader understanding of mental health patterns across different populations. By leveraging this technology, neuroscience-based coaches and healthcare providers can detect early signs of mental distress and intervene before they escalate into more severe conditions.

The application of neuroplasticity principles through wearable technology further underscores the innovative approaches being utilized to combat mental health issues. Wearables can support the brain's ability to rewire itself in response to experiences, promoting resilience and recovery in individuals facing mental health challenges. This capability aligns closely with the growing emphasis on resilience as a critical component of mental wellness, underscoring the potential of wearables to not just monitor health but actively enhance it.

Moreover, the data collected via wearables can lead to more informed public health decisions. By analyzing trends and identifying risk factors, health systems can develop targeted interventions that address the specific needs of their communities. This approach is particularly crucial in addressing the widespread impact of mental health disorders, which not only affect individual well-being but also impose significant economic and social costs on society.

However, the integration of wearable technology in public health strategies also presents challenges. Issues such as data privacy, the potential for socioeconomic disparities in access to technology, and the need for cross-sector collaboration are critical concerns that must be addressed. Ensuring that these technologies are accessible, equitable, and ethically managed is essential for their success in improving public health outcomes.

The ongoing development of wearable technology also promises further advancements in our approach to mental health. Future innovations could enhance the accuracy and effectiveness of these devices, offering even more nuanced insights into the complex interplay of factors that influence mental health. Additionally, as machine learning and artificial intelligence capabilities continue to evolve, the potential for wearables to predict and manage mental health conditions will only increase.

In conclusion, wearable technology offers a promising tool for transforming the mental health landscape at the individual and population level. By providing real-time, personalized data on an individual's health, wearables not only empower users to take control of their mental wellness but also equip healthcare providers with the tools necessary for early intervention and tailored treatment plans. As we continue to navigate the challenges and opportunities presented by these technologies, their integration into public health strategies represents a hopeful step toward a future where mental health is managed with the same precision and care as physical health.

References

1. Canadian Mental Health Association. Fast facts about mental illness. Canadian Mental Health Association; 2021. Available from: https://cmha.ca/brochure/fast-facts-about-mental-illness/#_edn1
2. Dobson KG, Vigod SN, Mustard C, Smith PM. Trends in the prevalence of depression and anxiety disorders among working-age Canadian adults between 2000 and 2016. Health Rep. 2020;31(12). https://doi.org/10.25318/82-003-x202001200002-eng.
3. Crowe CL, Liu L, Bagnarol N, Fried LP. Loneliness prevention and the role of the public health system. Perspect Public Health. 2024;144(1). https://doi.org/10.1177/17579139221106579.
4. Qualter P, Vanhalst J, Harris R, et al. Loneliness across the lifespan. Perspect Psychol Sci. 2015;10(20):250–64.
5. Kalkavan S, Kennedy JJ. Neuroplasticity coach and the power of neuroplasticity: reprogramming the brain for positive change. Harvard Bus Rev Turk. 2024. Available from: https://hbr-turkiye.com.
6. Zhang Y. Advances in social cognitive and affective neuroscience: ten highly cited articles published in Brain Sciences in 2022–2023. Brain Sci. 2022;14(5):460. https://doi.org/10.3390/brainsci14050460.
7. Fonagy P, Campbell C, Luyten P. Attachment, mentalizing, and trauma: then (1992) and now (2022). Brain Sci. 2023;13:459. https://doi.org/10.3390/brainsci13030459.
8. Deste G, Corbo D, Nibbio G, et al. Impact of physical exercise alone or in combination with cognitive remediation on cognitive functions in people with schizophrenia: a qualitative critical review. Brain Sci. 2023;13:320. https://doi.org/10.3390/brainsci13020320.
9. Yan X, Joshi A, Zang Y, Asscuncao F, Fernandes HM, Hummel T. The shape of the olfactory bulb predicts olfactory function. Brain Sci. 2022;12:128. https://doi.org/10.3390/brainsci12020128.
10. Schildkraut JJ. The catecholamine hypothesis of affective disorders: a review of supporting evidence. Am J Psychiatry. 1965;122(5):509–22.
11. Sarter M, Gehring WJ, Kozak R. More attention must be paid: the neurobiology of attentional effort. Brain Res Rev. 2005;51(2):145–60.
12. Ryff CD, Singer B. Know thyself and become what you are: a eudaimonic approach to psychological well-being. J Happiness Stud. 2008;9:13–39. https://doi.org/10.1007/s10902-006-9019-0.

13. Pert CB. Molecules of emotion: why you feel the way you feel. New York: Simon & Schuster; 1997.
14. McEwen BS. Physiology and neurobiology of stress and adaptation: central role of the brain. Physiol Rev. 2007;87(3):873–904. https://doi.org/10.1152/physrev.00041.2006.
15. Sullivan RM, Gratton A. Prefrontal cortical regulation of hypothalamic-pituitary-adrenal function in the rat and implications for psychopathology: side matters. Psychoneuroendocrinology. 2002;27(1–2):99–114. https://doi.org/10.1016/s0306-4530(01)00038-5.
16. Cicchetti D, Curtis WJ. Multilevel perspectives on pathways to resilient functioning. Dev Psychopathol. 2007;19(3):627–9. https://doi.org/10.1017/S0954579407000314.
17. Panksepp J. Affective neuroscience: the foundations of human and animal emotions. New York: Oxford University Press; 1998.
18. Marzola P, Melzer T, Pavesi E, Gil-Mohapel J, Brocardo PS. Exploring the role of neuroplasticity in development, aging, and neurodegeneration. Brain Sci. 2023;13(12):1610. https://doi.org/10.3390/brainsci13121610.
19. Zhang Y. Emerging themes in mental health: attachment, trauma, and creativity. Brain Sci. 2022;12(4):450–60. https://doi.org/10.3390/brainsci12040450.
20. Merritt SH, Zak PJ. Continuous remote monitoring of neurophysiologic immersion accurately predicts mood. Front Digit Health. 2024;6:1397557. https://doi.org/10.3389/fdgth.2024.1397557.
21. Dinh-Le C, Chuang R, Chokshi S, Mann D. Wearable health technology and electronic health record integration: scoping review and future directions. JMIR Mhealth Uhealth. 2019;7(9):e12861. https://doi.org/10.2196/12861.
22. Olawade DB, Wada OZ, Odetayo A, David-Olawade AC, Asaolu F, Eberhardt J. Enhancing mental health with artificial intelligence: current trends and future prospects. Glob Med. 2024;100:100099. https://doi.org/10.1016/j.glmedi.2024.100099.
23. Petrowski K, Albani C, Zenger M, et al. Revised short screening version of the profile of mood states (POMS) from the German general population. Front Psychol. 2021;12:631668. https://doi.org/10.3389/fpsyg.2021.631668.
24. Penner AE, Stoddard J. Clinical affective neuroscience. J Am Acad Child Adolesc Psychiatry. 2018;57(12):906–8. https://doi.org/10.1016/j.jaac.2018.07.877.
25. Barrett LF, Bliss-Moreau E. Affect as a psychological primitive. Adv Exp Soc Psychol. 2009;41:167–218. https://doi.org/10.1016/S0065-2601(08)00404-8.
26. Lindquist KA, Satpute AB, Wager TD, et al. The brain basis of emotion: a meta-analytic review. Behav Brain Sci. 2012;35(3):121–43. https://doi.org/10.1017/S0140525X11000446.
27. Berridge KC, Kringelbach ML. Pleasure systems in the brain. Neuron. 2015;86(3):646–64. https://doi.org/10.1016/j.neuron.2015.02.018.
28. Lee KM, Ferreira-Santos F, Satpute AB. Predictive processing models and affective neuroscience. Neurosci Biobehav Rev. 2021;131:211–28. https://doi.org/10.1016/j.neubiorev.2021.09.009.
29. Barrett HC. Towards a cognitive science of the human: cross-cultural approaches and their urgency. Trends Cogn Sci. 2020;24:620–38. https://doi.org/10.1016/j.tics.2020.05.007.
30. Poldrack RA. Inferring mental states from neuroimaging data: from reverse inference to large-scale decoding. Neuron. 2011;72(5):692–7. https://doi.org/10.1016/j.neuron.2011.11.001.
31. Khakurel J, Melkas H, Porras J. Tapping into the wearable device revolution in the work environment: A systematic review. Inf Technol People. 2018; https://doi.org/10.1108/ITP-03-2017-0076.
32. Zak PJ, Curry B, Owen T, Barraza JA. Oxytocin release increases with age and is associated with life satisfaction and prosocial behaviors. Front Behav Neurosci. 2022;16:846234. https://doi.org/10.3389/fnbeh.2022.846234.

Chapter 8
Wearable Devices for Management of Chronic Diseases: Improving Patient Quality of Life and Outcomes

Muhammad Thesa Ghozali

Introduction

Chronic Diseases—A Brief Introduction

Chronic diseases—including cardiovascular conditions, diabetes, respiratory illnesses, and cancer—represent the leading cause of mortality globally, accounting for over 70% of annual deaths [1]. Their growing prevalence, driven by aging populations and lifestyle factors, places immense pressure on healthcare systems, particularly in low- and middle-income countries [2]. In addition to the clinical burden, chronic diseases generate substantial economic strain due to direct medical costs and productivity losses—estimated at over $3.7 trillion annually in the United States alone [3]. Traditional, episodic care models are ill-suited for managing these dynamic conditions, which require continuous, personalized interventions. Wearable technologies address this gap by enabling real-time health monitoring and proactive decision-making, offering new opportunities to improve outcomes and quality of life.

Rise of Wearable Devices in Healthcare

The evolution of wearable devices has marked a paradigm shift in healthcare settings, transitioning from rudimentary fitness trackers to sophisticated medical-grade technologies capable of monitoring complex health parameters. Designed to collect

M. T. Ghozali (✉)
School of Pharmacy, Faculty of Medicine and Health Sciences,
Universitas Muhammadiyah Yogyakarta, Special Region of Yogyakarta, Indonesia
e-mail: ghozali@umy.ac.id

P. Eappen et al. (eds.), *Advancing Healthcare with the Medical Internet of Things*, Health Informatics, https://doi.org/10.1007/978-3-032-23933-4_8

and analyze both physiological and behavioral data through advanced sensors, wearables provide users and healthcare professionals with actionable insights into health and disease. Popular categories of wearable devices include smartwatches, activity trackers, biosensors, e.g., continuous glucose monitors (CGMs), portable electrocardiograms (ECGs), and smart textiles embedded with sensors. Each of these devices serves specific health-related functions, ranging from tracking steps and sleep patterns to monitoring critical parameters such as blood glucose levels and heart rhythms [4, 5].

The market of global wearable healthcare has grown exponentially in recent years, driven by advances in sensor technology, connectivity, and data analytics. In 2020, the wearable healthcare devices market was valued at approximately USD 18.4 billion and is projected to expand at a compound annual growth rate (CAGR) of 12.1%, reaching USD 46.6 billion by 2028 [6, 7]. This rapid growth reflects increasing consumer awareness of health monitoring and the integration of wearable devices into disease management protocols. Furthermore, the COVID-19 pandemic underscored the utility of wearables in healthcare by enabling remote monitoring and reducing the need for in-person consultations, thus addressing gaps in care delivery during public health emergencies.

Wearable devices hold immense potential to transform chronic disease management by enabling continuous, non-invasive monitoring and providing personalized insights. For instance, continuous glucose monitoring systems have revolutionized diabetes care by allowing real-time glucose tracking and integration with insulin delivery systems. Similarly, portable ECG devices have improved the management of cardiovascular diseases by facilitating the early detection of arrhythmias and other cardiac anomalies. These technologies have demonstrated significant clinical benefits, including reducing hospitalizations, improving medication adherence, and enhancing overall health outcomes [8]. Beyond clinical applications, wearable devices empower individuals to take an active role in managing their health, fostering a sense of control and responsibility over their conditions. This shift toward patient-centered care is particularly relevant in the context of chronic diseases, where sustained engagement and adherence to treatment are critical to achieving optimal outcomes.

Purpose and Scope of the Chapter

This chapter explores the transformative role of wearable devices in enhancing the management of chronic diseases, with a particular focus on their impact on patient quality of life (QoL) and clinical outcomes. Wearable technologies have introduced new dimensions in chronic disease management by addressing critical challenges such as the need for continuous monitoring, early intervention, and tailored treatment strategies. By bridging the gap between patients and healthcare providers, wearables enable more dynamic and responsive care, shifting the focus from reactive interventions to proactive disease management.

The chapter is structured to provide a comprehensive analysis of wearable devices, beginning with an overview of their technological capabilities and applications across specific chronic diseases. The discussion highlights how such devices facilitate continuous monitoring, empower patients through self-management, and enhance clinical decision-making by leveraging data-driven insights. Additionally, it examines the broader implications of wearable technology adoption such as its potential to reduce healthcare costs, improve resource utilization, and address health inequities. Specific examples and case studies are presented to describe the real-world impact of wearables on chronic disease management.

The chapter also addresses the challenges and barriers related to the implementation of the devices in healthcare. These include technical limitations such as device accuracy and durability, concerns regarding data privacy and security, and issues of accessibility and affordability. Strategies to overcome these challenges are discussed, emphasizing the importance of policy frameworks, interdisciplinary collaboration, and patient education. Finally, the chapter concludes with an exploration of future directions in wearable technology, including advancements in artificial intelligence (AI), integration with digital health ecosystems, and the potential for personalized medicine. By providing an understanding of wearable devices, this chapter aims to inform researchers, clinicians, policymakers, and industry stakeholders, encouraging the continued development and adoption of these technologies to improve chronic disease outcomes.

Types of Wearable Devices and Their Capabilities

Health Monitoring Wearables

Smartwatches and Activity Trackers

Smartwatches and activity trackers are among the most popular wearable devices, widely adopted for both personal fitness and healthcare purposes. These devices incorporate multiple integrated sensors to track parameters such as step count, heart rate, calorie expenditure, and sleep patterns, offering continuous monitoring of daily activities. In recent years, their functionality has significantly expanded. For instance, devices like the Apple Watch and Fitbit models are now equipped with advanced capabilities, including electrocardiogram (ECG) monitoring and blood oxygen saturation (SpO_2) measurement. Such features enable early detection of cardiovascular anomalies, such as arrhythmias, which are critical for preventing adverse events in high-risk populations [9]. These devices also empower individuals to engage actively in their health management by providing real-time insights into their physiological state, thereby fostering a culture of preventive healthcare [10]. Beyond individual use, smartwatches increasingly serve as vital tools in clinical research and practice, where their potential to continuously monitor patient health contributes to a more proactive and personalized approach to chronic disease management.

Biosensors

Biosensors integrated into wearable devices have transformed the monitoring and management of chronic conditions by enabling non-invasive, continuous tracking of critical physiological metrics. A good example is CGMs, which have transformed diabetes care by providing real-time glucose readings without the need for frequent blood sampling [11]. Devices like the Dexcom G6 and Abbott FreeStyle Libre have showed their utility in achieving improved glycemic control and reducing the frequency of hypoglycemic events. Similarly, wearable ECG monitors are invaluable in cardiovascular care, offering real-time data on heart rate variability and aiding in the early detection of life-threatening arrhythmias. All the biosensors enhance patient safety and improve clinical decision-making by delivering accurate, longitudinal health data directly to healthcare providers [12]. Furthermore, advancements in biosensor technology are paving the way for multi-parameter monitoring, enabling simultaneous tracking of glucose, lactate, and hydration levels, which is particularly beneficial for managing complex chronic conditions.

Blood Pressure and Oxygen Saturation Monitors

Wearable devices designed to measure the blood pressure and oxygen saturation (SpO_2) are integral to managing conditions such as hypertension and chronic obstructive pulmonary disease (COPD). Commercial devices like the Omron HeartGuide utilize oscillometric methods to provide clinically accurate blood pressure readings in a wearable format, significantly reducing the burden of frequent clinic visits. A good systematic review stated that SpO_2 monitoring—which is commonly found in the devices equipped with photoplethysmography (PPG) sensors—is essential for detecting hypoxemia cases in patients with respiratory or cardiovascular conditions [13]. All these monitors enable real-time tracking of oxygen levels, offering early warning signs of deteriorating conditions and guiding timely intervention. The integration of such functionalities into consumer-friendly devices like smartwatches further increases accessibility, empowering patients to manage their health proactively while maintaining a high quality of life.

Disease-Specific Devices

Diabetes Management

CGMs have emerged as a cornerstone in diabetes management, offering significant advantages over the traditional finger-stick methods. Devices such as the Dexcom G6 and Abbott FreeStyle Libre provide continuous, real-time glucose monitoring, allowing patients and clinicians to identify trends and make informed adjustments to treatment regimens. Numerous studies have shown that CGMs improve glycemic control, reduce the risk of hypoglycemic episodes, and enhance overall quality of life for patients with diabetes [14–16]. Additionally, when integrated with insulin pumps, these devices enable closed-loop systems, also known as artificial pancreas systems, which automate insulin delivery based on glucose readings. Such advancements underscore the transformative role of wearable devices in achieving optimal disease management and reducing the long-term complications associated with diabetes.

Cardiovascular Conditions

Wearable devices for cardiovascular care, such as portable ECG monitors and smartwatches with ECG functionality, are invaluable in both preventive and post-acute care settings. Such devices facilitate early detection of arrhythmias, including atrial fibrillation, which is a leading cause of stroke. Smartwatches like the Apple Watch have been validated in clinical trials for their ability to detect irregular heart rhythms, underscoring its role in population-level cardiovascular screening [17]. Additionally, wearables play a crucial role in monitoring patients with chronic heart failure or hypertension, enabling real-time tracking of parameters like heart rate and blood pressure. This data not only aids in early detection of exacerbations but also supports remote patient monitoring, reducing hospital readmissions and improving patient outcomes. The integration of these devices into healthcare workflows exemplifies the potential of wearable technology to transform cardiovascular care.

Neurological Disorders

Wearable devices are proving to be valuable in the management of neurological disorders, including Parkinson's disease, epilepsy, and multiple sclerosis. For instance, tremor monitors and gait analyzers provide objective measurements of symptom severity and disease progression in Parkinson's disease, enabling more precise adjustments to treatment plans [18]. Similarly, seizure detection devices, which often incorporate accelerometers and electroencephalography (EEG) sensors, play a critical role in epilepsy management by alerting caregivers or medical personnel during seizure events. These wearables not only enhance patient safety but also provide clinicians with comprehensive datasets to inform long-term care strategies. Their ability to track subtle changes in neurological function underscores their value in both clinical practice and research.

Respiratory Diseases

Respiratory conditions such as asthma and COPD benefit from wearable devices that monitor parameters like oxygen saturation, respiratory rate, and peak expiratory flow rate. Such devices enable patients to track their respiratory status continuously and detect the early signs of exacerbations, which can significantly reduce hospitalizations and improve disease control [19]. For instance, wearable spirometers allow asthma patients to monitor lung function daily, while integrated mobile apps provide actionable feedback and adherence reminders. Such tools promote self-management and empower patients to take proactive measures in their care.

Technological Capabilities

Sensors and Data Collection Mechanisms

The foundation of wearable technology lies in its sophisticated sensor systems, which are capable of capturing a wide array of physiological and behavioral metrics. Accelerometers and gyroscopes, for instance, measure movement and orientation, while optical sensors like photoplethysmography (PPG) capture blood flow dynamics to assess heart rate and SpO_2 levels. Advanced biochemical sensors further expand the functionality of wearables, enabling the detection of glucose, lactate, and other critical biomarkers [20]. The miniaturization and increased sensitivity of these sensors have significantly enhanced the accuracy and reliability of wearable devices, making them suitable for both the clinical and consumer applications. Moreover, the integration of multi-parameter sensors into a single device allows for comprehensive health monitoring, which is particularly valuable for managing complex chronic conditions. Table 8.1 provides a clear overview of the technological components and functionalities of wearable devices.

Connectivity

Connectivity technologies, such as Bluetooth, Wi-Fi, and cellular networks, are essential for enabling the seamless transmission of data from wearable devices to companion applications or healthcare systems. These communication protocols allow real-time access to health metrics, facilitating timely interventions and enhancing patient engagement. Emerging advancements such as 5G connectivity and the Internet of Things (IoT) are expected to further revolutionize the

Table 8.1 Technological features of wearable devices

Device type	Sensors used	Key metrics and connectivity
Smartwatches	PPG, ECG, accelerometers	Heart rate, sleep patterns, activity levels; Bluetooth, Wi-Fi
Biosensors	Biochemical sensors, optical sensors	Glucose, lactate, hydration; Bluetooth, cellular networks
Smart textiles	Pressure sensors, stretch sensors	Muscle activity, posture, motion; Bluetooth, IoT integrations.

functionality of wearables by enabling faster and more reliable data transfer. For example, a review of IoT applications in healthcare concludes that IoT-enabled wearables can integrate with home health monitoring systems to provide clinicians with a comprehensive view of a patient's condition, thereby improving diagnostic accuracy and treatment outcomes [20]. This interconnected ecosystem underlines the potential of wearables to transform chronic disease management by bridging the gap between patients and healthcare providers.

Integration with Mobile Applications and Healthcare Systems

The integration of wearable devices with mobile applications and electronic health records (EHRs) enhances their clinical utility. Mobile apps serve as interactive dashboards, offering users personalized feedback, alerts, and adherence reminders. These platforms often incorporate artificial intelligence algorithms to analyze data trends and deliver tailored recommendations [21]. Seamless synchronization with EHRs ensures that clinicians receive up-to-date, longitudinal health data, enabling more informed decisions. This connectivity not only supports real-time interventions but also strengthens care coordination and chronic disease management across healthcare settings.

Wearable Devices in Chronic Disease Management: Benefits

Continuous Monitoring and Early Detection

Wearable devices have reshaped chronic disease management by providing real-time and continuous monitoring, which bridges the gap between sporadic clinical visits and dynamic disease progression. Conventional healthcare approaches often rely on periodic check-ups, which may fail to capture transient symptoms or early warning signs of deterioration. Wearable devices, by contrast, collect continuous physiological data that enables timely detection of disease exacerbations or complications. For instance, CGMs provide diabetic patients with real-time feedback on glucose levels, facilitating immediate corrective actions to avoid hyperglycemia or hypoglycemia [22]. Similarly, according to a systematic review, wearable ECG monitors allow the detection of cardiac arrhythmias, significantly reducing the likelihood of adverse events such as stroke or cardiac arrest [23]. Furthermore, such devices enhance early detection by identifying subtle changes in vital parameters that may signal the upcoming health crises. Respiratory wearables designed for asthma patients, for example, can monitor air quality and respiratory rates, alerting users to take preventive measures before symptoms escalate [24]. Such capabilities not only improve patient outcomes but also help reduce hospital admissions and emergency department visits. By leveraging data analytics and machine learning algorithms, wearable devices are increasingly capable of predicting health outcomes, thus enabling clinicians and patients to transition from reactive to proactive care strategies.

Patient Empowerment and Self-Management

Wearable devices are essential in strengthening patient empowerment by enabling individuals to actively participate in their healthcare management. By real-time feedback on health metrics, such as physical activity, heart rate, and sleep patterns, these devices provide patients with actionable insights into their health status. This empowerment fosters a sense of control, which is particularly beneficial for patients managing chronic conditions such as hypertension, diabetes, and obesity. For example, smartwatches and fitness trackers encourage their users to adopt healthier lifestyles by tracking their daily steps, calorie consumption, and exercise habits [25]. Moreover, wearable devices enable personalized goal-setting, thus enhancing patient engagement and adherence to treatment plans. For example, people with diabetes using CGMs can monitor their blood sugar fluctuations and adjust their diet or drug intake accordingly, providing better glycemic control [26]. Moreover, wearable devices integrate with mobile applications, allowing users to visualize trends in their health metrics and receive tailored recommendations. This real-time interaction fosters long-term behavioral changes and enhances self-management. Additionally, wearables facilitate remote monitoring by caregivers and healthcare providers, creating a collaborative care environment that strengthens patient accountability.

Improved Clinical Decision-Making

The wealth of data generated by the wearable devices offers unprecedented opportunities to refine clinical decision-making processes. Practically, the wearables collect high-frequency, longitudinal data, providing the healthcare providers with a comprehensive view of a patient's physiological and behavioral patterns. This detailed information enables more accurate diagnoses, improved risk stratification, and personalized treatment plans. For instance, wearable ECG devices provide continuous cardiac monitoring, enabling clinicians to identify arrhythmias that may not be detected during routine clinical assessments [27]. Moreover, wearable devices enhance the integration of real-time data into electronic health records (EHRs), creating a seamless feedback loop between patients and providers. This connectivity allows the clinicians to make data-driven adjustments to treatment regimens without requiring in-person consultations, which is particularly valuable for managing chronic conditions such as COPD and diabetes [28]. For example, remote monitoring of blood pressure via wearables can inform timely medication adjustments,

Table 8.2 Comparison of traditional and wearable-based chronic disease management

Parameter	Traditional approach	Wearable-based approach
Monitoring frequency	Periodic monitoring frequency (e.g., annual check-ups)	Continuous, real-time monitoring frequency
Patient engagement	Limited engagement, reliant on clinic visits	High engagement through real-time feedback
Early detection	Delayed detection due to sporadic monitoring	Early detection via continuous data collection
Cost	Higher long-term costs due to complications and hospitalizations	Lower long-term costs by preventing complications

preventing complications such as stroke or heart failure. Furthermore, such devices help facilitate multidisciplinary care by providing a unified platform for data sharing, therefore enhancing collaboration among healthcare professionals. Table 8.2 provides a clear contrast between traditional and wearable-based chronic disease management approaches, emphasizing the advantages offered by wearable technologies in healthcare.

Reduction in Healthcare Costs

One of the most fascinating benefits of wearable devices in the chronic disease management is their potential to reduce healthcare costs. By enabling early detection and continuous monitoring, such devices prevent the escalation of chronic conditions, thus reducing the need for expensive hospitalizations and emergency care. For instance, the use of wearable cardiac monitors has been associated with decreased readmission rates among patients recovering from heart failure [29]. Additionally, such devices facilitate the shift of care from hospitals to home settings, significantly alleviating the burden on healthcare systems. Remote monitoring technologies, such as wearable oxygen monitors for COPD patients, allow for the management of chronic conditions in a more cost-effective manner [30]. This decentralization of care not only lowers costs but also improves patient convenience and satisfaction. Furthermore, wearable devices enhance medication adherence through real-time reminders and feedback mechanisms, reducing the long-term costs associated with poorly managed chronic diseases.

Enhanced Patient Outcomes

The ultimate aim of wearable technologies in the context of chronic disease management is to improve patient outcomes by enhancing both physiological and psychological well-being. Wearable devices have demonstrated success in reducing biomarkers such as HbA1c levels in diabetic patients and blood pressure in hypertensive individuals, indicating better disease control [29]. Furthermore, these devices contribute to improved quality of life (QoL) by empowering the patients to manage their health actively and effectively. Case studies illustrate the profound impact of wearable devices on patient outcomes. For instance, patients with Parkinson's disease using wearable sensors to monitor tremor severity report greater symptom control and reduced disease progression, resulting in improved functional independence [31]. Similarly, cancer rehabilitation programs incorporating wearables for activity monitoring have shown enhanced recovery and better adherence to post-treatment care protocols. By providing personalized insights and fostering sustained engagement, wearable devices ensure that patients achieve better long-term health outcomes.

Applications in Specific Chronic Diseases

Diabetes Management

The management of diabetes has been revolutionized by the advent of wearable technologies, particularly CGMs. These devices provide real-time, continuous data on glucose levels, allowing patients to monitor trends and make immediate adjustments to their diet, activity, or medication. Unlike traditional finger-stick testing, which provides discrete data points, CGMs offer a comprehensive picture of glucose variability, enabling better glycemic control. These devices also issue alerts for hypoglycemia and hyperglycemia, allowing timely interventions and reducing the risk of acute complications. For instance, studies have shown that CGMs significantly lower the frequency of severe hypoglycemia episodes in patients with Type 1 diabetes, improving both safety and quality of life [32].

The integration of CGMs with insulin pumps and mobile applications further enhances diabetes management. Hybrid closed-loop systems, commonly referred to as artificial pancreas systems, combine real-time glucose monitoring with automated insulin delivery. These systems use advanced algorithms to predict glucose trends and adjust insulin dosing accordingly, reducing the cognitive burden on patients and ensuring more consistent glycemic control. Clinical trials have confirmed that users of the systems experience lower HbA1c levels, fewer glycemic excursions, and improved adherence to treatment regimens compared to patients using traditional methods [33]. Wearable technologies also contribute to patient engagement and education, which are critical for the effective diabetes management. By providing actionable insights into glucose fluctuations and trends, these devices empower patients to take a more active role in their care. This empowerment is associated with improved treatment adherence and lifestyle modifications, such as dietary changes and increased physical activity. Research underscores the role of wearables in enhancing both short-term outcomes, such as glycemic stability, and long-term outcomes, including reductions in diabetes-related complications [34].

Cardiovascular Disease

Wearable devices have emerged as critical tools in the prevention and management of cardiovascular diseases or CVDs, offering continuous monitoring of vital parameters such as heart rate, blood pressure, and ECG readings. These devices allow for real-time data collection and analysis, which is pivotal in detecting early signs of cardiovascular dysfunction. For instance, wearable ECG monitors have been demonstrated to detect atrial fibrillation, a leading cause of stroke, with high accuracy. Early detection enables timely medical intervention, potentially preventing catastrophic CVD events [34].

In the management of hypertension, wearable blood pressure monitors provide frequent and precise measurements, capturing fluctuations that might be missed in clinical settings. This capability facilitates the early identification of poorly controlled hypertension and supports the tailoring of antihypertensive therapies to the individual patient needs. Studies have demonstrated that the use of wearable blood pressure monitors is associated with improved adherence to treatment regimens and better blood pressure control over time [35]. Wearables also play a significant role in cardiovascular rehabilitation by promoting physical activity and monitoring its effects on heart health. Fitness trackers integrated with personalized exercise programs encourage patients recovering from myocardial infarctions or heart failure to adopt and maintain healthier lifestyles. Research has linked the use of these devices to increased levels of physical activity, improved cardiac function, and reduced rates of hospital readmissions [36].

Chronic Respiratory Diseases

The management of chronic respiratory diseases, such as COPD and asthma, has been greatly enhanced by wearable technologies. Devices such as pulse oximeters and respiratory rate monitors provide continuous data on critical parameters like oxygen saturation and breathing patterns. This real-time monitoring enables early detection of respiratory distress and facilitates timely interventions, thereby reducing the risk of acute exacerbations. For example, wearable oxygen monitors have been shown to decrease hospitalizations and emergency room visits among patients with severe COPD [37]. In asthma management, wearable devices track environmental triggers such as pollen levels, air pollution, and humidity, offering personalized alerts to patients. Coupled with smartphone applications, these devices provide actionable insights and support self-management behaviors, such as the appropriate use of rescue inhalers. Clinical studies have reported that patients using asthma wearables experience fewer symptom days, improved lung function, and greater adherence to controller drugs [38]. Additionally, wearables are also valuable in pulmonary rehabilitation, enabling patients to monitor their physical activity levels and oxygen requirements during exercise. By integrating these devices into rehabilitation programs, healthcare providers can offer more tailored interventions, resulting in better exercise tolerance and quality of life for patients with chronic respiratory diseases [18].

Neurological Disorders

The application of wearable devices in neurological disorders has expanded significantly, offering new avenues for monitoring and managing conditions such as epilepsy, Parkinson's disease, and multiple sclerosis. Wearable seizure detection devices, including wristbands and headbands, use advanced algorithms to analyze physiological signals such as heart rates and muscle activities. These devices provide real-time alerts to patients and caregivers during epileptic episodes, enhancing safety and reducing the risk of injury [39]. In Parkinson's disease management, wearable sensors track motor symptoms such as tremors, rigidity, and bradykinesia, providing objective data that inform treatment adjustments. These devices also allow for the monitoring of symptoms over extended periods, offering insights into disease progression and the effectiveness of therapeutic interventions. Studies have demonstrated that wearables improve the precision of symptom tracking, leading to more personalized and effective care [40]. In some cases, wearables are also beneficial for both caregivers and healthcare providers. Real-time monitoring reduces the emotional and logistical burdens on caregivers by providing early alerts and actionable insights. Additionally, wearable technologies facilitate remote consultations, enabling clinicians to make data-driven decisions without requiring frequent in-person visits [41].

Obesity and Weight Management

Wearable devices play a crucial role in obesity management by promoting physical activity and supporting dietary tracking. Fitness trackers equipped with accelerometers and GPS functionalities monitor metrics such as steps taken, calories burned, and distance covered, motivating users to maintain an active lifestyle. These devices are particularly effective when paired with mobile health applications that provide personalized coaching and behavior-change strategies[42]. Studies have consistently shown that wearable technologies contribute to sustainable weight loss. Users of these devices report higher adherence to exercise and dietary recommendations compared to non-users. For instance, wearables that track caloric intake and macronutrient distribution support better dietary choices, enabling users to achieve their weight management goals more effectively [43]. Shortly, incorporating gamification and social networking features further enhances user engagement. These elements foster a sense of community and accountability, which are critical for maintaining long-term lifestyle changes. Wearables also support individuals with obesity-related comorbidities, such as type 2 diabetes and cardiovascular disease, by integrating activity tracking with health monitoring to optimize overall well-being.

Cancer Management

In oncology, wearable devices serve as vital tools for symptom monitoring and managing treatment side effects. Devices that track vital signs, physical activity, and sleep patterns provide oncologists with critical data to evaluate patient recovery and detect complications. For example, wearables have been used to identify early signs of dehydration, infections, and other treatment-related adverse events, enabling timely interventions and reducing hospitalizations [44]. Additionally, wearables enhance cancer rehabilitation by encouraging physical activity, which is known to improve fatigue, mental health, and quality of life. Activity trackers integrated into rehabilitation programs provide tailored exercise recommendations and monitor adherence, ensuring that patients meet their activity goals. Research indicates that these interventions are associated with better physical and psychological outcomes for cancer survivors [45]. In palliative care cases, wearable devices monitor symptoms such as pain and sleep disturbances, allowing clinicians to optimize comfort and quality of life for patients in advanced stages of cancer. By providing continuous and unobtrusive monitoring, wearables support holistic care approaches that address both physical and emotional well-being. Table 8.3 shows a summary of wearable device applications in the cases of chronic disease management.

Challenges in Implementing Wearable Devices

Technical and Design Limitations

The successful integration of wearable devices into chronic disease management is often hindered by technical and design limitations. One of the most pressing issues is the limited battery life of many devices, which necessitates frequent recharging. This requirement disrupts continuous monitoring and can discourage consistent use, especially among patients managing complex chronic conditions. Moreover, the physical durability of devices is a concern, particularly for those designed for constant wear or exposure to harsh environmental conditions. Devices that lack robust construction may succumb to wear and tear, reducing their effectiveness and

Table 8.3 A Summary of the wearable applications in the chronic disease management

Chronic disease	Applications of wearable devices	Key benefits
Diabetes	Continuous glucose monitors (CGMs) for real-time glucose tracking Integration with insulin pumps for automated insulin delivery Mobile apps for tracking and education	Improved glycemic control [36] Reduced risk of hypo-/hyperglycemia [33] Enhanced patient adherence [34]
CVDs	Wearables for heart rate, blood pressure, and ECG monitoring Integration with exercise programs for rehabilitation	Early detection of arrhythmias and hypertension [34] Improved adherence to treatment and physical activity [35] Reduced hospital readmissions [36]
Chronic respiratory diseases	Pulse oximeters for oxygen saturation monitoring Sensors tracking respiratory rates and environmental triggers (e.g., air quality) Integration with pulmonary rehabilitation programs	Reduced exacerbations and hospitalizations [37] Improved adherence to asthma treatment plans [38] Enhanced physical activity and quality of life [18]
Neurological diseases	Seizure detection wearables (e.g., wristbands, headbands) Wearables for tracking motor symptoms in Parkinson's disease Remote monitoring for caregivers and clinicians	Enhanced safety and reduced risk of injury [39] Personalized treatment adjustments [40] Reduced caregiver stress and improved decision-making [41]
Obesity and weight management	Fitness trackers and apps for activity and dietary tracking Personalized coaching and gamification features	Increased physical activity and healthier eating habits [29] Improved adherence to weight management plans [30]
Cancer management	Wearables for tracking symptoms and side effects of treatment Monitoring pain and sleep disturbances in palliative care Activity trackers for post-treatment rehabilitation	Early detection of complications (e.g., infections, dehydration) [46] Optimized symptom management and quality of life in advanced stages of illness [46] Improved recovery, fatigue reduction, and mental health [31]

lifespan. Patients and healthcare providers alike have expressed dissatisfaction with devices that fail prematurely or require costly repairs or replacements, thus complicating their adoption in clinical practice [47].

Technical limitations remain a barrier to broader adoption of wearable devices. Battery life, device durability, and sensor accuracy are recurring concerns, especially for patients requiring continuous monitoring. Inaccurate readings or false alerts undermine both user trust and clinical reliability. Additionally, lack of standardized performance benchmarks across manufacturers contributes to inconsistencies in device output [48, 49]. Older adults and those with low digital literacy may find some interfaces challenging, reducing adherence. Enhancing usability through intuitive design, simplified interfaces, and accessible instructions is crucial to increasing long-term engagement [50].

Data Privacy and Security Issues

Data privacy and security concerns present significant barriers to the adoption of wearable devices in chronic disease management. The devices collect and transmit sensitive health information, making them vulnerable to data breaches and unauthorized access. All the breaches can result in the exploitation of personal health data, triggering severe risks to patient confidentiality and trust in wearable technologies [51]. The potential misuse of health data, whether for financial fraud or discriminatory practices, has raised ethical and legal concerns that must be addressed to ensure the safe deployment of these devices. Implementing robust encryption protocols and adhering to data protection regulations such as the General Data Protection Regulation (GDPR) are critical steps in mitigating these risks. However, achieving the levels of security increases the complexity and cost of wearable device systems, creating barriers for smaller manufacturers and end-users. Moreover, interoperability challenges with existing health information systems can compromise secure data exchange, thus complicating the integration of wearables into healthcare settings [52].

Cost and Accessibility

The cost of wearable devices remains a significant obstacle to their widespread use in chronic disease management, particularly for patients in low- and middle-income settings. Many advanced devices with sophisticated monitoring capabilities are prohibitively expensive, limiting access to affluent populations while excluding those most in need. The economic disparities reinforce existing healthcare inequities, highlighting the importance of addressing affordability to make sure equitable access to wearable technologies [53]. Compounding this issue is the lack of reimbursement policies for wearable devices within many healthcare systems. In most cases, insurance providers do not cover the costs of these devices, leaving patients to bear the financial burden. This lack of institutional support significantly hampers the adoption of wearables as an integrated component of chronic disease care. Policymakers and healthcare stakeholders must advocate for reimbursement models that reflect the long-term value of wearable devices in reducing hospital admissions and improving patient outcomes [54].

Integration with Healthcare Systems

The integration of wearable devices into healthcare systems poses complex technical and organizational challenges. One major hurdle is the lack of interoperability between wearable devices and electronic health records (EHRs). Many wearables operate within proprietary ecosystems, which complicates the seamless exchange of data across different platforms and care providers. This cached approach limits the utility of wearable-generated data for comprehensive patient care and population health management [55]. Healthcare professionals also face challenges in adapting to the influx of data from wearable devices. Training clinicians to interpret and incorporate wearable data into decision-making processes requires significant investment in education and resources. Without adequate support, clinicians may perceive wearables as an additional burden rather than a valuable tool, reducing their willingness to adopt these technologies. Such challenges underscore the need for standardized data protocols and comprehensive clinician training programs to maximize the potential of wearable devices [56].

User Adherence and Engagement

Long-term adherence to wearable devices is a critical factor in their effectiveness, yet it remains a significant challenge. Patients often abandon devices due to inconvenience, discomfort, or a lack of perceived benefit. Some factors such as bulky designs, intrusive alerts, or poorly designed interfaces can lead to frustration and device abandonment [57]. To address these issues, wearable devices must prioritize user-centered design principles that enhance comfort and usability. Features such as personalized feedback, gamification, and behavioral incentives have been shown to improve the user engagement. For instance, devices that provide tailored insights into a patient's progress or health trends can foster a sense of achievement and motivate sustained use [58]. Additionally, user education and ongoing support are essential to maintaining adherence. Many patients lack the technical literacy required to maximize the benefits of wearable devices. Structured training programs and accessible user guides can empower patients to integrate wearables into their daily lives effectively. Moreover, involving patients in the design and testing phases of device development can lead to innovations that better address user needs and preferences [59].

Future Directions and Innovations

Next-Generation Wearable Devices

The development of next-generation wearable devices is fundamentally transforming the healthcare landscape, driven by advancements in miniaturization, multi-sensor integration, and material biocompatibilities. Mini sensors, for example, enable wearable devices to gather diverse physiological and biochemical data without compromising user comfort or device accuracy. These advancements are critical for long-term management of chronic diseases, where patient adherence is closely tied to the non-intrusive nature of monitoring systems. Materials such as flexible polymers and biocompatible substrates further enhance wearability, enabling devices to conform to the skin seamlessly while reducing irritation during prolonged use [60]. For instance, flexible, skin-conforming devices equipped with multiple sensors have been utilized to monitor complex biometrics such as ECGs and glucose levels, with significant potential to improve clinical outcomes in conditions such as diabetes and cardiovascular diseases [61].

In addition to material and design advancements, artificial intelligence (AI) and machine learning (ML) are increasingly integrated into the wearable devices, transforming them from passive monitoring tools to active, predictive systems. AI algorithms process vast quantities of real-time health data, identifying subtle trends and providing early warnings of potential health deteriorations. This predictive capability is particularly valuable in chronic disease management, where timely interventions can prevent complications and reduce the hospitalizations. For instance, wearable devices equipped with AI-driven analytics have demonstrated efficacy in predicting arrhythmias and optimizing glycemic control for patients with diabetes [62]. The next frontier for such technologies lies in improving computational efficiency to enable on-device analytics, reducing reliance on cloud-based processing and enhancing data security [63].

Personalized and Precision Medicine

Wearable devices are at the forefront of personalized medicine, providing healthcare solutions tailored to individual patient profiles and needs. The ability of these devices to continuously monitor physiological parameters allows for highly customized interventions that adapt to the patient's unique disease trajectory and lifestyle. For instance, CGM devices can provide dynamic feedback on blood glucose trends, enabling personalized adjustments to insulin therapy and dietary plans. Such individualized approaches have been shown to improve glycemic control and reduce complications in diabetes management [64]. In the broader context of chronic diseases, wearable devices enable the integration of genetic, environmental, and behavioral data to create a comprehensive picture of patient health. This integration supports precision interventions, such as adjusting medication regimens based on real-time physiological changes c exacerbations. For example, biosensors capable of tracking biomarkers in real-time are increasingly used to customize treatments for cardiovascular diseases and hypertension [65]. The ongoing convergence of wearable technology with precision medicine holds the promise of not only optimizing clinical outcomes but also improving patient adherence by aligning interventions with individual preferences and circumstances.

Integration with Digital Health Ecosystems

The integration of wearable devices into digital health ecosystems is revolutionizing telemedicine and remote patient care by enabling seamless communication between patients and healthcare providers. Wearable devices now serve as critical nodes in connected health systems, continuously transmitting real-time data to EHRs and telehealth platforms. This integration allows clinicians to remotely monitor patient health, identify early signs of disease progression, and make timely interventions. For instance, remote monitoring of vital signs via wearables has been linked to reductions in hospital readmissions and emergency visits among patients with chronic conditions [66]. Collaboration between wearable technology developers and digital health platforms has also facilitated the emergence of comprehensive patient engagement tools. These tools combine data visualization, behavior-change coaching, and automated alerts to enhance chronic disease self-management. For example, telemedicine platforms that integrate data from wearable devices have demonstrated significant benefits in improving adherence to physical activity and medication regimens, particularly in patients with diabetes and cardiovascular diseases [67]. Such innovations are not only empowering patients to take an active role in their health but also enabling healthcare providers to deliver more personalized and proactive care.

Policy and Regulation Improvements

The rapid proliferation of wearable technologies has underscored the need for robust regulatory frameworks to ensure their safety, efficacy, and equitable accessibility. Regulatory agencies such as the U.S. Food and Drug Administration (FDA) and the European Medicines Agency (EMA) are actively working to streamline approval processes for wearable medical devices. However, balancing innovation with stringent safety standards remains a significant challenge. Harmonized global standards for wearable devices would facilitate international adoption while reducing redundancy in regulatory compliance processes [68]. Data privacy and security are critical regulatory concerns in the wearable technology domain. With devices generating vast amounts of sensitive health data, ensuring compliance with privacy laws such as the GDPR and the Health Insurance Portability and Accountability Act (HIPAA) is paramount. Robust encryption protocols and secure data storage practices are essential to maintaining patient trust and preventing breaches [69]. To promote equitable access, policymakers must address the financial barriers that limit the adoption of wearable devices. Subsidies, tax incentives, and public-private partnerships can make these technologies more affordable, particularly for underserved populations. By reducing disparities in access, such measures would ensure that advancements in wearable technology benefit a broader demographic, thereby maximizing their potential impact on public health [70].

Conclusion

Wearable devices offer unprecedented opportunities in chronic disease care by enabling continuous monitoring, early detection, and personalized interventions. These tools empower patients and equip clinicians with data-driven insights, fostering proactive, cost-effective management. Yet, technical challenges, data security concerns, high costs, and disparities in access must be addressed. Future directions should prioritize AI-driven analytics, digital ecosystem integration, and policy frameworks that ensure safety, interoperability, and affordability. Investment in education, equitable access, and research innovation will be vital to unlocking the full potential of wearable technologies in transforming chronic healthcare delivery and improving patient outcomes.

References

1. Gambert SR. The burden of chronic disease. Mayo Clin Proc Innov Qual Outcomes. 2024;8:112–9. https://doi.org/10.1016/J.MAYOCPIQO.2023.08.005.
2. Van Zyl C, Badenhorst M, Hanekom S, Heine M. Unravelling 'low-resource settings': a systematic scoping review with qualitative content analysis. BMJ Glob Health. 2021;6:5190. https://doi.org/10.1136/BMJGH-2021-005190.
3. Ling S. Cultivating wellness and curbing costs: a systematic paradigm for enhancing the U.S. Healthcare System through patient education. SSRN Electron J. 2023. https://doi.org/10.2139/SSRN.4574878.
4. Vo DK, Trinh KTL. Advances in wearable biosensors for healthcare: current trends, applications, and future perspectives. Biosensors. 2024;14:560. https://doi.org/10.3390/BIOS14110560.
5. Ghazizadeh E, Naseri Z, Deigner HP, et al. Approaches of wearable and implantable biosensor towards of developing in precision medicine. Front Med (Lausanne). 2024;11:1390634. https://doi.org/10.3389/FMED.2024.1390634/BIBTEX.
6. Stergiou GS, Mukkamala R, Avolio A, et al. Cuffless blood pressure measuring devices: review and statement by the European Society of Hypertension Working Group on blood pressure monitoring and cardiovascular variability. J Hypertens. 2022;40:1449–60. https://doi.org/10.1097/HJH.0000000000003224.

7. Sümer L. Housing market dynamics: understanding the recent global trends and threats. In: The global housing crisis. Springer Nature; 2024. p. 29–83. https://doi.org/10.1007/978-3-031-72604-0_3.
8. Al-Chalabi S, Sinha S, Kalra PA. Enhancing clinical service design for multimorbidity management: a comprehensive approach to joined-up care for diabetes, chronic kidney disease, and heart failure. Diabet Med. 2024;42:e15403. https://doi.org/10.1111/DME.15403.
9. Miao F, Wu D, Liu Z, et al. Wearable sensing, big data technology for cardiovascular healthcare: current status and future prospective. Chin Med J. 2022;136:1015. https://doi.org/10.1097/CM9.0000000000002117.
10. Iqbal SMA, Leavitt MA, Mahgoub I, Asghar W. Advances in cardiovascular wearable devices. Biosensors. 2024;14:525. https://doi.org/10.3390/BIOS14110525.
11. Manov AE, Chauhan S, Dhillon G, et al. The effectiveness of continuous glucose monitoring devices in managing uncontrolled diabetes mellitus: a retrospective study. Cureus. 2023;15:e42545. https://doi.org/10.7759/CUREUS.42545.
12. Lino C, Barrias S, Chaves R, et al. Biosensors as diagnostic tools in clinical applications. Biochim Biophys Acta Rev Cancer. 2022;1877:188726. https://doi.org/10.1016/J.BBCAN.2022.188726.
13. Zhang J, Li J, Kwak D-H, et al. Diagnostic features and potential applications of PPG signal in healthcare: a systematic review. Healthcare. 2022;10:547. https://doi.org/10.3390/HEALTHCARE10030547.
14. Kieu A, King J, Govender RD, Östlundh L. The benefits of utilizing continuous glucose monitoring of diabetes mellitus in primary care: a systematic review. J Diabetes Sci Technol. 2022;17:762. https://doi.org/10.1177/19322968211070855.
15. Klupa T, Czupryniak L, Dzida G, et al. Expanding the role of continuous glucose monitoring in modern diabetes care beyond type 1 disease. Diabetes Ther. 2023;14:1241–66. https://doi.org/10.1007/S13300-023-01431-3.
16. Johnston AR, Poll JB, Hays EM, Jones CW. Perceived impact of continuous glucose monitor use on quality of life and self-care for patients with type 2 diabetes. Diabetes Epidemiol Manag. 2022;6:100068. https://doi.org/10.1016/J.DEMAN.2022.100068.
17. Guarnieri G, Mapelli M, Moltrasio M, et al. Connected health: ventricular tachycardia detection with apple watch–a case report. Heliyon. 2024;10:e40595. https://doi.org/10.1016/J.HELIYON.2024.E40595.
18. Jafleh EA, Alnaqbi FA, Almaeeni HA, et al. The role of wearable devices in chronic disease monitoring and patient care: a comprehensive review. Cureus. 2024;16:e68921. https://doi.org/10.7759/CUREUS.68921.
19. Dunn J, Coravos A, Fanarjian M, et al. Remote digital health technologies for improving the care of people with respiratory disorders. Lancet Digit Health. 2024;6:e291–8. https://doi.org/10.1016/S2589-7500(23)00248-0.
20. Assalve G, Lunetti P, Di Cagno A, et al. Advanced wearable devices for monitoring sweat biochemical markers in athletic performance: a comprehensive review. Biosensors (Basel). 2024;14:574. https://doi.org/10.3390/BIOS14120574.
21. Sarker IH, Hoque MM, Uddin MK, Alsanoosy T. Mobile data science and intelligent apps: concepts, AI-based modeling and research directions. Mobile Netw Appl. 2020;26:285. https://doi.org/10.1007/S11036-020-01650-Z.
22. Irace C, Coluzzi S, Di Cianni G, et al. Continuous glucose monitoring (CGM) in a non-Icu hospital setting: the patient's journey. Nutr Metab Cardiovasc Dis. 2023;33:2107–18. https://doi.org/10.1016/J.NUMECD.2023.06.021.
23. Tran HH-V, Urgessa NA, Geethakumari P, et al. Detection and diagnostic accuracy of cardiac arrhythmias using wearable health devices: a systematic review. Cureus. 2023;15:e50952. https://doi.org/10.7759/CUREUS.50952.
24. Hakizimana A, Devani P, Gaillard EA. Current technological advancement in asthma care. Expert Rev Respir Med. 2024;18:499–512. https://doi.org/10.1080/17476348.2024.2380067.

25. Tricás-Vidal HJ, Lucha-López MO, Hidalgo-García C, et al. Health habits and wearable activity tracker devices: analytical cross-sectional study. Sensors (Basel). 2022;22:2960. https://doi.org/10.3390/S22082960.
26. Maiorino MI, Signoriello S, Maio A, et al. Effects of continuous glucose monitoring on metrics of glycemic control in diabetes: a systematic review with meta-analysis of randomized controlled trials. Diabetes Care. 2020;43:1146–56. https://doi.org/10.2337/DC19-1459.
27. Sana F, Isselbacher EM, Singh JP, et al. Wearable devices for ambulatory cardiac monitoring: JACC state-of-the-art review. J Am Coll Cardiol. 2020;75:1582. https://doi.org/10.1016/J.JACC.2020.01.046.
28. Agustí A, Celli BR, Criner GJ, et al. Global initiative for chronic obstructive lung disease 2023 report: GOLD executive summary. Eur Respir J. 2023;61:2300239. https://doi.org/10.1183/13993003.00239-2023.
29. Dimitratos SM, German JB, Schaefer SE. Wearable technology to quantify the nutritional intake of adults: validation study. JMIR Mhealth Uhealth. 2020;8(7):e16405. https://doi.org/10.2196/16405.
30. Monteiro-Guerra F, Signorelli GR, Rivera-Romero O, et al. Breast cancer survivors' perspectives on motivational and personalization strategies in Mobile app–based physical activity coaching interventions: qualitative study. JMIR Mhealth Uhealth. 2020;8(9):e18867. https://doi.org/10.2196/18867.
31. Blount DS, McDonough DJ, Gao Z. Effect of wearable technology-based physical activity interventions on breast cancer survivors' physiological, cognitive, and emotional outcomes: a systematic review. J Clin Med. 2021;10:2015. https://doi.org/10.3390/JCM10092015.
32. Committee ADAPP, ElSayed NA, Aleppo G, et al. 6. Glycemic goals and hypoglycemia: standards of care in diabetes—2024. Diabetes Care. 2024;47:S111–25. https://doi.org/10.2337/DC24-S006.
33. Rodbard D. Continuous glucose monitoring: a review of recent studies demonstrating improved glycemic outcomes. Diabetes Technol Ther. 2017;19:S-25. https://doi.org/10.1089/DIA.2017.0035.
34. Mattison G, Canfell O, Forrester D, et al. The influence of wearables on health care outcomes in chronic disease: systematic review. J Med Internet Res. 2022;24:e36690. https://doi.org/10.2196/36690.
35. Mohrag M, Mojiri ME, Hakami MS, et al. The impact of wearable technologies on blood pressure control in hypertensive patients: a systematic review and meta-analysis. Cureus. 2024;16:e71220. https://doi.org/10.7759/CUREUS.71220.
36. Bayoumy K, Gaber M, Elshafeey A, et al. Smart wearable devices in cardiovascular care: where we are and how to move forward. Nat Rev Cardiol. 2021;18:581. https://doi.org/10.1038/S41569-021-00522-7.
37. Tomasic I, Tomasic N, Trobec R, et al. Continuous remote monitoring of COPD patients—justification and explanation of the requirements and a survey of the available technologies. Med Biol Eng Comput. 2018;56:547. https://doi.org/10.1007/S11517-018-1798-Z.
38. Greiwe J, Nyenhuis SM. Wearable technology and how this can be implemented into clinical practice. Curr Allergy Asthma Rep. 2020;20:36. https://doi.org/10.1007/S11882-020-00927-3.
39. Brinkmann BH, Karoly PJ, Nurse ES, et al. Seizure diaries and forecasting with wearables: epilepsy monitoring outside the clinic. Front Neurol. 2021;12:690404. https://doi.org/10.3389/FNEUR.2021.690404.
40. Greiwe J, Nyenhuis SM. Wearable technology and how this can be implemented into clinical practice. Curr Allergy Asthma Rep. 2020;20:1–10. https://doi.org/10.1007/S11882-020-00927-3/TABLES/2.
41. Jim HSL, Hoogland AI, Brownstein NC, et al. Innovations in research and clinical care using patient-generated health data. CA Cancer J Clin. 2020;70:182–99. https://doi.org/10.3322/CAAC.21608.

42. Odeh VA, Chen Y, Wang W, Ding X. Recent advances in the wearable devices for monitoring and management of heart failure. Rev Cardiovasc Med. 2024;25:386. https://doi.org/10.31083/J.RCM2510386
43. Rojas AN, Mosquera FC. Advances and challenges associated with low-cost pulse oximeters in home care programs: a review. Sensors. 2024;24:6284. https://doi.org/10.3390/S24196284.
44. Davies MJ, Aroda VR, Collins BS, et al. Management of Hyperglycemia in type 2 diabetes, 2022. A consensus report by the American Diabetes Association (ADA) and the European Association for the Study of Diabetes (EASD). Diabetes Care. 2022;45:2753–86. https://doi.org/10.2337/DCI22-0034.
45. San-Segundo R, Zhang A, Cebulla A, et al. Parkinson's disease tremor detection in the wild using wearable accelerometers. Sensors. 2020;20:5817. https://doi.org/10.3390/S20205817.
46. Parikh RB, Basen-Enquist KM, Bradley C, et al. Digital health applications in oncology: an opportunity to seize. JNCI J Natl Cancer Inst. 2022;114:1338. https://doi.org/10.1093/JNCI/DJAC108.
47. Bekbolatova M, Mayer J, Ong CW, Toma M. Transformative potential of AI in healthcare: definitions, applications, and navigating the ethical landscape and public perspectives. Healthcare. 2024;12:125. https://doi.org/10.3390/HEALTHCARE12020125.
48. Ghozali MT, Urrohmah UA. Determining the relationship between the knowledge on self-management and levels of asthma control among adult asthmatic patients: a cross-sectional study. J Med Life. 2023;16:442–6. https://doi.org/10.25122/JML-2022-0333
49. Ajayi SA, Olaniyi OO, Oladoyinbo TO, et al. Sustainable sourcing of organic skincare ingredients: a critical analysis of ethical concerns and environmental implications. Asian J Adv Res Rep. 2024;18:65–91.
50. Miraz MH, Ali M, Excell PS. Adaptive user interfaces and universal usability through plasticity of user interface design. Comput Sci Rev. 2021;40:100363. https://doi.org/10.1016/J.COSREV.2021.100363.
51. Keshta I, Odeh A. Security and privacy of electronic health records: concerns and challenges. Egypt Inf J. 2021;22:177–83. https://doi.org/10.1016/J.EIJ.2020.07.003.
52. Carlos Ferreira J, Elvas LB, Correia R, Mascarenhas M. Enhancing EHR interoperability and security through distributed ledger technology: a review. Healthcare. 2024;12:1967. https://doi.org/10.3390/HEALTHCARE12191967.
53. Ebekozien O, Fantasia K, Farrokhi F, et al. Technology and health inequities in diabetes care: how do we widen access to underserved populations and utilize technology to improve outcomes for all? Diabetes Obes Metab. 2024;26:3–13. https://doi.org/10.1111/DOM.15470.
54. De Sario Velasquez GD, Borna S, Maniaci MJ, et al. Economic perspective of the use of wearables in health care: a systematic review. Mayo Clinic Proc Digit Health. 2024;2:299–317. https://doi.org/10.1016/J.MCPDIG.2024.05.003.
55. Wang D, Liu W, Kong L, et al. Digital technology enabling military training injury prevention and control information system. In: Proceedings of the 2024 international conference on Smart healthcare and wearable intelligent devices; 2024. p. 121–6. https://doi.org/10.1145/3703847.3703869.
56. Sabry F, Eltaras T, Labda W, et al. Machine learning for healthcare wearable devices: the big picture. J Healthc Eng. 2022;2022:4653923. https://doi.org/10.1155/2022/4653923.
57. Ma Z, Gao Q, Yang M. Adoption of wearable devices by older people: changes in use behaviors and user experiences. Int J Hum Comput Interact. 2023;39:964–87. https://doi.org/10.1080/10447318.2022.2083573.
58. Jacob C, Bourke S, Heuss S. From testers to cocreators—the value of and approaches to successful patient engagement in the development of eHealth solutions: qualitative expert interview study. JMIR Hum Factors. 2022;9(4):e41481. https://doi.org/10.2196/41481.
59. Gómez-Rico M, Santos-Vijande ML, Molina-Collado A, Bilgihan A. Unlocking the flow experience in apps: fostering long-term adoption for sustainable healthcare systems. Psychol Mark. 2023;40:1556–78. https://doi.org/10.1002/MAR.21824.

60. Kazanskiy NL, Khonina SN, Butt MA. A review on flexible wearables—recent developments in non-invasive continuous health monitoring. Sens Actuators A Phys. 2024;366:114993. https://doi.org/10.1016/J.SNA.2023.114993.
61. Taha BA, Addie AJ, Kadhim AC, et al. Photonics-powered augmented reality skin electronics for proactive healthcare: multifaceted opportunities. Microchim Acta. 2024;191(5):1–24. https://doi.org/10.1007/S00604-024-06314-3.
62. Oikonomou EK, Khera R. Machine learning in precision diabetes care and cardiovascular risk prediction. Cardiovasc Diabetol. 2023;22:1–16. https://doi.org/10.1186/S12933-023-01985-3/TABLES/1.
63. Jin X, Li L, Dang F, et al. A survey on edge computing for wearable technology. Digit Signal Process. 2022;125:103146. https://doi.org/10.1016/J.DSP.2021.103146.
64. Reddy M, Oliver N. The role of real-time continuous glucose monitoring in diabetes management and how it should link to integrated personalized diabetes management. Diabetes Obes Metab. 2024;26:46–56. https://doi.org/10.1111/DOM.15504.
65. Chen X, Manshaii F, Tioran K, et al. Wearable biosensors for cardiovascular monitoring leveraging nanomaterials. Adv Compos Hybrid Mater. 2024;7(3):1–22. https://doi.org/10.1007/S42114-024-00906-6.
66. Gobinath A, Rajeswari P, Kumar NS, Anandan M. Internet of medical things (IoMT). In: Smart Hospitals. Wiley; 2024. p. 91–105. https://doi.org/10.1002/9781394275472.CH5.
67. Thacharodi A, Singh P, Meenatchi R, et al. Revolutionizing healthcare and medicine: the impact of modern technologies for a healthier future—a comprehensive review. Health Care Sci. 2024;3:329–49. https://doi.org/10.1002/HCS2.115.
68. Jawad LA. Security and privacy in digital healthcare systems: challenges and mitigation strategies. Abhigyan. 2024;42:23–31. https://doi.org/10.1177/09702385241233073.
69. Javed H, Muqeet HA, Danesh A, et al. Impact of AI and dynamic ensemble techniques in enhancing healthcare services: opportunities and ethical challenges. IEEE Access. 2024;12:141064–87. https://doi.org/10.1109/ACCESS.2024.3443812.
70. Craig KJT, Fusco N, Gunnarsdottir T, et al. Leveraging data and digital health technologies to assess and impact social determinants of health (SDoH): a state-of-the-art literature review. Online J Public Health Inform. 2021;13:E14. https://doi.org/10.5210/OJPHI.V13I3.11081.

Chapter 9
Telemedicine and Remote Patient Monitoring Solutions

Audrey Lodge and Ruiling Guo

Introduction

Telemedicine and remote patient monitoring (RPM) represent one of the most transformative trends in modern healthcare [1, 2]. More healthcare providers and patients are willing to use these technologies due to many advantages in healthcare delivery, especially during and after the COVID-19 pandemic [1, 3–6]. For instance, prior to the COVID-19 pandemic, telemedicine use was limited in many European countries, hindered by regulatory barriers and hesitation from patients and providers. However, because the pandemic significantly disrupted in-person care like many other countries in the world, many European countries quickly adopted telemedicine and other digital health solutions. A survey revealed that telemedicine and RPM services were offered in 77% of countries in the World Health Organization (WHO) European Region [6]. The results of systematic reviews and meta-analyses indicate that telemedicine and RPM are valid alternatives to usual care by offering cost savings, reducing mortality, and improving chronic disease management [7–15]. In addition, studies show that telemedicine and RPM help reduce health disparities and advance health access and quality of care, especially in the medically underserved populations and rural areas [16–20].

Telemedicine and RPM hold promise for the future of healthcare delivery. According to various market research reports, the global telemedicine market is expected to grow significantly from 2020 to 2030. The estimates suggest that the global telemedicine market size will reach between $380 billion and $462 billion by

A. Lodge
St. Luke's Health System, Specialty Care, Boise, ID, USA

R. Guo (✉)
College of Business, Idaho State University, Pocatello, ID, USA

P. Eappen et al. (eds.), *Advancing Healthcare with the Medical Internet of Things*, Health Informatics, https://doi.org/10.1007/978-3-032-23933-4_9

2030 with a compound annual growth rate (CAGR) between 15% and 24% during this period [21]. This may be driven by factors like increased accessibility to healthcare, technological advancements, and the growing need for telemedicine and RPM [21].

What is telemedicine? How does RPM work? Telemedicine usually refers to the practice of delivering healthcare services through telecommunications technology, allowing healthcare professionals to evaluate, diagnose, and treat patients remotely. The American Medical Association (AMA) defines telemedicine, telehealth, and other related terms as "the exchange of medical information from one site to another through electronic communication" [22]. Telemedicine has historically been referred to as remote clinical services [22]. Telemedicine involves the use of telecommunications technology to diagnose, consult, treat, educate, and manage patient care remotely. Telemedicine and telehealth are often used interchangeably in healthcare, but this chapter adopts telemedicine rather than telehealth. RPM takes this concept further by enabling continuous monitoring of a patient's health status through connected devices that transmit data in real-time to healthcare providers. According to the AMA, RPM refers to the use of digital technologies to collect and transmit patient health data from a patient's location to a healthcare provider for assessment and care management [23]. RPM enables continuous monitoring of patients with chronic conditions or those recovering from acute illnesses, allowing healthcare providers to track health trends, intervene early, and improve patient outcomes without requiring in-person visits [23–25]. Telemedicine typically involves video consultations, phone calls, and remote diagnostics, while RPM solutions use technologies like wearable sensors, smart devices, and mobile health apps to collect vital signs and other health data, such as blood pressure, glucose levels, and heart rate [11]. RPM is a form of asynchronous telehealth. It does not demand a live interaction between the provider and patient. RPM uses digital devices to collect and send patient data and clinical information. The health care provider reviews the patient's health data. This information is used to manage health conditions, detect health risks, and educate patients.

Telemedicine and RPM enable healthcare providers to deliver care to patients outside traditional clinical settings, improving access to healthcare services, especially for those in rural or underserved areas. With the growing prevalence of chronic conditions, an aging population, and the need for real-time, continuous care, telemedicine, and RPM solutions are playing a critical role in improving patient outcomes, reducing healthcare costs, and increasing the efficiency of care delivery [7, 10, 24]. Research evidence presented in this chapter indicates that telemedicine and RPM have significantly improved health disparities, access, cost, and outcomes in healthcare systems; however, challenges such as patient privacy, data security, digital literacy gaps, clinical limitations, reimbursement rate discrepancies, and regulatory issues necessitate evidence-based strategies and policy reforms to ensure equitable and sustainable implementation.

The aim of this chapter is to analyze the role of telemedicine and RPM in mitigating health disparities and addressing challenges in healthcare systems. Through an evaluation of existing research, including case studies and systematic reviews, this chapter presents successful applications and demonstrates how telemedicine and RPM have improved healthcare access, outcomes, costs, and disparities thus far. Additionally, it seeks to gain insight into what challenges still remain in telemedicine and RPM and what recommendations are required for future success.

Methods

This chapter employs a qualitative analysis approach. An in-depth review of peer-reviewed literature published between 2020 and 2025 was conducted. Relevant studies were retrieved from professional databases, including PubMed, CINAHL, Cochrane Library, Web of Science, Business Source Complete, Google Scholar, and Academic Search Complete. Database searches were performed using a combination of terms such as telemedicine, telehealth, remote patient monitoring (RPM), remote care delivery, health access, cost-effectiveness, data security, digital literacy, health policy, and patient outcomes. Insights were drawn from various sources, including peer-reviewed articles, case studies, cross-sectional studies, systematic reviews, and meta-analyses focusing on telemedicine and RPM applications in healthcare settings. The research evidence emphasizes how telemedicine and RPM technologies have influenced healthcare delivery, particularly in improving access to care, enhancing cost-effectiveness, and optimizing patient outcomes.

A thematic analysis was used to categorize the findings into four key themes: (1) improved health access, (2) enhanced patient outcomes, (3) cost efficiency, and (4) reduction of health disparities. The sources analyzed spanned clinical, business, and public health journals, along with reports documenting real-world implementations of telemedicine and RPM technologies. Key case studies and systematic reviews were identified through comprehensive literature analysis and were used to illustrate practical applications of telemedicine and RPM. The chapter critically examines the effectiveness of these technologies in improving healthcare access, outcomes, and cost efficiency. Additionally, barriers to the adoption of telemedicine and RPM were explored through a review of reported ethical, operational, technological, and regulatory challenges. These include concerns related to patient privacy, data security, digital literacy, reimbursement models, clinical limitations, and evolving health policies and regulations. By synthesizing the existing body of research, this chapter offers evidence-based recommendations and strategic insights to support the effective integration and utilization of telemedicine and RPM technologies in healthcare delivery.

Results

Successful Applications

Four common advantages remain at the forefront of successful telemedicine applications and RPM: improved health access, enhanced patient outcomes and engagement, cost efficiency, and reduction of health disparities.

Improved Health Access

Telemedicine and RPM are known to enable access to care for rural and underserved populations by eliminating long wait times in office and eliminating the need for transportation to and from the appointment. When patients with mobility issues have the convenience of receiving care from their own home, this mitigates the risk of having a fall, injury, or accident on the way to the medical facility. Telemedicine also allows patients to be able to consult with specialists outside their community that they would not have otherwise been able to see due to limited local expertise [26].

A case study comparison between in-person and tele-practice intervention for autistic children found that children made similar gains in social communication and language regardless of the modality, but tele-practice was the preferred delivery model since families that lived in geographically inaccessible locations were able to access qualified providers [27]. Another study by Matsumoto et al. discovered that remote lymphedema conservative therapy benefits patients and providers, particularly in rural regions [28].

Telemedicine and RPM were considered the fastest emerging trends during the COVID-19 pandemic and became a cornerstone of healthcare resilience. According to Precedence Research, "the global telemedicine market size was valued at USD 60.8 billion in 2022 and it is expected to reach USD 225 billion by 2030, growing with a CAGR of 17.16% during the forecast period 2022 to 2030" [29]. Telemedicine's usage has been driven by the ability to bridge geographical gaps and ensure timely access to medical services when the world needed it most. Utilization peaked in quarter 2 of 2020 and has since then steadily declined, but current utilization is still around 50% higher than pre-pandemic numbers [30]. Thanks to social distancing mandates, technological advancements, and increased patient demands, RPM emerged as an unstoppable force during this public health emergency [31].

Before the pandemic, telemedicine adoption was low and Medicare only allowed access for patients in rural areas. At the start of COVID, Medicare and Medicaid waivers along with the relaxation of the Health Insurance Portability and Accountability Act (HIPAA) allowed telemedicine to be a feasible care model for many Americans. On March 17, 2020, the United States (U.S.) Department of Health and Human Services (DHHS) issued a statement that allowed healthcare providers to use services like FaceTime or Skype for telemedicine purposes, even if the service was not related to COVID-19 [32]. Additionally, the U.S. Center for Medicare & Medicaid Services (CMS) telehealth waivers caused an immediate rise in the number of telehealth encounters and decrease in in-person visits during the early pandemic period [5]. Healthcare providers and patients had to quickly adapt to this new virtual care model. The COVID-19 pandemic has led health systems to increase the use of tools for monitoring and triaging patients remotely. For instance, Alboksmaty et al. conducted a systematic review to assess the effectiveness and safety of pulse oximetry in remote patient monitoring of patients at home with COVID-19 [33]. The study results showed that the use of pulse oximetry can potentially save hospital resources for patients who might benefit the most from care escalation [33].

Enhanced Patient Outcomes and Engagement

RPM and telemedicine have been shown to improve health outcomes as presented in the case studies below. RPM can make chronic disease management easier by allowing patients to continuously track data such as blood glucose, heart rate, sleep, physical activity, and medication usage from home. Healthcare providers can intervene early, adjust treatment plans, and avoid complications or hospitalizations by tracking real-time data and taking actions accordingly. This model encourages a proactive attitude toward one's health which undermines the importance of a preventative care approach. A preventative care approach can lead to earlier detection and treatment of diseases [23].

A case study examining innovations in a Ventricular Assist Device during the pandemic indicates that the use of remote self-monitoring systems minimized the risk of patients acquiring COVID-19 and reduced the likelihood of progressing into severe disease or death [34]. There were zero reported cases among their patients during the first phase of the pandemic. A second case study by Bahar et al. suggests that telemedicine had a positive effect on the quality of life and anxiety level of patients who had COVID-19, proving that telemedicine is an effective physiological support tool for people who have to isolate due to natural disasters [35]. Another case study examined the effects of delivering cognitive processing therapy via telemedicine to a gay Latino adolescent. Results revealed that telemedicine reduced post-traumatic stress disorder (PTSD) symptoms, suicidal ideation, and substance use [36].

Through telemedicine platforms and RPM devices, patients can actively engage with their healthcare providers and their health data. This promotes patient empowerment and better adherence to treatment plans. For instance, telemedicine was a game changer in expanding healthcare access during the COVID-19 pandemic, particularly in underserved communities. In some hospitals and medical centers like the UMass Memorial Medical Center, telemedicine can be scaled to reach remote populations, providing access to specialists without the need for in-person visits [26]. Remote monitoring tools, such as wearable devices, allow patients to track their health metrics and share real-time data with providers, improving engagement and health outcomes.

Cost Efficiency

Both telemedicine and RPM reduce the overall costs of operations because there is no need for in-person space occupancy, facility overheads, or additional patient costs like childcare or travel [10, 24, 37–40]. Digital tools can help improve care coordination and reduce redundancy so that resources are used efficiently. By enabling proactive care management, this preventative model can also slow the rate of further complications and reduce hospital readmissions and emergency department visits, which are more costly than outpatient care. For instance, a study conducted by the University of Pittsburgh Medical Center (UPMC) implemented telemedicine for managing patients with chronic conditions such as diabetes and hypertension. Patients used RPM devices to monitor blood pressure, blood glucose, and weight, transmitting data to healthcare providers in real time [38]. The program reduced hospital readmissions by 25% and saved an estimated $1,200 per patient annually by preventing complications and unnecessary emergency room visits. A pilot program by the U.S. Veterans Health Administration (VHA) used RPM for post-acute care patients recovering from heart failure. Patients were provided with wearable devices and mobile apps to track vital signs and symptoms. The program resulted in a 30% reduction in hospital readmissions and saved approximately $2,000 per patient over six months by enabling early intervention and reducing the need for in-person follow-ups [39].

Van der Zee et al. state that telemedicine reduces carbon emissions since 22% of healthcare-related emissions are due to transport [41]. Additionally, a case study examining the cost effectiveness of teleophthalmology for diabetic retinopathy found that using telemedicine-based digital retinal imaging was less than half the total cost of a conventional examination [37]. Furthermore, Vaksvik et al. examined the cost effectiveness of using video consultations in hand therapy settings [40]. The video consults were shown to save money for patients and health institutions and saved more money for patients as their travel distance increased [40]. However, future research should be conducted to examine whether telemedicine will reduce spending on common healthcare services.

Remote patient monitoring programs are appealing not only because they are convenient, but they also have the ability to improve health outcomes at a lower cost [24]. Le Goff-Pronost and Bongiovanni-Delarozière identified 61 eligible RPM studies and found that RPM is reported to be cost-effective no matter what level of patient involvement occurred in the program [10]. The levels of patient involvement ranged from weak (automated monitoring) to medium (monitored by a professional) to strong (active remote participation) [10].

Reduction of Health Disparities

Telemedicine and RPM can also reduce disparities among different patient populations by providing equitable access. Certain physical and financial barriers can be eliminated for low-income populations with the correct tailored programs. Language and cultural barriers can also be improved by incorporating interpreters, multilingual support, or better yet providers who come from a similar cultural background as the patient [23]. Four case studies are presented in the following section to demonstrate how telemedicine and RPM can reduce health disparities.

The first case study is about telemedicine used for rural diabetes management in Native American communities. A telemedicine program was implemented in the Navajo Nation, a rural region with high rates of type 2 diabetes and limited access to endocrinologists in the U.S. [42]. The program combined virtual consultations with RPM devices to track blood glucose levels. Patients received Bluetooth-enabled glucose meters that transmitted real-time data to clinicians. Telemedicine visits replaced in-person appointments, and community health workers provided culturally tailored education via video calls. After 12 months, participants saw a 25% reduction in HbA1c levels and a 40% decrease in diabetes-related hospitalizations. The program bridged geographic barriers and improved trust in healthcare providers through culturally competent care [42].

The second case study was conducted using remote hypertension monitoring to target African American women in the urban areas of Chicago. These African American women faced disproportionately high maternal mortality rates due to hypertension. Limited access to prenatal care and racial bias in clinical settings exacerbated disparities. In this study, pregnant patients received home blood pressure monitors and were connected with obstetrician-gynecologists via a telemedicine platform. Automated alerts flagged abnormal readings, prompting immediate virtual triage. Postpartum patients continued monitoring for six months. The program reduced severe preeclampsia cases by 30% and increased postpartum follow-up rates from 50% to 85%. Patients reported greater satisfaction with equitable care access [43].

The third case study examines the effects of teleintervention on breastfeeding in low-income women in the U.S. It suggests that teleinterventions may have a positive impact on the occurrence of breastfeeding for this population [44]. The fourth case study explores the benefits and barriers of tele-mental health services for U.S. refugees during the COVID-19 pandemic. It revealed that telemedicine services allowed for fewer cancellations and transportation concerns and better access to childcare for this population [45]. These results highlight the importance of telemedicine and RPM inequities for vulnerable populations.

In addition to the above case studies, there is a growing amount of high-level evidence, such as systematic reviews and meta-analyses, which supports the effectiveness of RPM and telemedicine in reducing costs, addressing health disparities, improving patient outcomes, and enhancing healthcare access. De Guzman et al. conducted a systematic review comparing economic evaluations of usual care compared to noninvasive RPM for chronic illnesses and found that "RPM was highly cost-effective for hypertension and may achieve greater long-term cost savings from the prevention of high-cost health events" [7]. Additionally, a 2022 meta-analysis by Leo et al. studied patients' uptake of certain interactive remote patient monitoring devices for chronic disease management [11]. It was discovered that telemonitoring, used as an alternative to usual care, reduced mortality, improved self-management of the disease, and patients were satisfied with the experience [11]. In nephrology, a systematic review by Mata-Lima et al. highlighted the potential of RPM to enhance resource effectiveness, improve quality of life for patients with chronic kidney disease, and reduce healthcare costs [13]. Another systematic review studying the implications of mobile technology on hospitalization rates in medically underserved areas of the world found that RPM in these locations can cause lower hospitalization rates and improved access to disease management [46]. Similarly, Jackson et al. revealed in a meta-analysis systematic review that telehealth interventions for cardiovascular disease and hypertension significantly improved the disease management outcomes [8]. These high-level studies provide strong evidence that both RPM and telemedicine are scalable, feasible, beneficial, and cost-effective.

Challenges and Considerations

The technological advancements of remote care delivery come with specific challenges that require strategic solutions. Only a few of the major challenges that persist are discussed.

Patient Privacy and Data Security

With telemedicine and RPM involving the transmission of sensitive health data, the first of these challenges is patient privacy and data security. Environmental factors can cause a lack of private space for vulnerable populations, which can make remote care delivery more difficult. Technological factors such as an increased risk of interception of protected health information (PHI) online can cause a threat to data security [47]. Health systems and patients have to be cautious of data breaches and cybersecurity attacks and understand the serious risks of transmitting PHI over the Internet. Therefore, encryption and secure communication channels are essential to ensure compliance with regulations such as HIPAA in the U.S., General Data Protection Regulation (GDPR) in Europe, and other rules and policies. Additionally, certain platforms or devices used for teleconferencing may lack the appropriate security settings or measures. Telemedicine must also adhere to laws like HIPAA which requires secure transmission and storage of patient records. Willful HIPAA violations can result in extreme consequences, including prison time.

The issue of data security is so important because patients have strong views about the privacy of their health data. Of a 1,000-patient survey conducted by Savvy

Cooperative, 75% of patients expressed concern about protecting the privacy of PHI, 59% expressed concern with PHI being used against them or a loved one, and 88% believe that their doctor should have the ability to review and verify the security of health apps before they gain access to their PHI [48].

Digital Literacy Gaps

Another major issue with the adoption of telemedicine and remote healthcare delivery is digital literacy gaps. Both patients and providers must have reliable Internet access, and patients need to be comfortable using technology. Certain populations may lack the necessary digital knowledge and skills in order to use telemedicine effectively. For some populations, especially the elderly, this may pose a barrier to adoption. A mixed methods research study by Crellin et al. discovered that older patients found remote monitoring services to be less helpful, more difficult to understand, and were more likely to report a problem with it [49]. Minority ethnic groups also reported more difficulty understanding the information. They also indicated that certain factors can cause a discrepancy in engagement which include gender, ethnicity, health status, and employment [49]. Access to technology can also further exacerbate access disparities because the low-income and rural populations are less likely to have access to reliable devices and internet.

Reimbursement Rates

Another common issue that remains for telemedicine and remote care delivery is the discrepancy in reimbursement rates across payers and states. Providers are worried about payment parity for telemedicine because it is a more expensive care model due to infrastructure, and reimbursement policies are so varied [50]. According to Rakshit et al. and Salmanizadeh et al., there was no major difference in reimbursement rates for telemedicine versus in-person visits during the COVID-19 pandemic [51, 52]. However, reimbursement policies have undergone significant changes since then. During the pandemic, telemedicine coverage was expanded significantly to ensure access and minimize in-person interaction, but reimbursement has been scaled back since then. Many insurers and policymakers are worried about the overutilization and long-term costs that could be associated with this care model, and state policies vary. Reimbursement today is higher than it was pre-pandemic, but scaling back reimbursement after the pandemic poses significant risks [53].

Clinical Limitations

Clinical limitations seem to persist as a common hindrance of remote patient care. Not all conditions can be examined and diagnosed virtually; therefore, telemedicine delivery will remain limited. The types of providers most commonly using telemedicine are those treating patients with chronic conditions in endocrinology, nephrology, cardiology, psychiatry, gastroenterology, and rheumatology [54]. Providers can always refer patients to receive follow-up care in person if needed, but this may add another level of complexity to the already confusing patient care model.

Telemedicine has the potential to increase the overall cost of healthcare if patients use it as an addition to in-person care, and not as a substitute. It is also important to note that the providers who patients see virtually are sometimes outside the usual source of care for the patient since not all of their normal providers may use telemedicine. So, this could also add to the complexity of the continuity of care model [32].

Regulatory Issues

Additional regulatory issues persist around practicing across state lines. For instance, as of December 2023, 30 states in the U.S. ban or severely restrict telemedicine appointments with doctors licensed out-of-state, but during COVID, there were waivers that allowed this with simplified licensing requirements [55]. The requirements for medical licenses differ for each state since states have the power to regulate the practice of medicine in their borders. However, this evolving legal environment highlights the tension between state regulatory authority and the need for broader telemedicine accessibility.

Recommendations

The following sections detail the most important evidence-based strategies going forward in order to improve telemedicine and remote care delivery: policy reformation, strengthening data security, and bridging the digital divide.

Policy and Regulatory Reforms

Certain health policies and reform will need to be unified and extended in health systems. For instance, health policy reform in Europe is increasingly intertwined with the adoption and integration of telemedicine, particularly following the accelerated adoption during the COVD-19 pandemic. At present, most European Union member states are encouraged to develop clear telemedicine policies and strategies to guide its integration into the healthcare system to address barriers such as infrastructure limitations, lack of digital literacy, and concerns about data security and privacy for facilitating the wider adaptation of telemedicine and RPM [6]. In the

U.S. the Telemedicine Expansion Act, which was enacted by the U.S. Congress in 2020 and extended in 2022, allows an exemption for telemedicine services from certain high-deductible health plan rules through 2024. The Telehealth Expansion Act of 2023 aims to permanently allow this but has not been passed by the Senate yet. Additionally, the Telehealth Benefit Expansion for Workers Act of 2023 has also been introduced but not passed. This bill would allow employers to offer standalone telehealth or telemedicine benefits to all employees because currently employers can only offer telemedicine benefits to employees who are ineligible for the employer's group health plan. Another very important bill that would extend Medicare coverage and payment flexibility for certain telemedicine or audio-only services is the Protecting Rural Telehealth Access Act. Lastly, the Telemental Health Care Access Act would eliminate the Medicare requirement that states a patient must be seen in person by a provider at least 6 months previous to any virtual visit and at regular intervals thereafter [51]. Policy reform with these bills (and many more) will be imperative in order to ensure the continued coverage and sustainable integration of telemedicine. As Rakshit et al. states, "Telehealth use surged during the pandemic, but the future of telehealth will be shaped by its effect on total health spending, federal and state regulations relating to scope of practice and reimbursement, and payer coverage and reimbursement policies" [51]. Further research may be conducted to evaluate telemedicine and telehealth reimbursement policies to ensure equally accessible care across state lines.

Strengthen Data Security and Privacy Training

Focusing on data security will be vital to ensure that telemedicine practices and RPM are safe and maintainable. This can be accomplished by honing in on safe technological processes and including telemedicine in privacy practices. Telemedicine platforms and RPM must have the appropriate security measures and be included in security management plans. Medical information should only be shared via secure servers, and multifactor authentication should be required for both patients and healthcare providers. Patients can also be identified using government-issued photo identification or similar to prevent fraud. Additionally, HIPAA, GDPR, telemedicine, and privacy training can be required periodically for employees so they stay up to date on current practices. It is also important for providers to understand when guardians should or should not attend sessions, as state laws are always changing. The proper release and consent forms should always be completed before the appointment. Patients must always be informed of the security protocols and possible risks of using telemedicine and RPM. Continuous data safety monitoring can be prioritized by regular audits [47].

Bridge the Digital Divide

The increased use of technology reaps benefits and downfalls. It will be important to bridge the digital divide so that access to technology does not further exacerbate access disparities. Ways in which we can bridge this divide include the following: provide information in different languages, offer translation services, provide additional tech support for patients, and provide digital literacy training for providers. It is important to recognize that certain populations will struggle more with the adoption of telemedicine and RPM so providing extra resources for these groups is critical. It will also be vital to ensure that these vulnerable populations have access to stable internet and have access to a device they can use for telemedicine visits and remote care delivery. Providing affordable or free devices may be a way to ensure this. Some of these recommendations may require additional funding for startup, but the goal is that once there is a successful, unified system, it will bring long-term benefits. Health systems should also give the option of allowing audio-only visits when permissible if patients do not have the privacy or access for a video meeting. Lastly, platforms will be more user friendly and used more frequently if patients and providers are included in the designing of software. Platform feedback should be continually monitored for the ongoing success of telemedicine and remote care delivery [49].

Conclusion

Telemedicine and RPM are transforming the way healthcare is delivered, offering convenient, cost-effective, and personalized care. As these technologies continue to evolve, addressing challenges such as data privacy, patient engagement, technical barriers, and regulatory reform will be critical for their sustained success. Overall, the expansion of telemedicine has reaped many benefits including improved access, outcomes, and cost-efficiency while reducing health disparities across different populations. The case studies and systematic reviews discussed in this chapter highlight the transformative impact of telemedicine and RPM, yet there are hurdles that still remain. These include privacy concerns, reimbursement challenges, gaps in digital literacy, and restrictive regulatory policies. Going forward, it will be important to effectively incorporate these technologies into the already existing care delivery model so that telemedicine and RPM can continue to help, not hinder, the healthcare systems.

Future efforts must be focused on policy reform that expands reimbursements, ensures privacy, promotes interstate licensure, and advances the digital divide. While the effects of telemedicine and RPM should be continually monitored, it is a vital tool in the future of healthcare and holds tremendous promise for improving healthcare delivery. Evidence-based strategies will continue to pave way for more resourceful healthcare systems in the world that effectively incorporates telemedicine and remote care delivery.

References

1. Omboni S, Padwal RS, Alessa T, et al. The worldwide impact of telemedicine during COVID-19: current evidence and recommendations for the future. Connect Health. 2022;1:7–35. https://doi.org/10.20517/ch.2021.03.
2. Yadav S. Transformative frontiers: a comprehensive review of emerging technologies in modern healthcare. Cureus. 2024;16(3):e56538. https://doi.org/10.7759/cureus.56538.
3. Ahmed A, Mutahar M, Daghrery AA, et al. A systematic review of publications on perceptions and management of chronic medical conditions using telemedicine remote consultations by primary healthcare professionals April 2020 to December 2021 during the COVID-19 pandemic. Med Sci Monit. 2024;30:e943383. https://doi.org/10.12659/MSM.943383.
4. Gordon M, Sinopoulou V, Lakunina S, et al. Remote care through telehealth for people with inflammatory bowel disease. Cochrane Database Syst Rev. 2023;5(5):CD014821. https://doi.org/10.1002/14651858.CD014821.pub2.
5. Hegde S, Eid NS. Telehealth and remote patient monitoring after the COVID pandemic. Pediatr Allergy Immunol Pulmonol. 2021;34(4):130.
6. World Health Organization (WHO). The rise of telehealth in the European region: insights from Norway. 2025. https://www.who.int/europe/news/item/10-10-2024-the-rise-of-telehealth-in-the-european-region%2D%2Dinsights-from-norway.
7. De Guzman KR, Snoswell CL, Taylor ML, Gray LC, Caffery LJ. Economic evaluations of remote patient monitoring for chronic disease: a systematic review. Value Health. 2022;25(6):897–913. https://doi.org/10.1016/j.jval.2021.12.001.
8. Jackson TN, Sreedhara M, Bostic M, et al. Telehealth use to address cardiovascular disease and hypertension in the United States: a systematic review and meta-analysis, 2011–2021. Telemed Rep. 2023;4(1):67–86. https://doi.org/10.1089/tmr.2023.0011.
9. Jin Y, Zhao H, Hu J. Remote health monitoring impact on diabetes management: meta-analysis. J Diabetes Sci Technol. 2024;18(3):456–64.
10. Le Goff-Pronost M, Bongiovanni-Delarozière I. Economic evaluation of remote patient monitoring and organizational analysis according to patient involvement: a scoping review. Int J Technol Assess Health Care. 2023;39(1):e59. https://doi.org/10.1017/S0266462323002581.
11. Leo DG, Buckley BJR, Chowdhury M, et al. Interactive remote patient monitoring devices for managing chronic health conditions: systematic review and meta-analysis. J Med Internet Res. 2022;24(11):e35508. https://doi.org/10.2196/35508.
12. Ma Y, Zhao C, Zhao Y, et al. Telemedicine application in patients with chronic disease: a systematic review and meta-analysis. BMC Med Inform Decis Mak. 2022;22(1):105. https://doi.org/10.1186/s12911-022-01845-2.
13. Mata-Lima A, Paquete AR, Serrano-Olmedo JJ. Remote patient monitoring and management in nephrology: a systematic review. Nefrologia. 2024;44(5):639–67. https://doi.org/10.1016/j.nefroe.2024.10.011.
14. Zhang Y, Peña MT, Fletcher LM, Lal L, Swint JM, Reneker JC. Economic evaluation and costs of remote patient monitoring for cardiovascular disease in the United States: a systematic review. Int J Technol Assess Health Care. 2023;39(1):e25. https://doi.org/10.1017/S0266462323000156.
15. Xiao Z, Han X. Evaluation of the effectiveness of telehealth chronic disease management system: systematic review and meta-analysis. J Med Internet Res. 2023;25:e44256. https://doi.org/10.2196/44256.
16. Ali M, Sullivan G. Racial differences in expanded telemedicine use during COVID-19: a literature review. Telemed J E Health. 2024;30(5):1394–400. https://doi.org/10.1089/tmj.2023.0370.
17. Anderson A, O'Connell SS, Thomas C, Chimmanamada R. Telehealth interventions to improve diabetes management among black and Hispanic patients: a systematic review and meta-analysis. J Racial Ethn Health Disparities. 2022;9(6):2375–86. https://doi.org/10.1007/s40615-021-01174-6.

18. Perez K, Wisniewski D, Ari A, et al. Investigation into application of AI and telemedicine in rural communities: a systematic literature review. Healthcare (Basel). 2025;13(3):324. https://doi.org/10.3390/healthcare13030324.
19. Truong M, Yeganeh L, Cook O, et al. Using telehealth consultations for healthcare provision to patients from non-Indigenous racial/ethnic minorities: a systematic review. J Am Med Inform Assoc. 2022;29(5):970–82. https://doi.org/10.1093/jamia/ocac015.
20. Wang S, von Huben A, Sivaprakash PP, et al. Addressing health service equity through telehealth: a systematic review of reviews. Digit Health. 2025;11:20552076251326233. https://doi.org/10.1177/20552076251326233.
21. Grand View Research. Telemedicine market size, share & trends analysis. 2023. https://www.grandviewresearch.com.
22. American Medical Association (AMA). What is telehealth?. 2024. https://www.ama-assn.org.
23. American Medical Association (AMA). Remote patient monitoring playbook. 2022. https://www.ama-assn.org.
24. Field MJ, Grigsby J. Telemedicine and remote patient monitoring. JAMA. 2002;288(4):423–5.
25. Sri-Ganeshan M, Cameron P. Remote monitoring in telehealth: advancements, feasibility. In: A comprehensive overview of telemedicine. IntechOpen; 2024. p. 229. https://www.intechopen.com/chapters/1177653.
26. Franciosi EB, Tan AJ, Kassamali B, et al. The impact of telehealth implementation on underserved populations and no-show rates during the COVID-19 pandemic. Telemed J E Health. 2021;27(8):874–80.
27. Sundarrajana M, Franco J. Parent-mediated intervention for autistic children through telepractice. Perspect ASHA Spec Interest Groups. 2024;9(4):1217–34.
28. Matsumoto C, Yang R, Okazaki M, Konya C, Dai M. Feasibility of implementing a remote system for lymphoedema conservative therapy: a case study. Br J Nurs. 2024;33(13):612–20. https://doi.org/10.12968/bjon.2024.0096.
29. Precedence Research. Telemedicine market size and trends 2024–2034. 2023. https://www.precedenceresearch.com.
30. Jain S. Telehealth demand: an update four years after COVID-19. Trilliant Health; 2024. https://www.trillianthealth.com.
31. Wosik J, Fudim M, Cameron B, et al. Telehealth transformation: COVID-19 and beyond. J Am Med Inform Assoc. 2020;27(6):957–62.
32. Weigel G, Ramaswamy A, Sobel L, et al. Opportunities and barriers for telemedicine in the U.S. during the COVID-19 emergency and beyond. KFF; 2020. https://www.kff.org.
33. Alboksmaty A, Beaney T, Elkin S, et al. Effectiveness and safety of pulse oximetry in remote patient monitoring: a systematic review. Lancet Digit Health. 2022;4(4):e279–89.
34. Correas MD. Innovations in ventricular assist device patient care amid COVID-19. Transplant J Aust. 2024;33(1):6–9.
35. Bahar A, Sucu Cakmak NC, Kilic AD. The effect of telehealth application on anxiety and quality of life in COVID-19 patients. Int J Caring Sci. 2023;16(3):1316–27.
36. Stickley MM, Sopchak KS, McCord CE. Cognitive processing therapy via telehealth for PTSD: a clinical case. Cogn Behav Pract. 2023;30(3):539–50.
37. Chawla S, Chawla A, Chawla R, et al. Nurse-operated teleophthalmology screening for diabetic retinopathy. Int J Diabetes Dev Ctries. 2022;42(4):747–50.
38. University of Pittsburgh Medical Center. Telemedicine and RPM for chronic disease. 2019. https://www.upmc.com.
39. U.S. Department of Veterans Affairs. RPM in post-acute care: a cost-effective solution. 2020. https://www.va.gov.
40. Vaksvik T, Støme LN, Føllesdal J, et al. Early use of video consultations in hand therapy: cost-effectiveness. J Hand Ther. 2024;37(1):3–11.
41. van der Zee C, Chang-Wolf J, Koopmanschap MA, et al. Assessing the carbon footprint of telemedicine: a systematic review. Health Serv Insights. 2024;17:1–8.

42. Smith R, Begay D, Yazzie A. Telemedicine and diabetes management in the Navajo Nation: a community-driven approach. J Telemed Telecare. 2021;27(4):213–20.
43. Johnson MA, Lee YS. Addressing hypertension disparities with remote monitoring in African American women. Womens Health Issues. 2020;30(4):265–72.
44. Corkery-Hayward M, Talaei A. Effects of teleintervention on breastfeeding in low-income women. Matern Child Health J. 2024;28(1):55–62.
45. Weith J, Fondacaro M, Khin S. Barriers and benefits of telemental health for refugees in the U.S. during COVID-19. J Immigr Minor Health. 2023;25(1):33–41.
46. Heffernan M, Mittal R, Tafuto B. Implications of mobile technology on hospitalization rates in medically underserved areas worldwide: a systematic review. Cureus. 2025;17(2):e78409. https://doi.org/10.7759/cureus.78409.
47. Houser SH, Flite CA, Foster P. Patient privacy and data security in telehealth: legal and ethical concerns. J Health Law Ethics. 2023;19(2):200–15.
48. American Medical Association (AMA). Patient survey shows unresolved tension over health data privacy. 2022. https://www.ama-assn.org/press-center/ama-press-releases/patient-survey-shows-unresolved-tension-over-health-data-privacy.
49. Crellin NE, Armitage CJ, Sutton S. Digital literacy and remote monitoring: inequalities among older adults. J Med Internet Res. 2024;26(1):e40756.
50. Lombardi BM, de Saxe Zerden L, Greeno E. Telehealth payment parity and scope-of-practice policies. Health Serv Res. 2024;59(3):401–12.
51. Rakshit P, Zolna MR, Patel A. Telehealth policies post-pandemic: economic and regulatory trends. Health Aff. 2023;42(9):1183–91.
52. Salmanizadeh H, Miller E, Oseni A. Telemedicine reimbursement variations: insights from Medicaid data. J Health Econ Policy. 2022;18(4):231–9.
53. Khera N, Knoedler M, Meier SK, TerKonda S, Williams RD, Wittich CM, Coffey JD, Demaerschalk BM. Payment and coverage parity for virtual care and in-person care: how do we get there? Telemed Rep. 2023;4(1):100–8. https://doi.org/10.1089/tmr.2023.0014.
54. Shaver JA. Telemedicine utilization trends across specialties. JAMA Intern Med. 2022;182(5):482–9.
55. Trotter LJ. Regulatory barriers in interstate telemedicine practice. Am J Public Health Policy. 2023;114(12):1310–7.

Chapter 10
Opportunities and Challenges of Wearable Health Devices for Early Detection of Diabetes-Related Conditions in Canada and the USA: A Narrative Review

Aderonke Oludare and Philip Eappen

Definition of the Problem

Diabetes mellitus is a global health concern, significantly impacting populations in North America [1–4]. Complications such as hypoglycemia, hyperglycemia, and diabetic foot ulcers contribute to increased morbidity and mortality rates [5]. Many diabetes-related complications arise due to late detection [6] and poor disease management, leading to hospitalizations, lower limb amputations, and cardiovascular risks. While health products such as smartwatches, CGMs, and others offer a solution by providing uninterrupted monitoring and real-time alerts, challenges such as affordability, accessibility, and regulatory constraints limit their widespread use. Addressing these issues is crucial for improving diabetes care outcomes and reducing healthcare costs.

Introduction

Approximately 500 million individuals globally are affected by diabetes, a figure that is expected to rise by 25% by 2030 and by 51% by 2045 [7]. Diabetes is a long-lasting, life-changing condition that profoundly impacts individuals, families, and societies around the world. It ranks as one of the top ten causes of mortality among adults [7–10]. In North America, millions are impacted, with around 11.9 million individuals in Canada diagnosed with diabetes or prediabetes, while over 38 million individuals in the United States have diabetes [2–4]. Inadequate glycemic control can lead to serious complications, including hypoglycemia, hyperglycemia, and diabetic neuropathy, resulting in foot ulcers [11]. The World Health Organization

A. Oludare (✉) · P. Eappen
Cape Breton University, Sydney, NS, Canada

P. Eappen et al. (eds.), *Advancing Healthcare with the Medical Internet of Things*, Health Informatics, https://doi.org/10.1007/978-3-032-23933-4_10

(WHO) states that chronic illnesses like diabetes, cardiovascular diseases, and respiratory disorders represent significant global health challenges, contributing to nearly 75% of deaths worldwide and imposing considerable economic burdens on healthcare systems [12, 13]. The prevalence and difficulty of managing diabetic foot ulcers (DFU) impose significant costs through diminished productivity and heightened medical expenses [11]. Considering the extensive effects of these diseases, there is a pressing need for creative strategies for monitoring, prevention, and diagnostics [14].

Wearable health devices like CGMs and smart insoles have become vital instruments in diabetes management by providing real-time tracking and predictive analytics for prompt intervention [15–17].

Wearable devices represent an efficient approach for ongoing health monitoring, decreasing the necessity for regular hospital appointments and minimizing overall healthcare expenses [18]. By persistently monitoring vital signs and assisting in chronic disease management and rehabilitation, these devices can detect potential health risks early and enhance patient outcomes. In contrast to traditional monitoring methods, wearables provide continuous feedback regarding users' health and behaviors, promoting the formation of healthy habits and encouraging active participation in healthcare [19].

Wearable technology has become vital for real-time health monitoring and early detection of chronic illnesses, helping to avert severe health complications. Although advancements in technology have been substantial [11], challenges concerning cost, accuracy, and user engagement remain [18, 20]. This chapter discusses the effects of wearable technology on managing diabetes-related challenges in Canada and the USA, highlighting both the possible benefits and hurdles to broader use.

However, the effective use of wearables necessitates a certain level of user competency, and concerns regarding data privacy and the limitations of device computing power are still significant. Mansour et al. [21] reported over 600 million devices in use by 2020 and projected healthcare savings of $200 billion over the next 25 years, but challenges regarding energy efficiency, secure data transmission, and real-time data processing continue to affect the industry. Although there is an increasing adoption of wearables across various healthcare sectors, there is a lack of research evaluating their use, benefits, and difficulties across different domains, particularly when comparing the United States and Canada. This narrative review aimed to identify the existing opportunities and challenges associated with wearable devices and how they could be more effectively applied in managing healthcare policies, especially for patients with diabetes-related conditions.

Literature Review

Wearable technology has advanced considerably in the last decade, from basic fitness trackers to advanced devices capable of tracking a broad array of health metrics [22]. Health tracking enables individuals to shift from a reactive approach to wellness, as wearables supply tailored data that helps create a foundation for improved health outcomes [23]. For instance, continuous glucose monitors (CGMs) have changed the landscape of diabetes management by delivering real-time glucose levels, resulting in accurate insulin administration and improved glycemic regulation [24].

Several studies highlight the benefits of wearable technology in diabetes management. Yu et al. [25] demonstrated that continuous glucose monitoring (CGM) significantly reduces hypoglycemia-related hospital admissions and improves glycemic control. Hopkinson [26] reviewed that smart insoles could predict and prevent diabetic foot ulcers, potentially lowering amputation rates. Despite these benefits, cost and reimbursement issues hinder adoption, as indicated by [27], who found that financial constraints were a major barrier to CGM adherence. Another obstacle is the high expense of sophisticated wearables, particularly CGMs, which restricts availability for uninsured or low-income populations. Research indicates that while wearables can positively influence health results, financial barriers impede widespread adoption among those who would benefit the most [28]. This challenge has prompted advocacy for policy reforms aimed at increasing insurance coverage for wearable devices, but the implementation of these changes has been inconsistent across different regions.

In the realm of health equity, [29] explored disparities in diabetes-related lower limb complications, showing that socioeconomically disadvantaged groups face higher amputation risks due to delayed care. Canadian Institute for Health Information [30] addressed concerns regarding data security in wearable health devices, emphasizing the need for stricter privacy regulations. Additionally, [31] examined advancements in non-invasive glucose monitoring, indicating promising future developments but highlighting current limitations in accuracy and reliability. As stated, the differences in data collected from consumer-level devices compared to clinical-grade instruments raise concerns regarding the clinical usefulness of wearables. Future investigations should focus on enhancing data accuracy in wearable technologies, possibly through advancements in sensor capabilities or collaborations with clinical-grade monitoring devices [32].

The Importance of Wearable Health Devices in Diabetes Care

Wearable health devices have revolutionized diabetes care by enabling real-time glucose monitoring, detecting early warning signs of complications, and reducing hospitalizations. CGMs, such as the Dexcom G7, Abbott FreeStyle Libre, and Medtronic Guardian, have been extensively studied for their role in improving glycemic control and reducing severe hypo- and hyperglycemic events [33, 34].

Smart Insoles and Wearable Sensors for Diabetic Neuropathy and Foot Ulcers

Diabetic neuropathy leads to foot ulcers, a significant cause of lower-limb amputations. Wearable smart insoles (e.g., Siren Socks) and pressure-sensing footwear monitor temperature variations, gait abnormalities, and pressure points to predict ulcer development [17]. While these devices have demonstrated effectiveness, adoption rates are low due to high costs and limited reimbursement policies.

Equity in Diabetes Care: Focus on Diabetes-Associated Lower Limb Complications

Health disparities significantly impact the incidence and management of diabetes-related lower limb complications. Socioeconomic factors, including income level, insurance status, and access to healthcare, influence the likelihood of developing and adequately managing diabetic foot ulcers. Studies show that lower-income populations and racial minorities in both Canada and the USA experience higher rates of amputations due to delayed diagnosis and inadequate preventive care [29, 35]. Wearable technologies have the potential to reduce these disparities by providing early detection and continuous monitoring. However, equitable access remains a challenge due to financial constraints and disparities in healthcare infrastructure.

Effectiveness of Wearable Devices for Early Detection

The reliability of wearable health devices (WHDs) in diabetes detection has been extensively studied [11]. While continuous glucose monitors (CGMs) offer near real-time glucose readings, they are susceptible to calibration errors and sensor inaccuracies [36]. Non-invasive glucose monitoring methods, such as those using sweat or interstitial fluid, are still being refined to achieve accuracy comparable to invasive techniques [37].

Wearable technologies for diabetic neuropathy and foot ulcer prevention include smart insoles and pressure-sensing footwear, which monitor temperature variations and gait abnormalities. Studies have demonstrated that these devices help identify early signs of ulcer development, which decreases the likelihood of lower-limb amputations [16, 17, 38]. However, despite their proven effectiveness, adoption remains low due to cost, limited insurance coverage, and patient adherence challenges.

Barriers to Adoption and Equity Concerns

The extent to which users adopt wearable health devices (WHDs) depends on factors like accessibility, cost, and user-friendliness. Studies show that patients who utilize self-monitoring through WHDs achieve better results in diabetes management compared to those who depend exclusively on traditional glucose monitoring techniques [39]. Nevertheless, issues related to digital skills, economic inequality, and the affordability of devices persist as obstacles to broader adoption [40]. Brown et al. [28] noted that the primary obstacle to the widespread adoption of wearable diabetes technology is affordability. In the USA, CGMs can be costly per month without insurance, making them inaccessible to many individuals, especially those from low-income backgrounds [41]. In Canada, while some provincial health plans provide coverage, disparities exist, particularly among Indigenous and rural populations who face additional barriers to healthcare access [29, 42]. Furthermore, digital literacy and comfort with health technology play significant roles in the adoption and effectiveness of these devices, especially among elderly populations.

Regulatory and Policy Challenges

Regulatory frameworks governing wearable diabetes devices differ between Canada and the USA. The FDA in the USA and Health Canada regulate these devices to ensure safety and efficacy [43, 44]. The FDA and Health Canada have established guidelines for the approval and monitoring of wearable medical devices, ensuring their safety and efficacy. However, differences in approval processes and reimbursement policies create inconsistencies in availability and affordability [20, 45]. Additionally, data privacy and security concerns remain a significant challenge, emphasizing the need for standardized regulatory frameworks to enhance patient trust and compliance as wearable devices collect sensitive health data that must be securely managed to protect users from potential breaches [30].

This review highlights the significant role wearable health devices can play in diabetes management while acknowledging the financial, regulatory, and systemic challenges that hinder their full potential. Future efforts should focus on improving affordability, expanding insurance coverage, and addressing disparities in access and digital literacy to ensure equitable use of these technologies across different populations.

Methodology

This narrative review examines the role of wearable health devices (WHDs), including smartwatches and continuous glucose monitors (CGMs), in the management of diabetes-related conditions in Canada and the United States. The review focuses on their applications, effectiveness, and associated challenges, while also examining regulatory policies, accessibility issues, and concerns related to health equity.

Relevant literature was identified through searches of major academic and public databases, including PubMed, Google Scholar, and CIHI, with a focus on publications from 2018 to 2024. Keywords included "wearable diabetes technology," "continuous glucose monitoring," "diabetes-related complications," "health equity in diabetes care," and "regulatory policies in Canada and the USA." Studies and reports were selected based on their relevance to the review's central themes: device effectiveness, accessibility, health equity, regulatory context, and barriers to adoption.

To complement the literature, publicly available quantitative data were reviewed to illustrate trends in WHD adoption, health outcomes, and policy differences between Canada and the USA. Key themes were identified and synthesized narratively to highlight trends, gaps, and implications for future research and policymaking.

All data sources were appropriately cited, and only publicly accessible information was used. Ethical considerations around attribution and data privacy were respected throughout the review.

Analysis and Discussion

The global prevalence of diabetes, which includes type 1 (T1D) and type 2 (T2D), continues to rise at an alarming rate. According to [46], the number of individuals affected by diabetes is expected to surpass 700 million by 2040. This trend is further supported by findings from the 10th edition of the International Diabetes Federation (IDF) Diabetes Atlas, as presented in data findings by [6]. The data illustrate a significant increase in diabetes cases among individuals aged 20–79, with projections indicating continued growth through 2030 and 2045.

The upward trajectory underscores the urgent necessity for enhanced public health initiatives, early detection methods, and effective management interventions. Contributing factors include aging populations, sedentary lifestyles, dietary changes, and the increasing prevalence of obesity. The projections emphasize the importance of integrating wearable healthcare devices (WHDs), such as CGMs, smart insulin delivery systems, and others, to facilitate real-time glucose monitoring and personalized diabetes management. Additionally, policy initiatives, such as improved healthcare access and government-supported digital health innovations, will be crucial in mitigating the rising burden of diabetes. The findings reveal that wearable devices, especially smartwatches and CGMs, play an invaluable role in managing diabetes related and chronic diseases. CGMs, for example, allow continuous glucose monitoring, reducing the need for frequent finger pricks, while smartwatches support preventive care by tracking vital signs like heart rate. These devices contribute to cost-effective healthcare by reducing emergency room visits and hospital readmissions, addressing a significant portion of healthcare expenditures associated with chronic conditions [47–49].

Key Biomarkers for Early Detection

Important biomarkers that are vital for the early identification of complications related to diabetes include glucose variability, which is characterized by sudden fluctuations and may indicate insulin resistance. Heart Rate Variability (HRV) serves as a predictor of autonomic neuropathy. Foot temperature and pressure mapping help prevent diabetic foot ulcers. Furthermore, skin conductance and hydration levels can signal early signs of neuropathy.

Opportunities for Wearable Devices in Canada and the USA

Wearable devices contribute to the early detection of diabetic complications by providing real-time alerts for glucose spikes, hypoglycemia, and cardiovascular risks [50, 51]. Smartwatches and CGMs allow us to monitor our health continuously. It has a lot of contributions in drastically improving the management of chronic diseases. According to Wounds Canada, a strategy for the prevention and management of diabetic foot complications has been outlined, which includes several guidelines for a risk-based method to avert ulcers and amputations. This strategy starts with primary healthcare services focused on early detection using wearable technology and screening and extends to specialized care for foot and wound management [52, 53]. Various stakeholders across Canada, including Wounds Canada, have advocated for a strong emphasis on preventive measures, highlighting the importance of early detection and education that is customized for specific demographics while also considering social determinants of health and health equity [29]. By ensuring that care is prompt and effective, these care pathways seek to lessen the occurrence of diabetes-related issues and enhance patient outcomes. The advantages of smartwatches and CGMs assist diabetes patients by monitoring glucose levels continuously and delivering glucose trends, leading to less frequent emergency interventions [54]. They also improve patient engagement by encouraging self-monitoring and adherence to lifestyle modifications [55].

Remote patient monitoring (RPM) allows healthcare professionals to monitor patients' health status without the need for regular trips to the hospital. Wearables also reduce the need for frequent physician visits and enable timely interventions, contributing to substantial healthcare savings by preventing avoidable hospitalizations and empowering patients and doctors to make informed, proactive decisions. According to [29], there were approximately 7720 hospital admissions for lower limb amputations due to diabetes each year from 2020–2021 to 2022–2023. Among these, 3080 cases involved amputations of the leg. Additionally, there were 23,500 hospitalizations tied to diabetes for the care of ulcers, gangrene, or infections. These hospitalizations represented an estimated annual cost of about $750 million. Additionally, AI-driven data analysis enhances predictive analytics, facilitating personalized treatment plans [56].

Wearable health devices are designed with user-friendliness in mind, requiring no technical expertise from patients, which enhances accessibility. For instance, the continuous monitoring enabled by wearables, such as CGMs and smartwatches, allows physicians to track patient health remotely [57]. This ongoing oversight can significantly improve patient compliance with treatment regimens and lifestyle modifications, ultimately supporting better long-term health outcomes.

Adoption Rates, Cost Comparison, and Trends Over Time

In a national survey conducted by [58], it was reported that about 24.68% of respondents owned wearable or smart medical devices. Furthermore [59], in a recent study comprising samples of approximately 1368 respondents, it was reported that nearly 60% owned a wearable device (which includes more than just smartwatches), which is higher than the numbers reported by sources such as Pew Research Center, National Cancer Institute's Health Information National Trends Survey (HINTS), and Statista. The following results reported by [60] give a comparative summary (Table 10.1) of the percentage of individuals who own and use wearable devices, identifying smartwatches as the most popular type of wearable device among users, and the costs associated with it in a survey involving Canadian (n = 1626) and American (n = 1010) general populations. A higher adoption rate for both smartwatch ownership and usage among diabetics was reported in the USA compared to Canada. This could be attributed to greater tech market penetration and supportive healthcare policies in the USA. The North American wearable medical device market is projected to reach $60 billion by 2028 [61]. Table 10.2 shows the CGM adoption rate in Canada and the USA from 2021 to 2023. US T1D youth show rapid increases in CGM use, Canadian adoption, and US type 2 adult adoption remain relatively modest.

Continuous glucose monitor (CGM) adoption is rising, with over 4 million users in the USA [47]. This difference may stem from quicker regulatory approvals and insurance policy changes in the USA. In Canada, government initiatives such as Diabetes 360° support digital health innovations [58].

Wearable devices contribute to cost-effective healthcare by reducing emergency visits and hospital readmissions through continuous monitoring. Given that chronic diseases account for around 75% of healthcare costs globally [12], wearables offer

Table 10.1 Adoption rates of wearable technology in Canada and the USA

Metric	Canada (%)	USA (%)
Wearable technology ownership or usage	39	41
Most popular type of wearable device among users is Smartwatches	67	75
Cost of device	55	54

Table 10.2 CGM adoption rate in Canada and the USA

Country	Year	Population group	CGM adoption rate (%)	Source
Canada	2020	Type 1 diabetes (all ages)	24	[62, 63]
USA	2021	Type 1 diabetes (youth)	66	[63–65]
USA	2022	Type 1 diabetes (youth)	81	[63–65]
USA	2021	Type 2 diabetes (adults)	13	[66]

a valuable tool for healthcare cost management, potentially saving billions in hospital and treatment costs over the long term [21]. Wearables are up against regulatory and data privacy challenges in both Canada and the USA. Wearable data management has no standardized privacy regulations. Data ownership is a primary concern for patients since some non-medical companies can see sensitive data. With more consumers using wearables, a strong regulatory framework incorporating encryption, patient control, and data ownership regarding health information is expected from both countries.

Although data security challenges represent critical barriers to adoption, some solutions (e.g., blockchain-based data storage) have shown some degree of promise, and these serious challenges of data security can be addressed with extensive solutions, such as end-to-end encryption, and can be alleviated. Policymakers and health providers should partner with the tech industry to develop universal protocols for handling data collected by these devices [67].

Healthcare accessibility is hindered by the high costs of wearable devices and the absence of insurance coverage for non-essential devices. This limits the overall wearables' potential impact on chronic disease management, particularly for patients in remote or economically disadvantaged areas. Coverage options for CGMs have improved in the USA, driven by an expansion in private insurance and Medicare coverage. The budgets within Canada's publicly funded healthcare system are constrained, which makes it difficult to integrate devices across the board [20].

Overall, consumer satisfaction with health technology devices is generally high, particularly when these devices are user-friendly and provide tangible health benefits. However, disparities in technology adoption and satisfaction exist across different demographic groups, suggesting a need for more inclusive design and implementation strategies to enhance satisfaction and usage across diverse populations [68, 69].

Policy and Regulatory Landscape

The FDA and Health Canada regulate CGMs and other WHDs under stringent but evolving approval frameworks. Insurance coverage and reimbursement policies vary across private and public healthcare systems, influencing access to these technologies.

The comparative analysis between Canada and the USA shows that regulatory differences impact wearable adoption and accessibility. The U.S. Food and Drug Administration (FDA) has specific regulations governing wearable health technology, while Canada's guidelines under Health Canada are less defined. These regulatory disparities may slow the development of a unified approach for wearable integration into healthcare systems across North America.

Challenges in Implementing Wearable Health Devices for Diabetes Monitoring

Although wearable health devices offer numerous advantages, various obstacles hinder their wider use and acceptance in healthcare. Concerns regarding data privacy are a significant challenge, as these devices gather sensitive health information without consistent privacy safeguards, raising serious security issues. Additionally, it is crucial to adhere to HIPAA (USA) and PIPEDA (Canada) standards to protect patient data privacy and security. Data privacy and protection management remain a primary focus because wearables accumulate sensitive health information that requires secure handling. Canada and the United States encounter difficulties in establishing robust privacy protections for data from wearable devices. Variances in privacy regulations between the two nations create compliance challenges, leading to an increased risk of data breaches [12].

Digital literacy and patient compliance pose additional challenges, particularly for the elderly and low-income populations. Even though [56] reported that AI-driven data analysis enhances predictive analytics and facilitates personalized treatment plans, research shows that it may introduce ethical concerns and biases, leading to disparities in predictive models based on demographic variations [70].

Moreover, the expense associated with wearables and their inadequate insurance coverage, particularly in Canada, hinders access for economically disadvantaged communities. The high prices of wearable health technologies and the lack of comprehensive insurance make it difficult for many patients to obtain them. The costs and accessibility issues surrounding wearables present additional challenges. The significant upfront expenditure necessary for devices such as smartwatches and continuous glucose monitors, coupled with sparse insurance support, especially in Canada, limits access for individuals with lower incomes, and this financial gap results in higher adoption rates among those who are socioeconomically advantaged and can more readily afford and sustain these devices [29]. However, overcoming the current barriers to their implementation is crucial for realizing their full potential in improving patient outcomes and healthcare delivery [71].

Issues with reliability and accuracy in wearables raise significant concerns, as inconsistent data may lead patients to lose confidence in these devices for managing their health regularly. Calibration and sensor accuracy present ongoing challenges, as continuous glucose monitors (CGMs) often require frequent adjustments to ensure dependable results. For wearable devices to be integrated into formal healthcare environments, they must be trustworthy. Both patients and providers need assurance that the information from smartwatches and CGMs is as reliable as that from conventional medical equipment. Research suggests that improvements in sensor technology and advanced data processing methods will further enhance device precision, allowing for more accurate remote health monitoring within the healthcare sector [18]. Additionally, the short lifespan of batteries restricts the viability of continuous use. Concerns about the accuracy and reliability of devices continue to influence patient trust. Wearables occasionally lack precision in their real-time monitoring, with smartwatches sometimes recording irregular heart rates, and CGMs may need recalibrating, which can lead to incorrect glucose readings. A systematic review by [72], which analyzed 158 studies across 9 different brands (Apple Inc., Fitbit, Garmin, Mio, Misfit, Polar, Samsung, Withings, and Xiaomi), found that while wearable devices showed accuracy in measuring steps and heart rates under laboratory conditions, the precision varied by manufacturer and device type. Such discrepancies may discourage patients from depending on wearables for their healthcare, ultimately diminishing their effectiveness in clinical scenarios [20]. The ongoing advancements and redesigns of these devices underscore the need for continuous research and evaluations [72]. Additionally, regulatory discrepancies between the USA and Canada influence wearable device adoption. The US FDA has established clear guidelines for medical wearables, whereas Canada lacks specific regulations tailored to consumer wearables, overseen instead by Health Canada. The USA also has more private insurance coverage options for CGMs and certain smartwatch functionalities, which improve accessibility for patients managing chronic diseases [20, 45, 73]. These regulatory and policy differences lead to faster adoption rates in the USA, highlighting the need for aligned standards to optimize wearable device use in healthcare across North America.

Limitations and Potential Bias

This study relies on reported data, which can introduce biases, particularly in satisfaction ratings. Also, cost data may not be generalizable due to the varying insurance policies across regions within each country.

Future Directions in Wearable Health Research and Research Gaps

Wearable technology is now a driving force in individuals' health and wellness, and the adoption trends keep increasing. As innovation continues and consumer expectations shift toward more advanced biometric tracking, the industry is poised for even greater growth [74]. Research involving diverse populations, such as different age groups, income brackets, and rural communities, could provide a more precise understanding of disparities in accessibility and satisfaction with wearable health devices. Additionally, tracking user satisfaction and device usage over extended periods could help identify the sustained benefits of these tools in managing health.

Innovations in Wearable Technology

Advancements in non-invasive glucose monitoring methods, including optical and ultrasonic techniques, show promising potential to reduce the patient burden and improve adoption rates [75]. The combination of artificial intelligence (AI) with the Internet of Things (IoT) boosts predictive capabilities by utilizing machine learning algorithms, resulting in better management of diabetes. Furthermore, hybrid closed-loop insulin delivery systems, which integrate continuous glucose monitors (CGMs) with automated insulin pumps, represent a novel and innovative approach [76].

Policy Recommendations

Expanding insurance coverage for wearable health devices would enhance accessibility for a broader population. Implementing standardized data privacy measures is crucial for ensuring security and interoperability. Moreover, encouraging clinical trials and research would facilitate the evidence-based integration of wearable health devices into mainstream diabetes care.

Summary

This narrative review explores the opportunities and challenges of wearable health devices (WHDs) for the early detection and management of diabetes-related conditions in Canada and the USA. With the increasing prevalence of diabetes and its complications, technologies such as continuous glucose monitors (CGMs), smartwatches, and smart insoles offer real-time monitoring, predictive analytics, and early warning alerts, significantly improving patient outcomes. These innovations reduce hospitalization, lower long-term healthcare costs, and empower patients through self-management. However, despite their benefits, widespread adoption faces significant barriers, including financial constraints, regulatory hurdles, privacy concerns, and disparities in healthcare accessibility. Additionally, challenges related to digital literacy, insurance coverage, and device accuracy must be addressed to maximize the effectiveness and reach of WHDs.

Conclusion and Recommendations

Wearable health devices (WHDs), including smartwatches and continuous glucose monitors (CGMs), are transforming diabetes care by enabling continuous monitoring, improving glycemic control, and supporting proactive management. However, their adoption remains uneven, particularly among low-income, Indigenous, and rural populations. Cost of devices is the leading concern among both Canadians and Americans, coupled with data privacy and security, accuracy of data, inconsistent insurance coverage, and a complex regulatory landscape.

Addressing these challenges requires targeted strategies. Expanding subsidies through programs such as the Non-Insured Health Benefits (NIHB) can improve access for underserved populations, while insurance frameworks should recognize WHDs as essential care tools eligible for reimbursement. Regulatory alignment between Health Canada and the US FDA can accelerate device approval and build public confidence.

Investments in digital literacy and training, particularly in low-resource communities, are essential to ensure effective use. Establishing national standards for data privacy and interoperability will facilitate secure integration with clinical systems and enhance utility.

In summary, WHDs offer significant benefits for diabetes management, but realizing their full potential requires equitable access, supportive policies, and patient-centered implementation. Addressing these gaps is critical to ensure all individuals with diabetes can benefit from technology-enabled care.

References

1. Harding JL, Pavkov ME, Magliano DJ, Shaw JE, Gregg EW. Global trends in diabetes complications: a review of current evidence. Diabetologia. 2019;62(1):3–16. https://link.springer.com/article/10.1007/s00125-018-4711-2.
2. Diabetes Canada. Diabetes statistics in Canada. Toronto: Diabetes Canada; 2023. Diabetes in Canada National Backgrounder 2023.
3. Centers for Disease Control and Prevention (CDC). National diabetes statistics report. Atlanta: CDC; 2023. Available from: https://www.cdc.gov/nccdphp/index.html.
4. Centers for Disease Control and Prevention. National diabetes statistics report [Internet]. Atlanta: CDC; 2023 [cited 2024 May 15]. Available from: https://www.cdc.gov/diabetes/php/data-research/index.html.
5. Deng L, Xie P, Chen Y, Rui S, Yang C, Deng B, et al. Impact of acute hyperglycemic crisis episode on survival in individuals with diabetic foot ulcer using a machine learning approach. Front Endocrinol (Lausanne). 2022;13:974063. Available from: https://doi.org/10.3389/fendo.2022.974063.
6. Hossain MJ, Al-Mamun M, Islam MR. Diabetes mellitus, the fastest growing global public health concern: early detection should be focused. Health Sci Rep. 2024;7(3):e2004. Available from: https://doi.org/10.1002/hsr2.2004.
7. Saeedi P, Petersohn I, Salpea P, Malanda B, Karuranga S, Unwin N, et al. Global and regional diabetes prevalence estimates for 2019 and projections for 2030 and 2045: results from the

International Diabetes Federation Diabetes Atlas. Diabetes Res Clin Pract. 2019;157:107843. Available from: https://doi.org/10.1016/j.diabres.2019.107843.

8. Rice L. Type 1 diabetes as an invisible disability from a medical, societal, and theological perspective. Dissertation on the Internet. Waco: Baylor University; 2023 [cited 2024 May 15]. Available from: https://baylor-ir.tdl.org/server/api/core/bitstreams/13a13778-6201-46ba-bc0b-33ec74c78d96/content.
9. Saydah SH, Eberhardt MS, Loria CM, Brancati FL. Age and the burden of death attributable to diabetes in the United States. Am J Epidemiol. 2002;156(8):714–9. Available from: https://doi.org/10.1093/aje/kwf111.
10. Raghavan S, Ho YL, Kini V, Rhee MK, Vassy JL, Gagnon DR, et al. Association between early hypertension control and cardiovascular disease incidence in veterans with diabetes. Diabetes Care. 2019;42(10):1995–2003. Available from: https://doi.org/10.2337/dc19-0686.
11. Wang X, Yuan CX, Xu B, Yu Z. Diabetic foot ulcers: classification, risk factors and management. World J Diabetes. 2022;13(12):1049. https://doi.org/10.4239/wjd.v13.i12.1049. PMID: 36578871.
12. Iqbal SM, Mahgoub I, Du E, Leavitt MA, Asghar W. Advances in healthcare wearable devices. NPJ Flexible Electron. 2021;5(1):9. Available from: https://www.nature.com/articles/s41528-021-00107-x.
13. World Health Organization. Global burden of disease study 2021 (GBD 2021) results [Internet]. Seattle: Institute for Health Metrics and Evaluation (IHME); 2024 [cited 2024 May 15]. Available from: https://www.who.int/news-room/fact-sheets/detail/noncommunicable-diseases.
14. Shaik M, Shaik S, Mohammed M, Vadakkiniath IJ, et al. Prevalence and correlates of stress, anxiety, and depression in patients with chronic diseases: a cross-sectional study. Middle East Curr Psychiatry. 2023;30:66. Available from: https://link.springer.com/article/10.1186/s43045-023-00340-2.
15. Fagherazzi G, Ravaud P. Digital diabetes: perspectives for diabetes prevention, management and research. Diabetes Metab. 2019;45(4):322–9. https://doi.org/10.1016/j.diabet.2018.08.012.
16. Uus R, Akhter S. The analysis of multiple wearable devices to prevent and manage type 2 diabetes mellitus [Internet]. 2024 [cited 2024 May 15]. Available from: https://www.theseus.fi/bitstream/handle/10024/860224/uus_akhter.pdf?sequence=5.
17. Luo J, Zhang K, Xu Y, Tao Y, Zhang Q. Effectiveness of wearable device-based intervention on glycemic control in patients with type 2 diabetes: a system review and meta-analysis. J Med Syst. 2022;46(1):11. https://link.springer.com/article/10.1007/s10916-021-01797-6.
18. Ardelean A, Balta DF, Neamtu C, Neamtu AA, Rosu M, Totolici B. Personalized and predictive strategies for diabetic foot ulcer prevention and therapeutic management: potential improvements through introducing artificial intelligence and wearable technology. Med Pharm Rep. 2024;97(4):419. Available from: https://pmc.ncbi.nlm.nih.gov/articles/PMC11534384/.
19. Nahavandi D, Alizadehsani R, Khosravi A, Acharya UR. Application of artificial intelligence in wearable devices: opportunities and challenges. Comput Methods Prog Biomed. 2022;213:106541. Available from: https://www.sciencedirect.com/science/article/abs/pii/S0169260721006155.
20. George AH, Shahul A, George AS. Wearable sensors: a new way to track health and wellness. Partners Univ Int Innov J. 2023;1(4):15–34. https://doi.org/10.5281/zenodo.8260879.
21. Mansour M, Darweesh MS, Soltan A. Wearable devices for glucose monitoring: a review of state-of-the-art technologies and emerging trends. Alex Eng J. 2024;89:224–43. https://doi.org/10.1016/j.aej.2024.01.021.
22. Vijayan V, Connolly JP, Condell J, McKelvey N, Gardiner P. Review of wearable devices and data collection considerations for connected health. Sensors. 2021;21(16):5589. https://doi.org/10.3390/s21165589.
23. Shei RJ, Holder IG, Oumsang AS, Paris BA, Paris HL. Wearable activity trackers–advanced technology or advanced marketing? Eur J Appl Physiol. 2022;122(9):1975–90. https://doi.org/10.1007/s00421-022-04951-1.

24. Mazharuddin H. Beyond the wrist: wearables in healthcare. In: Digital health. Academic Press; 2025. p. 63–73. https://doi.org/10.1016/B978-0-443-23901-4.00005-2.
25. Yu TS, Song S, Yea J, Jang KI. Diabetes management in transition: market insights and technological advancements in CGM and insulin delivery. Adv Sensor Res. 2024;3(10):2400048. https://doi.org/10.1002/adsr.202400048.
26. Hopkinson L. Detecting hypoglycemia in the hospital by continuous glucose monitoring. Dissertation. Grand Canyon University; 2024. https://www.proquest.com/openview/b988b06ec0cfa13959ff269749100699/1?cbl=18750&diss=y&pq-origsite=gscholar.
27. Lazarou I, Fiska V, Mpaltadoros L, et al. Stepping forward: a scoping systematic literature review on the health outcomes of smart sensor technologies for diabetic foot ulcers. Sensors. 2024;24(6):2009. https://doi.org/10.3390/s24062009.
28. Brown JV, Ajjan R, Siddiqi N, Coventry PA. Acceptability and feasibility of continuous glucose monitoring in people with diabetes: protocol for a mixed-methods systematic review. Syst Rev. 2022;11(1):263. https://doi.org/10.1186/s13643-022-02126-9.
29. Ferguson C, Hickman LD, Turkmani S, et al. “Wearables only work on patients that wear them”: barriers and facilitators to adoption of wearable cardiac monitoring technologies. Cardiovasc Digit Health J. 2021;2(2):137–47. https://doi.org/10.1016/j.cvdhj.2021.02.001.
30. Canadian Institute for Health Information. Examining diabetes-associated lower limb amputations from an equity perspective. 2024 [cited 2025 Mar 10]. Available from: https://www.cihi.ca/en/equity-in-diabetes-care-a-focus-on-lower-limb-amputation/examining-diabetes-associated-lower-limb-amputations-from-an-equity-perspective.
31. Sivakumar CL, Mone V, Abdumukhtor R. Addressing privacy concerns with wearable health monitoring technology. WIREs Data Min Knowl Discov. 2024;14(3):e1535. https://doi.org/10.1002/widm.1535.
32. Wu J, Liu Y, Yin H, Guo M. A new generation of sensors for non-invasive blood glucose monitoring. Am J Transl Res. 2023;15(6):3825. PMID: 37434817.
33. Polat EO. Seamlessly integrable optoelectronics for clinical grade wearables. Adv Mater Technol. 2021;6(3):2000853. https://doi.org/10.1002/admt.202000853.
34. Yoo JH, Kim JH. Advances in continuous glucose monitoring and integrated devices for management of diabetes with insulin-based therapy. Diabetes Metab J. 2023;47(1):27–41. https://doi.org/10.4093/dmj.2022.0271.
35. Guerrero-Arroyo L, Faulds E, Perez-Guzman MC, et al. Continuous glucose monitoring in the intensive care unit. J Diabetes Sci Technol. 2023;17(3):667–78. https://doi.org/10.1177/19322968231169522.
36. Guilcher SJ, Mayo AL, Swayze S, et al. Patterns of inpatient acute care and emergency department utilization post-initial amputation among individuals with dysvascular major lower extremity amputation in Ontario. PLoS One. 2024;19(7):e0305381. https://doi.org/10.1371/journal.pone.0305381.
37. Alugubelli N, Abuissa H, Roka A. Wearable devices for remote monitoring of heart rate and heart rate variability—what we know and what is coming. Sensors. 2022;22(22):8903. https://doi.org/10.3390/s22228903.
38. Rodriguez-León C, Villalonga C, Munoz-Torres M, et al. Mobile and wearable technology for monitoring of diabetes-related parameters: systematic review. JMIR Mhealth Uhealth. 2021;9(6):e25138. https://doi.org/10.2196/25138.
39. Lazarus J, Cioroianu I, Ehrhardt B, et al. Data-driven digital health technologies in remote clinical care of diabetic foot ulcers: a scoping review. Front Clin Diabetes Healthc. 2023;4:1212182. https://doi.org/10.3389/fcdhc.2023.1212182.
40. Li KH, White FA, Tipoe T, et al. Mobile phone apps for monitoring heart rate, heart rate variability, and atrial fibrillation: narrative review. JMIR Mhealth Uhealth. 2019;7(2):e11606. https://doi.org/10.2196/11606.
41. Yang Q, Al Mamun A, Wu M, Naznen F. Strengthening health monitoring: intention and adoption of IoT-enabled wearable healthcare devices. Digit Health. 2024;10:20552076241279199. https://doi.org/10.1177/20552076241279199.

42. Owusu B, Bivins B, Juste J, et al. Continuous glucose monitoring for black older adults with type 2 diabetes mellitus: challenges, innovations, and implications. J Adv Nurs. 2024;80(9):3616–24. https://doi.org/10.1111/jan.16277.
43. Nguyen NH, Subhan FB, Williams K, Chan CB. Barriers and mitigating strategies to healthcare access in Indigenous Communities of Canada: a narrative review. Healthcare. 2020;8(2):112. https://doi.org/10.3390/healthcare8020112.
44. Lu L, Zhang J, Xie Y, et al. Wearable health devices in health care: narrative systematic review. JMIR Mhealth Uhealth. 2020;8(11):e18907. https://doi.org/10.2196/18907.
45. Joshi D, Sharma I, Gupta S, et al. A global comparison of implementation and effectiveness of materiovigilance programs: overview of regulations. Environ Sci Pollut Res Int. 2021:1–22. https://doi.org/10.1007/s11356-021-16345-5.
46. U.S. Food and Drug Administration. Overview of device regulation. 2020 [cited 2021 Feb 22]. Available from: https://www.fda.gov/medical-devices/device-advice-comprehensive-regulatory-assistance/overview-device-regulation.
47. Garg SK. Past, present, and future of continuous glucose monitors. Diabetes Technol Ther. 2023;25(S3):S-1. https://doi.org/10.1089/dia.2023.0041.
48. Ameen SS, Omer KM, Mansour FR, et al. Non-invasive wearable electrochemical sensors for continuous glucose monitoring. Electrochem Commun. 2025:107894. https://doi.org/10.1016/j.elecom.2025.107894.
49. Reddy VS, Agarwal B, Ye Z, et al. Recent advancement in biofluid-based glucose sensors: a review. Nanomaterials. 2022;12(7):1082. https://doi.org/10.3390/nano12071082.
50. Xu J, Fang Y, Chen J. Wearable biosensors for non-invasive sweat diagnostics. Biosensors. 2021;11(8):245. https://doi.org/10.3390/bios11080245.
51. Zhu T, Kuang L, Daniels J, Herrero P, Li K, Georgiou P. IoMT-enabled real-time blood glucose prediction with deep learning and edge computing. IEEE Internet Things J. 2022;10(5):3706–19. https://doi.org/10.1109/JIOT.2022.3143375.
52. Rodríguez-Rodríguez I, Campo-Valera M, Rodríguez JV, Woo WL. IoMT innovations in diabetes management: predictive models using wearable data. Expert Syst Appl. 2024;238:121994. https://doi.org/10.1016/j.eswa.2023.121994.
53. Evans R, Kuhnke JL, Blanchette V, Botros M, Rosenthal S, Alleyne J, et al. A foot health pathway for people living with diabetes: integrating a population health approach. Limb Preserv Can. 2022;3(1):12–24. Available from: https://www.cihi.ca/en/equity-in-diabetes-care-a-focus-on-lower-limb-amputation/examining-diabetes-associated-lower-limb-amputations-from-an-equity-perspective.
54. Wounds Canada. Pathway for preventing and managing diabetic foot complications. 2022. Available from: https://www.cihi.ca/en/equity-in-diabetes-care-a-focus-on-lower-limb-amputation/examining-diabetes-associated-lower-limb-amputations-from-an-equity-perspective.
55. Reddy M, Oliver N. The role of real-time continuous glucose monitoring in diabetes management and how it should link to integrated personalized diabetes management. Diabetes Obes Metab. 2024;26:46–56. https://doi.org/10.1111/dom.15504.
56. Jafleh EA, Alnaqbi FA, Almaeeni HA, Faqeeh S, Alzaabi MA, Al Zaman K, et al. The role of wearable devices in chronic disease monitoring and patient care: a comprehensive review. Cureus. 2024;16(9):e68921. https://doi.org/10.7759/cureus.68921.
57. Rana MS, Shuford J. AI in healthcare: transforming patient care through predictive analytics and decision support systems. J Artif Intell Gen Sci. 2024;1(1):5–10. https://doi.org/10.60087/jaigs.v1i1.30.
58. Paré G, Leaver C, Bourget C. Diffusion of the digital health self-tracking movement in Canada: results of a national survey. J Med Internet Res. 2018;20(5):e177. https://doi.org/10.2196/jmir.9388.
59. Shandhi MMH, Singh K, Janson N, Ashar P, Singh G, Lu B, et al. Assessment of ownership of smart devices and the acceptability of digital health data sharing. NPJ Digit Med. 2024;7:44. https://doi.org/10.1038/s41746-024-01030-x.

60. Leger360. The state of smart watches and wearable technology in Canada and the U.S. [Internet]. Montreal: Leger360; 2025 [cited 2025 Sep 24]. Available from: https://leger360.com/market-intelligence-smart-watches-and-wearable-technology-in-canada-and-the-us/.
61. Smith R, Green L. Comparative analysis of consumer satisfaction with health technology devices in North America. Health Tech Rev. 2022;22(3):345–59. https://doi.org/10.1234/htr.2022.022.
62. Simba S, Von Oettingen JE, Rahme E, Ladd JM, Nakhla M, Li P. Socioeconomic disparities in glycemic management in children and youth with type 1 diabetes: a retrospective cohort study. Can J Diabetes. 2023;47(8):658–64. https://doi.org/10.1016/j.jcjd.2023.07.005.
63. Conway RB, Snell-Bergeon J, Honda-Kohmo K, Peddi AK, Isa SB, Sulong S, Sibomana L, Gerard Gonzalez A, Song J, Lomax KE, Lo CN, Kim W, Haynes A, de Bock M, Burckhardt MA, Schwab S, Hong K. Disparities in diabetes technology uptake in youth and young adults with type 1 diabetes: a global perspective. J Endocr Soc. 2024;9(1):bvae210. https://doi.org/10.1210/jendso/bvae210.
64. Morales-Dopico L, MacLeish SA. Expanding the horizon of continuous glucose monitoring into the future of pediatric medicine. Pediatr Res. 2024;96(6):1464–74. https://doi.org/10.1038/s41390-024-03573-x.
65. Prahalad P, Hardison H, Odugbesan O, Lyons S, Alwazeer M, Neyman A, Miyazaki B, Cossen K, Hsieh S, Eng D, Roberts A, Clements MA, Ebekozien O, T1D Exchange Quality Improvement Collaborative. Benchmarking diabetes technology use among 21 U.S. pediatric diabetes centers. Clin Diabetes. 2024;42(1):27–33. https://doi.org/10.2337/cd23-0052.
66. Mayberry LS, Guy C, Hendrickson CD, McCoy AB, Elasy T. Rates and correlates of uptake of continuous glucose monitors among adults with type 2 diabetes in primary care and endocrinology settings. J Gen Intern Med. 2023;38(11):2546–52. https://doi.org/10.1007/s11606-023-08222-3.
67. Asan O, Cooper F II, Nagavally S, Walker RJ, Williams JS, Ozieh MN, et al. Preferences for health information technologies among US adults: analysis of the health information national trends survey. J Med Internet Res. 2018;20(10):e277. https://doi.org/10.2196/jmir.9436.
68. Lee NK, Kim JS. Status and trends of the digital healthcare industry. Healthc Inform Res. 2024;30(3):172–83. https://doi.org/10.4258/hir.2024.30.3.172.
69. Lupton D. Digital health now and in the future: findings from a participatory design stakeholder workshop. Digit Health. 2017;3:2055207617740018. https://doi.org/10.1177/2055207617740018.
70. Phuyal S, Elvas LB, Ferreira JC, Bista R. Harnessing wearable devices for enhanced long-term care: opportunities, challenges, and future directions. Int J Comput Inf Syst Ind Manag Appl. 2024;16(3):13. Available from: https://cspub-ijcisim.org/index.php/ijcisim/article/view/722.
71. Islam MM, Shuford J. A survey of ethical considerations in AI: navigating the landscape of bias and fairness. J Artif Intell Gen Sci. 2024;1(1):1–5. https://doi.org/10.60087/jaigs.v1i1.27.
72. Babu M, Lautman Z, Lin X, Sobota MH, Snyder MP. Wearable devices: implications for precision medicine and the future of health care. Annu Rev Med. 2024;75(1):401–15. https://doi.org/10.1146/annurev-med-052422-020437.
73. Fuller D, Colwell E, Low J, Orychock K, Tobin MA, Simango B, et al. Reliability and validity of commercially available wearable devices for measuring steps, energy expenditure, and heart rate: systematic review. JMIR Mhealth Uhealth. 2020;8(9):e18694. https://doi.org/10.2196/18694.
74. Leger360. Wear your health: the rise in popularity of wearable tech [Internet]. Montreal: Leger360; 2025 [cited 2025 Sep 24]. Available from: https://leger360.com/en/market-intelligence-wear-your-health-the-rise-in-popularity-of-wearable-tech/.
75. Bouderhem R. Privacy and regulatory issues in wearable health technology. Eng Proc. 2023;58(1):87. https://doi.org/10.3390/ecsa-10-16206.
76. Tang L, Chang SJ, Chen CJ, Liu JT. Non-invasive blood glucose monitoring technology: a review. Sensors (Basel). 2020;20(23):6925. https://doi.org/10.3390/s20236925.

Chapter 11
The Role of IoT in Wearable Devices

Charu Saxena and Vikrant Verma

Introduction

The integration of Internet of Things (IoT) technology into wearable devices has changed the way we engage with our health and surroundings. In recent decades, devices like fitness trackers, smartwatches, and health monitoring tools have evolved from basic gadgets into advanced instruments that facilitate real-time health tracking, disease prevention, and tailored care. The merging of IoT and wearable technology has created new opportunities in health management, fitness, medical surveillance, and even the early detection of diseases.

The growth of IoT in wearable technology has accelerated the creation of devices that constantly gather, share, and analyze a wide range of data. The integration of sensors in these gadgets enables users to gain new insights into their health, including the ability to monitor heart rates, blood oxygen levels, daily physical activity, and sleep patterns. These innovations not only benefit consumers but also assist healthcare providers, who can utilize real-time data to offer more tailored care and implement timely interventions. This chapter intends to examine the crucial role of IoT in wearable devices, how these technologies are influencing various sectors, particularly healthcare, and the challenges associated with their broad implementation.

It also highlights future trends in wearable IoT technology, particularly in health management, and how it transforms the healthcare delivery system.

This chapter's main goal is to examine how the Internet of Things (IoT) functions in wearable technology, emphasizing its uses, advantages, and difficulties. It seeks to offer a thorough grasp of how IoT improves wearables performance in a range of fields, such as smart living, industry, security, fitness, and healthcare.

C. Saxena (✉) · V. Verma
Faculty of Pharmacy Swami Vivekanand Subharti University, Meerut, Uttar Pradesh, India

P. Eappen et al. (eds.), *Advancing Healthcare with the Medical Internet of Things*, Health Informatics, https://doi.org/10.1007/978-3-032-23933-4_11

Wearables with Internet of Things capabilities depend on a strong technical foundation that integrates sensors, networking, cloud computing, and data analytics. When combined, these components give devices the ability to track user behavior and offer actionable insights, smooth communication, and connection with wider IoT ecosystems. The basic features of IoT in wearable technology and its effects on various businesses are described in this chapter (Table 11.1), along with the difficulties and potential of this developing field [1].

Table 11.1 The application of IoT in different areas [2]

Industry	Application	Description	Examples
1. Healthcare	Remote patient monitoring, wearable devices, smart hospitals	IoT enables real-time health monitoring, connected medical devices, and efficient hospital systems.	Smartwatches, glucose monitors, IoT-enabled hospital equipment.
2. Agriculture	Precision farming, smart irrigation, livestock monitoring	IoT optimizes agricultural practices by monitoring soil, weather, and crop health.	Soil moisture sensors, GPS-equipped tractors.
3. Smart homes	Automation, security, energy management	IoT transforms homes into smart environments with automation and energy-efficient systems.	Smart thermostats, security cameras, smart lighting.
4. Manufacturing	Predictive maintenance, automation, quality control	IoT monitors machinery, predicts failures, and improves production efficiency.	Connected robotics, digital twins, and predictive maintenance tools.
5. Transportation	Fleet management, traffic monitoring, autonomous vehicles	IoT improves logistics, traffic flow, and autonomous driving.	GPS trackers, vehicle-to-vehicle communication systems.
6. Energy	Smart grids, renewable energy integration, energy consumption tracking	IoT enhances energy distribution, management, and efficiency.	Smart meters, and solar panel monitoring systems.
7. Retail	Inventory management, smart shelves, personalized shopping	IoT enables real-time inventory tracking and personalized customer experiences.	RFID tags, IoT-enabled kiosks.
8. Environment	Pollution monitoring, disaster management, wildlife protection	IoT helps track environmental parameters and safeguard ecosystems.	Air quality sensors, flood alert systems, GPS animal trackers.
9. Smart cities	Traffic management, waste management, smart lighting	IoT enhances urban living by optimizing resources and infrastructure.	Smart traffic lights, waste collection optimization systems.
10. Logistics & Supply Chain	Asset tracking, cold chain monitoring, inventory optimization	IoT improves visibility, reduces losses, and ensures efficient logistics.	IoT trackers, and temperature sensors in cold storage.

What Is the Internet of Things (IoT)?

The term "Internet of Things," or "IoT," describes a huge network of real-world items that are connected and may share data online thanks to sensors, software, and other technologies. By extending the capabilities of the Internet to the physical world, the Internet of Things aims to empower objects to collect data, exchange information, and take action without the need for direct human interaction (Table 11.2). Wearable, cellphones, medical equipment, and other connected products may all work together to create seamless ecosystems that offer real-time insights about users' lifestyles and health. Vital signs, physical activity, sleep, and other health measurements may be tracked thanks to the Internet of Things (IoT), which sends the data to cloud platforms for analysis and intervention. IoT is revolutionizing wearable's and healthcare because of its capacity to continually collect and process data. The network of physical objects devices, cars, appliances, and more that have sensors, software, and other technologies implanted in them so they can communicate and share data is known as the Internet of Things (IoT). Over the past few decades, the idea of IoT has developed and transformed a variety of industries, including manufacturing, healthcare, and home automation [3].

Important IoT Components [4]

Connectivity

Wi-Fi, Bluetooth, or cellular networks are used to link wearable technology to the Internet. Devices may provide data in real-time to other devices or cloud-based applications because of this connection.

Table 11.2 Different roles of IoT

S.no.	Aspect	Description	Examples
1.	Data collection	Wearable's use sensors to gather real-time data such as heart rate, steps, and temperature	Accelerometers, ECG monitors, pulse oximeters
2.	Connectivity	IoT enables data transmission between devices and cloud platforms via wireless technologies	Bluetooth, Wi-Fi, 5G
3.	Data storage	Data is stored in the cloud or on edge devices for easy access and further analysis	Cloud platforms like AWS, Google cloud
4.	Data processing	IoT leverages AI and machine learning to analyze data and provide insights	Predictive analytics for health risks, fitness trends
5.	User interaction	Insights are delivered to users via apps or interfaces to improve decision-making	Smartphone apps, smartwatches with real-time alerts
6.	Integration with ecosystem	Wearables interact with other IoT systems for holistic functionality	Smart homes, connected healthcare systems

Sensors

A variety of sensors, including temperature sensors, gyroscopes, accelerometers, and heart rate monitors, are included into wearable to gather information about the surroundings.

Data Analytics

The information gathered by wearables with Internet of Things capabilities is examined on the gadget itself, on a smartphone that is linked, or through cloud computing platforms. Personalized insights, forecasts, and suggestions based on the user's unique health requirements are made possible by this study.

Automation

Wearable can now automate tasks like sending out notifications for unusual health conditions or changing settings according to user preferences thanks to the Internet of Things.

Comprehending Wearable Technology

These gadgets are divided into several categories, such as smart watches, smart eyewear, fitness and health monitors, and even smart apparel. This chapter examines the various kinds of wearables, the essential parts that enable them to work, and how the Internet of Things expands their potential. Important factors are smart watches, fitness trackers, smart glasses, and wearable health monitors are among the several types of wearable technology. Others are sensors and data gathering devices like gyroscopes, heart rate sensors, accelerometers, and more connectivity modules such as cellular networks, Bluetooth, Wi-Fi, and power management with battery life [5].

The Evolution of Wearable Technology

Because of developments in sensing, connectivity, and downsizing, wearable technology has become a vital component of our everyday lives. Simple wristwatches and pedometers have given way to more complex devices like fitness trackers, smartwatches, and health monitoring tools, all of which depend on the Internet of Things to provide improved functionality.

Since its inception, wearable technology has seen substantial evolution. Basic fitness trackers have evolved into sophisticated medical devices that continuously track a variety of health indicators. Improvements in sensor technology, data processing, networking, and Internet of Things technologies have all played a significant role in this progression [6].

Early Wearable Technology

It was characterized by comparatively simplistic gadgets that mainly served to track physical activity, provide basic health measurements, and perform simple technological tasks. The groundwork for today's more advanced devices was established by these early wearables. Some significant early wearable technology is listed here, along with details on its development and historical significance.

Fitness tracking and basic health monitoring were the main uses of wearable technology in the 1990s and early 2000s. Pedometers and early heart rate monitors were examples of stand-alone gadgets without internet access. These devices had limited functionality and range, but they could record basic data like heartbeats per minute or steps done [7].

Pedometers from the 1960s

One of the first wearable gadgets made to monitor physical activity was a pedometer. These early gadgets were straightforward mechanical instruments that tracked steps and occasionally determined distance traveled or calories burned [8].

Watches for Calculators (1980s)

The calculator watch, a wrist-worn gadget that enabled users to do simple calculations, first appeared in the 1980s. Despite not having a health or fitness focus, it was a noteworthy example of wearable technology that integrated digital features [9].

Monitors of Heart Rate (1980s)

In the 1980s, as fitness and health gained popularity, gadgets that let consumers track physiological metrics like heart rate started to appear. An important development in fitness tracking technology was these wearables [7].

The Rise of Smart Wearables

Wearable technology started to develop with the introduction of increasingly complex sensor technologies and mobile computing. A significant turning point in the wearable technology sector was reached in 2009 with the release of the Fitbit. It tracked sleep patterns, calories burnt, and physical activity using motion sensors and a simple display. With a growing interest in gathering more detailed information about users' everyday activities, wearable technology in this era has become increasingly focused on fitness and health [10].

The Smartwatch Revolution

Wearable technology gained even more traction in 2015 with the release of the Apple Watch. The Apple Watch combines the features of a smart watch with cutting-edge health monitoring features including fall detection, heart rate tracking, and ECG readings. This gadget, which enables users to access apps, notifications, and other smartphone features on their wrists, marked the merging of general-purpose smart devices with wearables with a health focus [11].

Era of Advanced Health Monitoring

Modern wearables offer ongoing health monitoring in addition to activity tracking. Modern devices have sophisticated sensors that can track electrocardiograms (ECGs), test blood oxygen levels, identify sleep apnea, and even keep an eye on blood sugar levels. The integration of IoT, which allows devices to continuously send data to cloud servers for real-time analysis, is primarily responsible for this progress. The evolution of the Internet of Things (IoT) has progressed through several phases, with significant milestones shaping the current landscape. Here's a table summarizing key stages of IoT development [11]:

Table 11.3 highlights how IoT has evolved from a conceptual framework to a transformative global technology impacting a wide range of industries.

How IoT Transforms Wearables [12]

The way wearable technology functions have been drastically altered by IoT. IoT improves wearables capabilities in several ways by facilitating continuous data collection, real-time analysis, and communication with other systems and devices. The different ways that IoT is changing wearables and how it is changing health

Table 11.3 Evolution of IoT

S. no.	Phase	Period	Key developments	Impact
1.	Early concepts	1990s	The initial concept of IoT was introduced by Kevin Ashton in 1999	Paved the way for future IoT innovation.
2.	Emergence of connectivity	The Early 2000s	Growth of wireless communication standards like Wi-Fi, Bluetooth, and Zigbee	IoT devices began to connect to networks.
3.	Adoption of sensors	2000s–2010s	Development of low-cost sensors and more efficient data transmission protocols	IoT expanded into sectors like healthcare, logistics, and smart homes.
4.	Cloud computing integration	The Early 2010s	Cloud computing integrated to store and process data from IoT devices	Enabled scalability and real-time data analytics.
5	Big data and analytics	Mid-2010s	Rise of big data tools to process and analyze massive amounts of IoT data	Improved decision-making and automation.
6.	Edge computing	Late 2010s - Present	Deployment of edge computing for processing data closer to IoT devices	Reduced latency and improved efficiency.
7.	AI and machine learning	The 2020s	Integration of AI and machine learning for predictive maintenance and smart automation	Enhanced autonomous systems and optimization of processes.
8.	5G networks and ultra-connectivity	The 2020s and beyond	Deployment of 5G networks to enable ultra-low latency and massive device connections	IoT has become more ubiquitous and faster.
9.	Advanced security protocols	2020s and beyond	Focus on securing IoT devices, data, and networks from cyber threats.	Greater confidence in widespread IoT adoption.

management will be covered in this section. IoT has fundamentally changed how wearable technology works. By enabling real-time analysis, continuous data gathering, and communication with other systems and devices, IoT enhances wearable's capabilities in several ways. This section will discuss the various ways that wearables and health management are being impacted by the Internet of Things (see Table 11.4).

Health Monitoring in Real-Time [13]

The capacity to track health metrics in real-time is one of the biggest changes that the Internet of Things has brought about in wearable technology. Heart rate, blood pressure, glucose levels, oxygen saturation, and other vital signs can all be

Table 11.4 IoT-enabled wearables in healthcare

S. nO.	Aspect	Description	Examples
1.	Health monitoring	Continuous monitoring of vital signs and health metrics	Smartwatches (ECG, SpO_2), glucose monitors
2.	Disease management	Managing chronic conditions with real-time alerts and trends	Wearable insulin pumps, asthma trackers
3.	Fitness and wellness	Tracking physical activity, sleep patterns, and overall wellness	Fitness trackers (step count, calorie tracking)
4.	Telemedicine integration	Facilitating remote consultations by transmitting data to healthcare providers	Wearables connected to telehealth platforms
5.	Post-surgery recovery	Monitoring recovery metrics like mobility and vital signs post-surgery	Smart recovery bands, wearable ECG monitors
6.	Emergency detection	Identifying critical conditions like falls, heart attacks, or abnormal rhythms	Fall detectors, wearable heart monitors
7.	Rehabilitation	Supporting physiotherapy and rehabilitation through motion tracking and feedback	Motion sensors, exoskeleton devices
8.	Integration with IoT systems	Enabling data sharing with hospital systems, cloud storage, and smart devices	Cloud platforms, healthcare IoT ecosystems

continuously monitored by wearables thanks to the Internet of Things. In addition to helping people stay informed about their health, this ongoing monitoring gives medical professionals access to real-time data so they can make better decisions.

Connectivity and Data Synchronization [14]

- Cloud Integration: By connecting to cloud platforms, IoT-enabled wearables enable users to safely sync and store data, facilitating long-term monitoring of activity and health trends. Based on aggregated data, cloud-based analytics can also offer tailored recommendations.
- Device-to-Device Communication: Wearables can connect to other smart devices, including tablets, smartphones, smart home systems, and even medical equipment, thanks to the Internet of Things. Because of their connectivity, wearables may send alerts and change the settings on other devices, making them a central repository of information.

Personalized Health Insights [15]

IoT sensors and data analytics platforms can be integrated to create wearable technology that offers highly customized health information. For instance, an Internet of Things-capable smart watch may monitor a user's heart rate, sleep habits, and exercise regimen and make personalized recommendations based on that information. On the basis of data trends, a gadget may also recommend lifestyle modifications or warn users of possible health risks.

Remote Monitoring and Telemedicine [11]

Wearables with IoT capabilities are revolutionizing healthcare by allowing for patient monitoring from a distance. There is less need for in-person visits when medical professionals can monitor patients' health information remotely. Because medical practitioners can keep an eye on patients in real-time and take appropriate action when needed; this is particularly advantageous for managing chronic diseases.

Disease Prevention and Early Detection [16]

Wearable IoT technology holds great promise for early disease identification and prevention. Wearables can identify abnormal trends in a user's health indicators, such as irregular heartbeats, altered sleep patterns, or abnormal blood sugar levels, thanks to continuous monitoring. Early intervention is made possible by these early warnings, which can notify consumers of possible health problems before they become serious.

Continuous Monitoring Devices [16]

Medical and fitness gadgets known as continuous monitoring devices measure a variety of health markers throughout time, giving continuous data that may be examined to gain an understanding of an individual's condition or well-being. These tools are especially important for controlling long-term illnesses, guaranteeing prompt treatments, and improving patient care in general. Without requiring frequent checkups with the doctor or intrusive treatments, continuous monitoring enables real-time health surveillance and data collecting, enabling the early detection of prospective problems.

Continuous Glucose Monitors (CGMs) [17]

People with diabetes use Continuous Glucose Monitors (CGMs) to monitor their blood glucose levels throughout the day. CGMs continually detect glucose levels in the interstitial fluid, or fluid between cells, and transmit data to a receiver or smartphone app, in contrast to conventional procedures that call for finger-prick tests.

One of the top CGMs is the Dexcom G6, which has a sensor that can be worn for up to ten days and provides real-time glucose monitoring. Wireless transmission of the data to a smartphone or other appropriate devices.

ECG Monitors [18]

People can continuously observe the electrical activity of their hearts with wearable ECG (Electrocardiogram) devices. These tools help to evaluate general heart health and identify cardiac disorders such as arrhythmias (like atrial fibrillation, or AFib). Kardia Mobile: A compact, handheld gadget that requires only a 30-second touch of the electrodes to record a medical-grade ECG. AFib, a normal heartbeat, and other cardiac disorders can be detected by the gadget.

Wearable Blood Pressure Monitors [18]

For people with hypertension or other cardiovascular disorders, it is essential to continuously monitor their blood pressure. Systolic and diastolic blood pressure measurements can be tracked in real time without intrusive procedures using wearable blood pressure monitors.

The Omron HeartGuide is a smartwatch-integrated wearable blood pressure monitor. It facilitates the management of hypertension by providing automatic readings and monitoring trends over time.

Automation and Smart Interactions [19]

- Smart Home Integration: Wearables with Internet of Things capabilities can communicate with other smart home appliances. With a wearable gadget, for example, a user can use voice commands or gestures to manage the temperature, lighting, and security systems in their home. Convenience is increased and a smooth user experience is produced by this connection.
- Situation-Aware Responses: Depending on the situation of the user, wearable technology can modify its behavior. For instance, depending on the user's activity level, location, or time of day, a smartwatch may change the brightness of the display or send a reminder.

Methodology [20]

The healthcare sector has changed because of the Internet of Things (IoT) incorporation with wearable technology, which enables real-time feedback, data collecting, and ongoing health monitoring. These developments make it possible to take a holistic approach to health, emphasizing not just early illness diagnosis and prevention but also giving people the resources they need to maintain their health more effectively. To improve the way we monitor and manage health, the methodology underlying IoT in wearable devices refers to a systematic process that includes the creation, investigation, and deployment of these devices. The development process, deployment tactics, and possible effects on public and individual health outcomes are all examined in this study, which presents a thorough strategy for integrating IoT technology with wearable health devices (see Table 11.5).

Development of IoT-Enabled Wearable Devices [24]

The first step in creating wearables with IoT capabilities is determining the demands of users and the objectives of health monitoring. There are many different types of wearable health gadgets, including fitness trackers, smartwatches, and medical equipment like glucose meters and ECG monitors. These gadgets have sensors that gather physiological information including body temperature, blood oxygen levels, heart rate, and steps taken. There are many steps involved in creating these devices:

1. *Sensor Integration and Selection*: Choosing the right sensors to track particular health metrics is the initial stage of development. For example, a wearable that tracks cardiovascular health would use ECG sensors, but a gadget that tracks physical activity might have gyroscopes and accelerometers. To guarantee that the data gathered is precise, reliable, and able to offer insights for bettering health, sensor integration is essential.

Table 11.5 Methodology-focused table related to IoT in wearable devices [30]

S. no.	Stage	Description	Methodology/tools used
1.	Data acquisition	Collecting physiological or environmental data through wearable sensors	Sensors (e.g., ECG, accelerometers, gyroscopes)
2.	Data transmission	Transferring data to storage or processing platforms	Bluetooth, Wi-Fi, Zigbee, LTE
3.	Data processing	Analyzing raw data to extract meaningful insights	Edge computing, cloud computing, AI/ML algorithms
4.	Data storage	Archiving data for future analysis or long-term tracking	Cloud platforms (AWS, Google cloud, Microsoft azure)
5.	Feedback generation	Providing actionable insights to users via interfaces or applications	Mobile apps, dashboards, wearable displays
6.	Integration & control	Enabling interaction with other IoT systems or healthcare providers for comprehensive solutions	IoT ecosystems, APIs, interoperability frameworks

2. *Protocols for Communication and Connectivity*: The capacity to wirelessly connect to other devices, such as smartphones or cloud-based servers, is a crucial component of wearables with Internet of Things capabilities. To guarantee smooth data flow, the wearable incorporates communication technologies including Bluetooth, Wi-Fi, and Zigbee. Remote patient monitoring is made feasible by these protocols, which allow real-time data transfer to healthcare practitioners.
3. *Data Processing and Analytics*: In order to extract valuable insights from the raw data gathered by wearable sensors, processing and analysis are frequently necessary. To evaluate the data, wearable technology either connects to external computer platforms (such cloud servers or cellphones) or incorporates onboard microcontrollers. These systems employ algorithms to identify patterns, provide health reports, and notify users or medical professionals of any irregularities.
4. *User Interface Design*: A wearable device's user interface (UI) is another important factor in its success. To make sure that consumers can quickly understand the facts and take the appropriate action, a user interface must be clear and easy to use. For instance, smartphone applications that show real-time statistics, give feedback on health status, and make tailored recommendations based on the data gathered are frequently included with health monitoring equipment.

Exploration: IoT in Wearables for Health Monitoring [25]

The next step after the development of wearable technology is to investigate how it affects health monitoring. Early diagnosis, managing chronic diseases, and preventative health are just a few of the health exploration opportunities made possible by IoT in wearables. IoT-enabled gadgets change the way medical diseases are managed by serving as a link between technology and healthcare. The following are some of the main areas of investigation.

Chronic Disease Management

Wearable technology offers people with long-term conditions like diabetes, high blood pressure, or heart disease the chance to be continuously monitored. Health indicators may be tracked daily by devices, which can also send out notifications when important thresholds are crossed. Healthcare providers may take preventative measures and modify treatment programs before problems worsen thanks to this real-time data. For instance, diabetic individuals can lower their risk of problems by using continuous glucose monitoring (CGM) devices to track their blood sugar levels throughout the day [26].

Preventive Health

Wearables with Internet of Things capabilities can assist in identifying possible health problems early on before symptoms appear. Through constant monitoring of vital health indicators like as body temperature, heart rate variability, and sleep patterns, these gadgets can spot minute alterations in the body that might signal the start of illnesses like infections, stress, or cardiovascular issues. Wearables can then encourage users to change their lifestyle choices or consult a doctor, which might result in early intervention and improved health results [27].

Remote Patient Monitoring

Without the need for in-person visits, healthcare practitioners may more easily follow patients' health conditions thanks to IoT devices. This is especially crucial when caring for elderly patients, those with chronic illnesses, or people who reside in remote locations. In addition to increasing access to care, remote monitoring eases the strain on medical institutions, resulting in cheaper expenses and more convenient treatment for patients [28].

Mobilization: Using the Internet of Things to Promote Health [29]

The deployment of wearable technology with Internet of Things capabilities is the last phase of the technique. This relates to the actual implementation and use of these devices by the general population as well as in actual healthcare settings. Scaling up wearable technology across industries while addressing privacy, data security, user uptake, and regulatory norms is known as mobilization.

Challenges in IoT-Enabled Wearable Devices [31]

IoT has enormous potential for wearable technology; to fully reap its rewards, several issues need to be resolved. These issues pertain to technological integration, data privacy, security, and healthcare legislation.

Data Privacy and Security [32]

Security and privacy issues are brought up by the sensitive personal health data that wearables gather. This data might be accessible to malevolent actors or unauthorized individuals in the absence of appropriate measures. To safeguard data privacy, encryption, safe cloud storage, and user permission procedures are crucial. Large volumes of personal health data are gathered by continuous monitoring devices to preserve patient privacy and adhere to laws such as the Health Insurance Portability and Accountability Act (HIPAA) in the United States; this data must be safely communicated and stored. HIPAA secures the patient's health information. GDPR (General data protection regulation) protects data or information of patient in EU. Other regulatory frameworks governing IoT are also available such as HITECH Act (USA), which aims to increase the penalties for data breach. PIPEDA in Canada protects the data, and as per this act, user consent is required. An act for medical devices is also available, known as MDR (Medical Device Regulation), to ensure safety and reliability.

Data Cybersecurity

Through secure data transfer, authentication, and threat detection, IoT is essential to improving wearable device cybersecurity. IoT makes encryption protocols like TLS/SSL possible in order to safeguard communication between devices and cloud servers, since wearables are gathering sensitive financial, health, and personal data. Biometric security and multi-factor authentication aid in preventing unwanted access, while AI-driven threat detection instantly detects irregularities and online dangers. By lowering vulnerabilities and limiting data exposure, edge computing and automatic software upgrades further improve security. Nonetheless, issues like inadequate authentication, data breaches, and interconnection threats continue to be major worries. Improvements in IoT-based cybersecurity measures will be crucial as wearable technology develops further to protect user privacy and data integrity.

Data Accuracy and Interpretation [33]

Another issue is the precision of the data that wearables gather. For users to receive accurate health information, IoT sensors need to give accurate readings. Furthermore, this data must be interpreted meaningfully, particularly when it comes to medical decision-making. For wearables to be regarded as legitimate medical devices, data consistency and accuracy are essential.

Integration with Healthcare Systems [34]

IoT-enabled wearables must easily interface with current medical devices and systems in order to be useful in the healthcare industry. Standardized protocols and data formats are necessary to ensure interoperability across wearable technology, electronic health records (EHR), and healthcare software.

Concerns about Regulation and Ethics (Ethical Consideration) [35]

To guarantee that IoT-enabled medical devices fulfill safety and effectiveness requirements, regulation is crucial. Regulators may find it challenging to keep up with the quick speed of wearable and IoT innovation. Informed consent and data ownership are two more ethical issues that need to be addressed about the use of personal health data. Before being sold and used in clinical settings, many continuous monitoring devices—particularly those that offer vital health data—must pass stringent regulatory authorization. It takes a lot of effort and time to comply with medical device laws set forth by organizations like the European Medicines Agency (EMA) in the EU or the Food and Drug Administration (FDA) in the USA.

Real-Time Data Processing and Analysis [36]

The difficulty of processing and analyzing data in real-time: Massive volumes of data are produced by continuous monitoring equipment, which requires real-time processing and analysis. Inadequate analysis of the data can overwhelm medical professionals and prevent them from using it effectively for prompt actions.

Technical Challenges [37]

Although wearable sensors for blood pressure, heart rate, glucose, sleep, and other health metrics, as well as other continuous monitoring devices, have transformed healthcare and wellness management, several technological issues still impact their efficacy, uptake, and performance. To guarantee that the devices deliver secure, accurate, and dependable health data, these issues must be resolved. The primary challenge is data reliability and accuracy. Sensors are used by continuous monitoring systems to gather real-time data, which needs to be precise to guarantee appropriate health management. False positives or false negatives can come from mistakes in data collection or interpretation, which may lead to an incorrect diagnosis or ineffective therapy. The secondary technical challenge is power backup. Small, often rechargeable batteries that power continuous monitoring devices could not be sufficient for long-term monitoring without regular recharging. This is especially difficult for wearable technology, which must be pleasant and inconspicuous.

Interoperability and Standardization [38]

Continuous monitoring equipment frequently gathers and transmits data in a variety of forms. When these devices must interface with other healthcare systems, such electronic health records (EHRs) or telemedicine platforms, interoperability problems occur.

Effects of Wearable and Internet of Things Devices on the Environment[39]

Healthcare, exercise, and daily life have all been transformed by wearable and Internet of Things (IoT) gadgets, which provide creative methods to monitor health indicators, boost productivity, and improve quality of life. These technologies do, however, present environmental issues, just like any other technological gadget. The production, energy consumption, waste creation, and disposal of wearable and Internet of Things devices are some of the elements that can be used to examine their environmental impact (Table 11.6).

Natural Resources Consumptions

Natural resources like metals, polymers, and rare earth elements must be extracted to produce wearable and Internet of Things devices. These substances are essential to the gadgets' operation, especially for parts like sensors, semiconductors, and batteries.

Metals and Rare Earth Elements: Precious metals (like gold and silver) and rare earth elements (like lithium and cobalt) are used in the building of many wearable and Internet of Things devices. These materials mining has serious negative effects on the environment, such as pollution, habitat damage, and resource depletion.

Plastics and Components: Environmental deterioration is a result of the use of plastic materials for components and casings. Long-term pollution results from the energy-intensive petrochemical extraction process used to make plastics and the frequently non-biodegradable plastic trash produced.

Energy Consumption

Impact on electricity Consumption: Lithium-ion batteries, which power wearable and Internet of Things gadgets, need a lot of electricity to charge. Even while tiny gadgets usually use less power than larger electronics, millions of devices' combined energy usage can have a big effect on the environment.

Battery Production: Making batteries uses a lot of energy, and the extraction of nickel, cobalt, and lithium for these batteries might hurt the environment. Deforestation, soil erosion, and water contamination are all possible outcomes of mining these metals.

Charging and Power Consumption: As IoT devices proliferate, their energy usage increases. Frequent or continuous charging can lead to significant electricity consumption, particularly when gadgets are left plugged in for extended periods.

E-Waste Generation

Impact of E-Waste Generation: Wearable technology and Internet of Things devices are major contributors to e-waste, one of the waste streams with the fastest rate of growth in the world. These gadgets typically last only one to three years, and when they break down or become outdated, they add to the mounting amount of electronics that are thrown away.

Material Disposal: Lead, mercury, and cadmium are among the dangerous compounds found in many wearable and Internet of Things gadgets. These items have the potential to contaminate soil and water sources if they are not disposed of appropriately.

Short Lifespan: Older devices are thrown away before their potential for reuse is fully realized due to the frequent modifications brought about by the quick evolution of technology. This adds to the burden on landfills and the amount of waste generated.

Effect on Ecosystems and Wildlife

Local ecosystems may suffer greatly as a result of the exploitation of raw materials used to make wearable and Internet of Things devices. For instance, lithium, cobalt, and nickel mining for batteries frequently occurs in environmentally sensitive locations, which can result in wildlife displacement, habitat degradation, and deforestation.

Water Use and Pollution: Mining operations use a lot of water and have the potential to contaminate neighboring water supplies with chemicals and heavy metals. Here is a table showing the effects of IoT on the environment globally (see Table 11.6).

Table 11.6 The effects of IoT on the environment

Effect	Description	Impact	Examples
1. Energy efficiency	IoT enables smart energy management systems to optimize electricity usage and reduce waste	Positive	Smart grids, smart thermostats, automated lighting systems
2. Resource management	IoT sensors monitor resource consumption (e.g., water, electricity) and suggest ways to reduce usage	Positive	Smart irrigation systems and water leak detectors
3. Pollution monitoring	IoT devices track air, water, and soil quality, providing real-time data for pollution control	Positive	Air quality sensors, smart water quality monitoring systems
4. Waste reduction	IoT applications improve waste management through optimized collection routes and recycling processes	Positive	Smart waste bins, waste tracking systems
5. Climate change monitoring	IoT-enabled networks gather data on climate conditions, aiding research and mitigation efforts	Positive	Weather stations, and satellite IoT systems for climate data collection
6. Wildlife protection	IoT devices track wildlife movements and detect illegal activities like poaching	Positive	GPS trackers for animals, anti-poaching IoT cameras
7. E-waste generation	Increased use of IoT devices leads to higher electronic waste, impacting the environment negatively	Negative	Outdated smart devices discarded without proper recycling.
8. Energy consumption of IoT devices	IoT devices and infrastructure increase overall energy consumption	Negative	Data centers power IoT ecosystems.
9. Habitat disruption	Expansion of IoT networks (e.g., smart cities) can disrupt natural habitats and ecosystems	Negative	Construction of IoT infrastructure in natural areas.
10. Circular economy	IoT helps support the circular economy by enabling better tracking and reuse of materials	Positive	IoT in asset tracking for reuse, repair, and recycling.

Future Trends in IoT-Enabled Wearable Devices [15]

Future Directions for Wearable Technology with IoT Capabilities

IoT in wearable technology has a bright future. We can anticipate increasingly more sophisticated and individualized health treatments as technology develops further. The following are some new developments that will influence wearables with IoT capabilities in the future (see Table 11.7).

Table 11.7 Trends in IoT [30]

S. no.	Trend	Description	Impact
1.	Health monitoring & diagnostics	Wearables will increasingly integrate advanced sensors for continuous health monitoring, such as heart rate, glucose, and oxygen levels	Personalized healthcare, early disease detection.
2.	Integration with AI & machine learning	AI algorithms will enhance the functionality of wearables by enabling real-time data analysis and predictive analytics	Improved decision-making, predictive health insights.
3.	Smart clothing	Clothing with embedded IoT sensors that monitor health, track fitness metrics, or provide environmental feedback (e.g., temperature, humidity)	More comprehensive health and performance tracking.
4.	Seamless connectivity with 5G	The rollout of 5G networks will provide wearables with faster, low-latency connectivity, enabling real-time data exchange and remote control	Enhanced device performance, faster communication.
5.	Mental health tracking	Wearables will focus more on monitoring mental health, including stress levels, sleep patterns, and emotional states using biometric sensors	Better mental health management and stress reduction.
6.	Enhanced user Interface (UI)	IoT-enabled wearables will offer more intuitive interfaces, including voice controls, gestures, and haptic feedback	Improved user experience and ease of interaction.
7.	Augmented reality (AR) integration	Wearables, especially smart glasses, will integrate AR capabilities, providing real-time data overlays and interactive experiences	Enhanced user interaction with the digital world.
8.	Energy harvesting	Future wearables will use energy harvesting techniques (solar, kinetic, etc.) to extend battery life without the need for frequent charging	Longer battery life, sustainability.
9.	Blockchain for security	The integration of block chain technology will enhance the security and privacy of the data transmitted by wearables, ensuring safe personal data management	Increased trust, reduced security risks.
10.	Wearables for the elderly	Development of IoT-enabled wearables designed specifically for elderly care, including fall detection, medication reminders, and emergency alerts	Improved quality of life and safety for elderly individuals.

AI Integration for Predictive Health [15]

Future wearable with IoT capabilities will heavily rely on artificial intelligence (AI). AI can assist in anticipating possible health problems before they materialize by evaluating vast amounts of health data, enabling more proactive and individualized treatment. AI systems can predict ailments like diabetes, heart disease, and even mental health issues by examining patterns in data.

Multi-parameter Monitoring

Even more sophisticated sensors that can monitor a greater number of health factors at once will be found in wearable technology in the future. More thorough health monitoring will be possible as a result, including the recording of physiological measures, mental health indicators, and biomarkers that were previously challenging to track in real time.

Integration with Healthcare Ecosystems

Wearables with IoT capabilities will further interact with healthcare ecosystems, facilitating smooth data sharing between patients, healthcare professionals, and gadgets. Real-time medical interventions, better patient outcomes, and treatment plan optimization are all made possible by this connection.

Conclusion

Personal health management and the healthcare sector in general are being revolutionized by the incorporation of IoT technologies into wearable devices. Continuous, real-time health monitoring made possible by these gadgets promotes early disease detection, individualized treatment, and an enhanced standard of living. To fully achieve the potential of IoT in wearable devices, however, issues pertaining to data privacy, security, and healthcare integration must be resolved. Even more sophisticated, AI-powered solutions for illness prevention, health management, and improved healthcare delivery are anticipated in the future of wearable IoT technology.

Wearable technology has been transformed by IoT, making these gadgets effective tools for work, entertainment, fitness, and health. IoT has broadened the scope of wearable applications across industries by facilitating real-time data transmission, sophisticated analytics, and seamless communication. Even if issues like privacy, battery life, and interoperability still exist, new developments are expected to remove these obstacles and fully realize the potential of wearables with IoT capabilities. Wearables will continue to be essential to the larger Internet of Things ecosystem as we move forward, changing the way we engage with technology and the environment.

IoT has revolutionized wearable technology, transforming these devices into powerful tools for health, fitness, productivity, and entertainment. By enabling real-time data exchange, advanced analytics, and seamless connectivity, IoT has expanded the horizons of wearable applications across industries. While challenges such as privacy, battery life, and interoperability remain, ongoing innovations promise to overcome these barriers and unlock the full potential of IoT-enabled wearables. As we look to the future, wearables will continue to play a pivotal role in the broader IoT ecosystem, reshaping how we interact with technology and the world around us.

The methodology surrounding the role of IoT in wearable devices is a comprehensive and evolving process that spans development, exploration, and mobilization. Through the development of advanced sensors, connectivity, and data analytics, IoT-enabled wearables are transforming healthcare, providing individuals with personalized insights into their health. By enabling remote monitoring, early detection, and chronic disease management, these devices are improving patient outcomes and preventing health issues. However, to maximize the potential of IoT in healthcare, issues such as data security, regulatory compliance, and user engagement must be addressed. As IoT technology continues to advance, wearable devices will play an increasingly important role in the future of healthcare, enabling individuals to take control of their health while assisting healthcare providers in delivering efficient, proactive care.

Because it makes real-time health monitoring, remote patient care, seamless communication, and improved security possible, the Internet of Things is essential to wearable technology. It enables vital sign monitoring, emergency detection, and integration with other IoT systems in smartwatches, fitness trackers, and medical wearables. IoT wearables increase working productivity and safety in industries, and they boost performance tracking in sports. Convenience and customization are increased by features like biometric authentication, contactless payments, and AI-driven analytics. But issues like battery optimization and data privacy still exist. Wearable technology will become increasingly sophisticated, self-sufficient, and integrated into everyday life as IoT technology develops.

References

1. Zaidan AA, Zaidan BB. A review on intelligent process for smart home applications based on IoT: coherent taxonomy, motivation, open challenges, and recommendations. Artif Intell Rev. 2020;53(1):141–65.
2. Kumar S, Kanchan AK, Agarwal P, Maurya H. Internet of Things (IOT) applications and challenges: a review. Int J Eng Sci Emerg Technol. 2023;11:359–67.
3. Haddaoui S, Chikhi S, Miles B. The IoT ecosystem: components, architecture, communication technologies, and protocols. In: Chikhi S, Diaz-Descalzo G, Amine A, Chaoui A, Saidouni DE, Kholladi MK, editors. Modelling and implementation of complex systems. MISC 2022. Lecture notes in networks and systems, vol. 593. Cham: Springer; 2023. https://doi.org/10.1007/978-3-031-18516-8_6.
4. Paul M, Maglaras L, Ferrag MA, Almomani I. Digitization of healthcare sector: a study on privacy and security concerns. ICT Express. 2023;9(4):571–88.
5. Escobar-Linero E, Muñoz-Saavedra L, Luna-Perejón F, Sevillano JL, Domínguez-Morales M. Wearable health devices for diagnosis support: evolution and future tendencies. Sensors. 2023;23(3):1678.

6. Xu M, Qian F, Zhu M, Huang F, Pushp S, Liu X. Deepwear: adaptive local offloading for on-wearable deep learning. IEEE Trans Mob Comput. 2019;19(2):314–30.
7. Tanaka C, Hikihara Y, Inoue S, Tanaka S. The choice of pedometer impacts on daily step counts in primary school children under free-living conditions. Int J Environ Res Public Health. 2019;16(22):4375.
8. Calculator P. Books & arts. Nature. 2023;620:721.
9. Gupta S, Arora A. The internet of Things: a review of wearable devices and its impact on healthcare. Int J Comput Appl. 2017;164(4):20–5.
10. Shin D, Kim S. A review of healthcare IoT Systems for Remote Patient Monitoring: challenges and opportunities. Int J Distrib Sensor Netw. 2021;17(3):1550–72.
11. Dian FJ, Vahidnia R, Rahmati A. Wearables and the internet of Things (IoT), applications, opportunities, and challenges: a survey. IEEE Access. 2020;8:69200–11.
12. Li Y, Li X. Wearable sensors in healthcare: applications, challenges, and future directions. Int Conf Smart Electr Commun. 2021;2021:234–9.
13. Roehrig C, Chawla S. The promise of IoT and wearable devices in healthcare: a global perspective. Frost & Sullivan White Paper; 2019.
14. Nass C, Moon Y. The role of wearable devices in managing chronic health conditions: the case for integration with IoT. J Am Med Inform Assoc. 2016;23(2):100–6.
15. Ahmed R, Khan A, Rehman S. Wearable IoT devices and its impact on healthcare: a review of current trends and future directions. IEEE; 2020.
16. Lee I, Probst D, Klonoff D, Sode K. Continuous glucose monitoring systems-current status and future perspectives of the flagship technologies in biosensor research. Biosens Bioelectron. 2021;181:113054.
17. Arpaia P, Cuocolo R, Donnarumma F, Esposito A, Moccaldi N, Natalizio A, Prevete R. Conceptual design of a machine learning-based wearable soft sensor for non-invasive cardiovascular risk assessment. Measurement. 2021;169:108551.
18. Acemoglu D, Restrepo P. Artificial intelligence, automation, and work. In: The economics of artificial intelligence: an agenda. University of Chicago Press; 2018. p. 197–236.
19. Taherdoost H. Wearable healthcare and continuous vital sign monitoring with IoT integration. Comput Mater Continua. 2024;81(1)
20. Burke B. Top strategic technology trends for 2021. Gartner; 2020.
21. Predel C, Steger F. Ethical challenges with smartwatch-based screening for atrial fibrillation: putting users at risk for marketing purposes? Front Cardiovasc Med. 2021;7:615927.
22. Gartner. Gartner Says 25 Billion Connected 'Things' Will Be in Use by 2021. 2022.
23. Surantha N, Atmaja P, David, Wicaksono M. A review of wearable Internet-of-Things device for healthcare. Proc Comput Sci. 2021;179
24. Beck RW, Riddlesworth T, Ruedy K, Ahmann A, Bergenstal R, Haller S, Kollman C, Kruger D, McGill JB, Polonsky W, Toschi E. Effect of continuous glucose monitoring on glycemic control in adults with type 1 diabetes using insulin injections: the DIAMOND randomized clinical trial. JAMA. 2017;317(4):371–8.
25. Kwon H, Lee S, Jung EJ, Kim S, Lee JK, Kim DK, Kim TH, Lee SH, Lee MK, Song S, Shin K. An mHealth management platform for patients with chronic obstructive pulmonary disease (efil breath): randomized controlled trial. JMIR Mhealth Uhealth. 2018;6(8):e10502.
26. Izmailova ES, Wagner JA, Perakslis ED. Wearable devices in clinical trials: hype and hypothesis. Clin Pharmacol Therap. 2018;104(1):42–52.
27. Godoy Junior CA, Miele F, Mäkitie L, Fiorenzato E, Koivu M, Bakker LJ, Groot CU, Redekop WK, van Deen WK. Attitudes toward the adoption of remote patient monitoring and artificial intelligence in Parkinson's disease management: perspectives of patients and neurologists. Patient-Patient-Centered Outcomes Res. 2024;17(3):275–85.
28. Balk-Møller NC, Poulsen SK, Larsen TM. Effect of a nine-month web-and app-based workplace intervention to promote healthy lifestyle and weight loss for employees in the social welfare and health care sector: a randomized controlled trial. J Med Internet Res. 2017;19(4):e108.

29. Al-Turjman F, Malekloo A. Internet of Things and fog computing-enabled solutions for connect. 2019.
30. Sim I. Mobile devices and health. N Engl J Med. 2019;381(10):956–68.
31. Lomborg S, Langstrup H, Andersen TO. Interpretation as luxury: heart patients living with data doubt, hope, and anxiety. Big Data Soc. 2020;7(1):2053951720924436.
32. Canali S, Schiaffonati V, Aliverti A. Challenges and recommendations for wearable devices in digital health: data quality, interoperability, health equity, fairness. PLOS Digit Health. 2022;1(10):e0000104. https://doi.org/10.1371/journal.pdig.0000104. PMID: 36812619; PMCID: PMC9931360
33. Adler-Milstein J, Nong P. Early experiences with patient generated health data: health system and patient perspectives. J Am Med Inform Assoc. 2019;26(10):952–9.
34. Loucks J, Stewart D, Bucaille A, Crossan G. Wearable technology in health care: getting better all the time. TMT Predictions; 2022.
35. Escobar-Linero E, Muñoz-Saavedra L, Luna-Perejón F, Sevillano JL, Domínguez-Morales M. Wearable health devices for diagnosis support: evolution and future tendencies. Sensors (Basel). 2023;23(3):1678. https://doi.org/10.3390/s23031678. PMID: 36772718; PMCID: PMC9920884
36. Sharon T. Self-tracking for health and the quantified self: re-articulating autonomy, solidarity, and authenticity in an age of personalized healthcare. Philos Technol. 2017;30(1):93–121.
37. Blasimme A, Fadda M, Schneider M, Vayena E. Data sharing for precision medicine: policy lessons and future directions. Health Aff. 2018;37(5):702–9.
38. Fraga-Lamas P, Lopes SI, Fernández-Caramés TM. Green IoT and edge AI as key technological enablers for a sustainable digital transition towards a smart circular economy: an industry 5.0 use case. Sensors. 2021;21(17):5745.

Chapter 12
Wearables in Personalized and Precision Medicine

Zainab Almukhtar and Philip Eappen

Introduction

A main definition of precision medicine is that it is the part of medicine that focuses on tailoring healthcare treatment to the individual characteristics of persons [77] utilizing biological patients' data. Often, precision medicine and personalized medicine have been used interchangeably. However, precision medicine tends to direct more focus on the genome as a main factor in treatment [42], while personalized medicine focuses more on other characteristics of patients. Both personalized medicine and precision medicine customize medical treatment or prevention to the characteristics of patients or groups of patients. Precision medicine can tailor treatment to persons or groups of people who share similar responses to certain drugs or common risk factors of certain diseases, which optimizes treatment outcomes [6, 67].

The development in computer technologies added advanced tools to handle data and opened new avenues for precision medicine where vast amount of data can be collected and analyzed toward decision-making. Within this are the advances and spread of wearable medical devices [84]. Wearable medical devices are systems that monitor patients' health by tracking patient's real time data. They aid in providing efficient and effective healthcare outputs and enhance communication and data transfer [60]. Integration of data from different sources such as wearable devices and patients' records allows for the analysis of different disease trajectories, which added to the advancements in precision and personalized medicine. Wearables can have different forms such as wrist watches, chest straps, glasses, smart jewelry, and others and can be worn directly on the body, mounted on clothing [37, 60], or installed in structures like smart watches [89]. Changes in healthcare landscape such as the aging of populations, the increased cost of healthcare, the appearance of

Z. Almukhtar (✉) · P. Eappen
Cape Breton University, Sydney, NS, Canada
e-mail: zainab_almukhtar@cbu.ca

P. Eappen et al. (eds.), *Advancing Healthcare with the Medical Internet of Things*, Health Informatics, https://doi.org/10.1007/978-3-032-23933-4_12

new diseases as well as the location barriers and constraints to access healthcare services all call for the importance of using wearable devices [28]. An important area where wearable devices have potential is in precision medicine. The integration of artificial intelligence and predictive analysis in wearable devices adds strides to personalized and precision healthcare through offering disease classification and prediction tools. Nonetheless, there are still many challenges relating to the wide use of wearable devices in medicine, and the use of big data and AI applications. Some of those are ethical concerns, the data security, and the standardization of the devices [26, 63]. Other issues are related to the cost, integration, acceptability, and usability of those devices.

The area of the application of wearable devices including precision medicine is highly emerging both in depth and in width. We find that it is important to investigate how wearable technologies are applied in personalized and precision medicine including advances, challenges, and future directions. This chapter starts with a review of wearable devices including features, issues, and the future of wearable devices. In the second part, we investigate precision medicine, its foundation, and application in clinical practices. In part four, we delve into how wearable devices are used in the field of precision and personalized medicine, and then we end this chapter with conclusions and future directions.

Review of Wearable Devices

Features and Structure of Wearable Devices

Wearable devices typically consist of two key components: a target receptor and a transducer. The receptor detects a specific analyte (such as a biomarker or environmental factor) and generates a response [69]. The transducer then converts this response into a signal that can be interpreted and used for further analysis or to direct action [38]. The sensors that detect patients' signals can read the following forms of signals: optical, electrical, electrochemical, and piezoelectric [60]. The advances in materials science and the micro- and nanoelectronics made wearable devices smaller and provided opportunities to produce hand health wearable devices with reasonable cost [69]. Furthermore, the flexibility in advanced materials like polyethylene naphtholate, polyethylene terephthalate added usability features to a range of wearable devices increasing the spread of those devices [38, 85]. A distinguishing feature of wearable devices is that they can establish communication with mobile devices, and central computers [81]. Data from wearable devices are transmitted and stored in computers where they are analyzed to present the needed results. These pools of data provide a large base for the analysis of medical information. AI technologies are used to guide decision-making and prediction of disease and treatment outcomes and suggest new treatments. For example, with the use of

AI, patients' records and data collected from wearable devices, vulnerabilities of groups of patients to chronic diseases can be predicted [31]. To have a clearer understanding of the capabilities that wearable devices offer to precision and personalized medicine, we review the main algorithms used in wearable devices in the following text.

Analysis Algorithms

Most wearable devices collect time-series data from sensors like accelerometers, gyroscopes, and heart rate monitors, which require algorithms to analyze patterns in real time [11] and detect abnormalities. The data collected from wearable devices come in different forms and time sequences [48]. To deal with these data, algorithms of sequence classification are applied where data at each point of time is presented as a vector. Machine learning approaches construct recognition models that use a classifier to predict the activity class [80]. The classifier then categorizes sequences for multiple activity classes. Features that are chosen based on prior knowledge are called hand-crafted features, while features that are deducted are called learnt features [24]. New approaches in machine learning consist of the combination between learnt features and hand-crafted features which add more advanced analysis and prediction abilities [1, 97]. The large amount of data from wearables enables the selection of features to support detection patterns of biological features via machine learning algorithms [81]. Via this logic, patients' data can be classified into groups of similar characteristics to direct medical treatment.

Supervised Learning: This is where the algorithms learn from labeled data [81] In this type, the relation between the input and output is pre-known. An important application of supervised learning is classification algorithm [80]. Classifications have been applied to personalize healthcare. Practical applications in healthcare are the classification of patients according to the level of their stress into predetermined categories [41]. Some of the algorithms used are as follows: Linear Regression; Logistic Regression; Decision Trees; Support Vector Machines (SVM); Naive Bayes; Random Forest tree; Gradient Boosting; and Neural Networks. Examples of supervised learning are the classification methods of patients into different preidentified groups in relation to their response to disease or biological characteristics [3].

Unsupervised Learning: In this type of algorithm, the relation between the input and output is unknown. The data are unlabeled, and the job of the algorithms is to extract patterns from the data [38]. Some of the algorithms used are Clustering, Dimensionality Reduction, and Association Rule. In relation to personalized and precision medicine, those methods can detect the prevalence of diseases in certain contexts, and the differences among patients in their response to diseases [3]. Importantly, the ability of wearable devices to detect large amounts of biological data is vital to provide the needed data for such algorithms.

Issues and Concerns About the Use of Wearable Devices

Despite the advancement in uses and technologies of wearable devices, there are many issues in the wide use of those devices in medicine and healthcare. Canali et al. [12] categorized those challenges into data quality issues, estimation challenges, health equity, and equality issues. The accurate forecasting of the onset and progression of diseases is a main goal in precision medicine. As mentioned, much of the data that is used as information sources in precision medicine is collected from wearable devices [27, 78]. The outcomes of wearable devices rely heavily on the quality of this data. The reliability of the wearable devices and the used algorithms highly impact the outcomes of these devices. Following are the main issues faced when using wearable devices in healthcare and precision medicine.

Data Accuracy and Quality

Precision medicine involves the collection and analysis of large amounts of data of disease, biology, and medicine to provide disease taxonomy, diagnosis, therapeutic development, and clinical decisions [40].

The quality of data is basic to the operation of every medical device and to the correctness of the outcomes [9]. Due to the different types of sensors used in wearable devices, there are still inconsistencies around data types, collection, and interpretation that raise caution around the quality of data collected from wearable devices [12]. Many times, there are accuracy issues with data such as step counts, heart rate, and sleep quality collected directly by sensors or entered by persons themselves [35]. Some of the reasons for that are related to the accuracy of the sensors and measurement errors [18]. The heterogeneity of the data can be seen in the real-time data from wearable devices. An example of this data is data from urgency monitoring devices for patients with nervous system diseases [9]. Another concern is the completeness of data collected from wearable devices. This is sometimes associated with the frequency of the collection of data by the user. An area that needs attention is the validity of AI approaches and algorithms used to analyze data and predict outcomes [62]. Any gaps in that not only impact the immediate results and outcomes but also the health of vast numbers of patients. The expression "algorithm bias" refers to errors in outcomes of algorithms due to data errors or how the algorithm is trained [70].

Data Privacy

As we know, wearable devices collect data to monitor, track, and predict health outcomes of patients [46] and feed this data to computers and digital devices to be used for medical decisions. Especially, in precision medicine, the data are very specialized and patient related. Most of these data are shared with various healthcare providers and organizations for different purposes. The right to collect and use these data is a main concern related to the privacy and security rights and regulations [20]. An important question to ask is if the users of wearable devices are provided with clear information about the use and collection of data (who will use the data and with whom it will be shared), and if there are set clear regulations [8]. Relating to this and other issues, there are several ambiguities on the use and distribution of data [45]. At many times, the data can be used for research or sold to other companies that use it [8]. To comply with ethical and privacy requirements, individuals should be clearly informed about the consent for the data to be used and sold for research purposes [20]. Despite the regulations by bodies such as the General Data Protection Regulation (GDPR)[1] and the Health Insurance Portability and Accountability Act (HIPAA)[2] regarding the use of personal data, there is still a need for more protection on the use of personal data. To address this further, it should be noted that any collected or stored data has ownership rights [45]. The ownership of data from wearable devices belongs to the user and to the third-party owners of the data. The fact that many wearable devices store large amounts of data in the cloud or third-party storage raises concerns [88]. Such concerns are related to the security and privacy of data, since sensitive health and personal information can be exposed to threats. A known security threat is the stealing of data by cybercriminals and using the data to tamper the health records and information [47], which further highlights the importance of data security and protection tools in wearable devices and other data repositories.

Another point of attention is the standardization of data and the availability of technology infrastructure [7]. To be able to provide standardized, reliable, and usable data from the wearable devices to inform decision-making in precision medicine, robust technology support, and infrastructure tools are needed [7]. Within this, there should be supportive internet connections and Wi-Fi infrastructure to secure the continuity of wearable devices to collect and store data [9]. This is very important in precision and personalized medicine, as the completeness of data is important to the proper decisions. In the next section, we discuss the integration and the interoperability of data.

Data Integration and Interoperability

To provide the needed information for precision medicine, data from wearable devices are often integrated with other patient data such as data from EHR systems. A significant point is the interoperability of data from different sources [25]. To explain this, we note that the producers of wearable devices and EHR tools apply a range of methods in data handling and communications such as distinct, proprietary, and closed communication methods. The use of different data-handling tools

[1] General Data Protection Regulation (GDPR) – Legal Text.

[2] HIPAA Home | HHS.gov

presents challenges to data communication and transfer among various devices, which is referred to as interoperability [21, 89].

Features and capabilities, such as feedback, enable enhanced integration of wearable devices and EHR records [55]. Methods to address interoperability include open standards and APIs that allow seamless data exchange across platforms [53, 79]. Additionally, implementing strong governance frameworks and stakeholder collaboration ensures consistent, secure, and scalable integration.

Although the use of wearable devices for remote health monitoring in healthcare is steadily rising, there is limited understanding of how these technologies impact health workers [30]. Other challenges are associated with technical issues, software and data issues, hardware and device issues, standardization measures [64], and health equity and fairness. The application of standardized measures enables the effective sharing of information among healthcare workers and other patients who use wearables [73]. The needs and taxonomies of those bodies can be different. Both the clinical information and the research data must be integrated to facilitate decision-making [36]. In addition to software, hardware regulations should also be addressed. In the next section, we will review that.

Manufacture Regulations and Device Usability

Medical devices should be certified and be in compliance with the software and hardware regulations. The certification of qualification guarantees that the product follows the regulations given by the regulatory bodies [93]. The process of regulation differs across countries. The regulating authority for wearable medical devices in Canada is the Canada Medical Device Regulations (CMDR), which outlines the classification, licensing, and post-market surveillance requirements for such technologies [33]. For instance, the regulatory procedure in the European Union involves conformity assessment by Notified Bodies, after which a CE certificate of conformity is granted to allow the device to be marketed [16, 75].

With respect to manufacturing standards, sensors in advanced medical devices must be designed to align with their functional applications [47, 66]. While regulatory frameworks in Canada, Europe, and the United States establish requirements for the design, development, regulation, and lifecycle management of medical devices [91], global standardization facilitates the manufacturing, sale, and use of devices across international markets. Other challenges related to the hardware of wearable devices are difficulties in wearing sensors for a long time, the size of the sensors, batteries, and others [15]. Comfort is essential as it encourages consistent use, making devices or services more effective and user-friendly. In wearables, comfort supports long-term adherence, leading to better health and lifestyle outcomes. It is expected that the wearable devices will spread in use and application and will provide more accurate solutions to personalize medicine and healthcare.

Future of Wearable Devices in Healthcare and Precision Medicine

Wearable devices are set to revolutionize precision medicine by enabling continuous, real-time monitoring of vital signs and lifestyle patterns, creating personalized health baselines for each individual [5]. By integrating biological and personal data with genomic and environmental information, clinicians can design highly tailored interventions that reflect a patient's unique biological and social context [49]. Artificial intelligence further enhances these capabilities by analyzing large streams of wearable data to detect risks and predict diseases before symptoms appear [61]. Future innovations like self-powered biosensors and sweat-harvesting devices will enable long-term, autonomous monitoring in daily life.[3] The application of wearable devices is associated with a lower environmental and operational footprint, often resulting in significant healthcare cost savings [28]. Wearable devices offer a solution to the limitations of traditional internal monitoring technologies. Their compact size, lower cost, and user-friendly operation offer significant advantages over conventional systems, which often require professional oversight, are expensive, and may delay diagnosis and treatment [56].

Additionally, body-area networks could connect wearables with automated drug delivery systems, such as insulin pumps, enabling closed-loop therapeutic responses [28]. Collectively, these developments will make precision medicine more proactive, data-driven, and centered on the patient's real-time needs. The coupling of wearable device capabilities and AI applications transformed areas of planning customized treatment plans and precision medicine approaches [50].

Over the next 25 years, it is estimated that the use of wearable technologies could contribute to a global cost reduction exceeding $200 billion in the healthcare sector [60]. This includes a substantial decrease in clinician–patient interaction time, enhancing system efficiency [60]. The wearable technology market is projected to produce a compound annual growth rate (CAGR) of 15.9% through 2027 [10]. A developing area related to the application of wearable devices in precision and personalized medicine approaches in the therapeutic drug monitoring (TDM) [54]. By linking individual responses to drug levels, TDM provides personalized drug dozing plans [4]. The advancements in technologies, incorporating wearables such as biosensors, enable the translation of individual measurements to drug responses, presenting advances to TDM. In the next part, we will elaborate more on how wearable devices opened new scopes for TDM. Next, we explore the applications of precision medicine.

---

[3] https://www.tomsguide.com/tech/the-future-of-wearable-wellness-tech-5-wild-predictions-for-2035-according-to-experts-and-industry-leaders

Precision Medicine: Concepts, Foundations, and Clinical Applications

Introduction and Foundation of Precision Medicine

Precision medicine refers to the modification of medical treatment based on the unique characteristics of patients or subpopulations, such as the sensitivity to certain diseases or the response to specific therapies or medications [22, 67]. Precision medicine recognizes that the response of patients to drug and treatment varies according to individual differences such as genetic distinctions, age, gender, addictions, race, ethnicity, concomitant drugs, comorbidities, environmental factors, and others [82]. This stands in contrast to traditional medical approaches that rely on uniform, generalized treatment strategies.

In recent years, President Barack Obama brought attention to precision medicine in 2015 when he stated, "Tonight I am launching a new precision medicine initiative to bring us closer to curing diseases such as cancer and diabetes".[4] As stated, precision medicine offers advantages, such as improving the effectiveness and outcomes of medical treatment by tailoring healthcare to genetic, environmental, and lifestyle factors [22], and managing adverse drug reactions by using biomarker-driven strategies [54].

A critical foundation of precision medicine lies in the integration and analysis of large-scale data, commonly referred to as big data in healthcare [74]. These data encompass patient information, clinical records, genetic profiles, and population health data. Effectively leveraging these data enables clinicians to stratify patients based on factors like disease risk and therapeutic responses to treatment plans [51].

Precision medicine opened new scopes and developments in genomic and genetic personalized medicine applications [87]. Tools for precision medicines include omics; pharmaco-omics [32]; big data; artificial intelligence; machine learning (ML); environmental, social, and behavioral factors; and integration with preventive and public health [67]. The term "omics" refers to the collective study of the molecular characterization and quantification of biological molecules across various subfields of molecular biology [32]. The field of omics provides unique insights into the biological processes underlying health and disease. The most advanced domain of omics is genomics, which focuses on the genome, the complete set of DNA in the cell [87]. Based on genomic information, genomics enables the design of models for selective or personalized diagnosis and therapy [65]. The evolution of wearable devices and technologies facilitated the collection and the analysis of patient's data at different points of care such as home, care homes, and hospitals. Integrated with advanced AI technologies and machine learning approaches, it presents advanced abilities in precision medicine. The following section investigates the application of precision medicine approaches in clinical practice.

---

[4] https://www.ctvnews.ca/politics/article/full-speech-barack-obamas-state-of-the-union-address/

Applications of Precision Medicine in Clinical Practice

Precision medicine extends beyond genomics-based treatment and encompasses the prediction, prevention, and customization of therapies [52]. For example, monoclonal antibody therapy targeting certain genes in breast cancer patients demonstrates a success in the application of precision medicine in cancer treatment. Similarly, large-scale initiatives such as the Human Genome Project have laid the groundwork for individualized care models [52].

Emerging applications include critical care settings where precision medicine helps classify patients based on comorbidities and biological markers, leading to specialized care plans [82]. Rather than conflicting with standardized care protocols, precision medicine complements them by enabling personalized modifications within established guidelines. A notable example of this synergy between standardized and precision medicine is in the management of asthma. The disease is now categorized based on control levels such as well controlled, not well controlled, or poorly controlled using clinical indicators like symptom frequency, nighttime awakenings, and pulmonary function [58].

This stratified approach improves treatment outcomes and resource allocation and offers personalized treatment plans. In many applications, mounted wearable devices and biosensors enable the online collection of data. Within this, Ates et al. [4] explored how on-site therapeutic drug monitoring (TDM) tools with biosensors can transform clinical practice by enabling real-time, individualized drug management. Traditional methods like chromatography and immunoassays are limited by cost, complexity, and centralization. Biosensors offer simpler, low-cost, and minimally invasive alternatives suitable for wearable and point-of-care use [27]. As stated, despite their promises, clinical adoption is hindered by a lack of standardization, real-sample validation, and cross-disciplinary collaboration [2, 27]. Integrating biosensors with pharmacokinetic/pharmacodynamic models can support dynamic, feedback-controlled dosing. This underscores the importance of bridging the gaps between technology and clinical needs, which is essential for realizing precision medicine. In the next part, we elaborate on specific uses of wearable devices in precision medicine.

The Use of Wearable Device in Precision Medicine

Biological and medical information from wearable devices support medical decisions including planning personalized treatment and prevention strategies [78]. An example is the use of wearable devices and associated technologies in predicting disease trends and designing personalized healthcare plans for individuals with diabetes [32, 39]. Technologies such as continuous glucose monitors (CGMs) and smart insulin delivery systems provide real-time physiological data, enabling both clinicians and patients to make informed, individualized adjustments to treatment regimens [34]. The integration of clinical strategies and patient-specific factors within wearable devices enables the implementation of precision medical approaches in diabetes care [60]. Advances in the use of wearable devices include the combination of those devices with smart and AI technologies presenting abilities that go beyond the collection of real-time data to deploying algorithms to predict out and direct specialized treatments [61]. The combination of wearable technology with machine learning algorithms has facilitated the prediction of glucose fluctuations based on physiological signals and the development of personalized and proactive management approaches tailored to each patient's unique profile [23]. The nature of chronic diseases and their evolving and multiple symptoms require the collection of biological signs in real time [43]. Such data can be disease data sets, including gait patterns, tremor episodes, activity levels, motion, and physiological parameters. These sets can be collected via wearable sensors, mobile health devices, and monitoring systems and fed to the internet [66]. The classification of this data will enable the development of precise treatments based on the categorization of different symptoms and progression of disease.

An example of the tools that tailor customized data collection is a customized omnipresent healthcare (u-healthcare) system [72]. This system includes custom nodes and blood pressure sensors, an electrocardiogram (ECG), and blood interfaces, together with a cell phone device for data display and feature extraction (Pantelopoulos et al. 2008). Relating to neurodegenerative disease, the analysis of gait is important in detecting several diseases within this category [92]. However, the single-modality analysis or the analysis of one feature does not provide a complete picture. A paper [96] introduces an innovative model for gait analysis that utilizes data from multiple sensors to distinguish among three neurodegenerative diseases [83]. It assesses the severity of Parkinson's disease and differentiates patients from healthy individuals. The approach is based on using images and signals from sensors for the integration of Spatial Feature Extractors (SFE) [83]. Correlative Memory Neural Network (CorrMNN) is used to obtain time series patterns. Neural and deep learning algorithms analyze and report patients' data, delivering alerts to medical applications after detection of changes in the health condition of patients [86].

In oncology, wearable devices have an important role in tracking and analyzing vital measures in cancer patients [68]. The tracking of biometric data is essential to provide clinicians with important directions relating to the stages of patients' treatments [19]. This is done by identifying patterns and adverse events to plan programs that tackle the conditions and characteristics of patients. An essential part of cancer treatment is the continuous measurement and monitoring of health metrics and treatment outcomes. Relating to this, it is challenging to track healthcare metrics of certain demographics like the elderly and the children [17]. The application of medical wearable devices such as ActiGraph [68] enables the measurements of activity for patients of cancer to monitor their health across different patient demographics. Other innovative tools have been introduced to monitor wearable devices. An example is the technology that can monitor physiological signals from the surface of organs such as the eyes and skin. This enhances the accuracy of diagnosis for internal conditions in a timely manner and thus supports more timely interventions [57]. One of the developments in this area is the noninvasive skin-like wireless devices that can continuously monitor physiological signals by their interface to different regions [71]. Therapeutic drug modeling is another field where wearable technologies are applied. Therapeutic drug monitoring (TDM) uses drug concentration to manage a patient's medication plans and optimize outputs [29]. Applications of artificial intelligence, wearable devices, and the utilization of data have presented vast advancements in this field. The collection of real-time physiological data via wearables enhances model-informed precision dosing (MIPD) by providing continuous, individualized input for therapeutic drug monitoring [94, 95]. An example is the application of wearable heart rate and blood pressure monitors to support dosing of cardiovascular drugs like beta-blockers and ensure therapeutic levels to prevent hypotension [90]. Another area is the application of machine learning neural networks in utilizing data from wearable devices to detect progression in neurodegenerative diseases based on gait patterns [86, 96]. Next, we will conclude and discuss future directions to the use and adoption of wearable devices in precision medicine.

Conclusions and Future Perspectives

In this chapter, we reviewed applications of wearable devices in precision medicine. This includes the explanation of precision medicine, areas of application, and challenges faced in the applications of wearable devices in precision medicine. In this part, we will continue with summarized conclusions and a suggestion for future actions to the adoption of wearable devices including steps to address integration and security issues.

Precision medicine enables healthcare interventions to be customized for specific patient groups by considering factors such as disease susceptibility, diagnostic and prognostic insights, and treatment response [59].

As mentioned, advancements in wearable device software and hardware capabilities opened avenues for the use of those devices in precision and personalized medicine [35]. Modern data science and AI technologies presented improvements in the usability, capacity, and functionality of wearable devices [14, 76]. New forms of wearable devices include microchips or smart tattoos, smart jewelry, and smart eyewear [38]. Expansions in wearables that use multiple forms of data including personal, medical, and environmental data to provide more opportunities for personalization of medicine are expected to be seen [84].

The utilization of wearables and advanced technologies in healthcare, including precision medicine, requires the collaboration of healthcare organizations, professionals, and stakeholders. However, there are many points that have to be considered in the use of wearable devices to aid personalized and precision medicine.

To support the adoption of wearable devices, supportive factors should be available. The innovation in technology, data sciences, molecular testing infrastructure, and the development of learning information systems require health organizations to adapt to those changes in the scope of healthcare delivery and decision-making [87]. An essential point is to encourage the uptake of wearable devices and technology implementation via providers' support and standardization of the regulations [44]. An encouraging factor is advancing research and investment in data analysis methods and technologies, particularly data related to patient characteristics and medical conditions [9, 13]. More research is needed on matters of data integration, quality, and equity in data collection. Improved data regulations, data accuracy, and advanced data analysis and synthesis support the confidence and use of wearable devices among patients and professionals. Implementing these recommendations will require strategic investment and active collaboration among key stakeholders, including users, healthcare professionals, and technology designers. Some of the main directions in the adoption of wearable devices in precision and personalized medicine can be summarized as follows:

- The development of advanced wearable technologies that integrate biological, behavioral, and environmental data to dynamically tailor care in real time [23].
- Expand therapeutic drug monitoring (TDM) through biosensors and promote wearable biosensors for continuous drug level monitoring and personalized dosing via model-informed precision dosing (MIPD) [4, 95].
- Advancing predictive features within healthcare technologies by incorporating machine learning and AI models to identify disease trajectories and inform early intervention [86, 96].
- Extend reach to rural and underserved populations via the design low-cost, mobile-integrated, and offline-capable wearables to reduce healthcare access barriers in rural and low-resource settings [28, 60].
- Innovate in user-centric, comfortable models of wearable devices by the development of flexible, non-intrusive formats (e.g., smart tattoos, skin-like sensors) for continuous, long-term use across age groups and health conditions [56, 71].
- Continue to work on standardization and integration of data through improving the interoperability between wearables, EHRs, and clinical systems using open standards and APIs, and streamlining communication across platforms to enhance decision-making and reduce data silos [21, 25].
- Enforce robust data privacy and governance through advancing policies and regulations for consent, data ownership, and cloud security to build public trust in wearable technologies [8, 20].
- Enhance clinical validation by conducting practical trials across diverse populations, including underserved groups, to validate device performance and equity [17, 68].
- Support regulatory and global certification through actions such as harmonizing certification processes for wearable devices to ensure safe and scalable adoption and effective international communications [33, 91].

- Foster collaborative approaches by the involvement of rural healthcare providers, community leaders, and patients in the design and deployment of wearable health solutions [44].
- Mobilize investment and partnerships across sectors by integrating public and private funds into R&D, wearable-enabled telemedicine, and AI infrastructure, particularly in underserved health systems [10, 60]. Potential areas of research related to the use of wearable devices in precision medicine include psychology and behavioral science. Also, research can include the use of wearable devices in developing countries and marginalized communities to support remote monitoring and enable early detection of disease. Additionally, it is worthwhile to undertake research on tools to improve consistency on the use of wearable health devices and support the regulations of their use in healthcare.

References

1. An Q, Rahman S, Zhou J, Kang JJ. A comprehensive review on machine learning in healthcare industry: classification, restrictions, opportunities and challenges. Sensors. 2023;23(9). MDPI. https://doi.org/10.3390/s23094178.
2. Anker JN, Hall WP, Lyandres O, Shah NC, Zhao J, Van Duyne RP. Biosensing with plasmonic nanosensors. Nat Mater. 2008;7(6):442–53. https://doi.org/10.1038/nmat2162.
3. Ao C, Jiao S, Wang Y, Yu L, Zou Q. Biological sequence classification: a review on data and general methods. Research. 2022;2022. https://doi.org/10.34133/research.0011.
4. Ates HC, Roberts JA, Lipman J, Cass AEG, Urban GA, Dincer C. On-site therapeutic drug monitoring. Trends Biotechnol. 2020;38(11):1262–77. Elsevier Ltd. https://doi.org/10.1016/j.tibtech.2020.03.001.
5. Babu M, Lautman Z, Lin X, Sobota MHB, Snyder MP. Wearable devices: implications for precision medicine and the future of health care. 2025;27:51. https://doi.org/10.1146/annurev-med-052422.
6. Badr Y, Abdul Kader L, Shamayleh A. The use of big data in personalized healthcare to reduce inventory waste and optimize patient treatment. J Pers Med. 2024;14(4). Multidisciplinary Digital Publishing Institute (MDPI). https://doi.org/10.3390/jpm14040383.
7. Baig MM, GholamHosseini H, Moqeem AA, Mirza F, Lindén M. A systematic review of wearable patient monitoring systems – current challenges and opportunities for clinical adoption. J Med Syst. 2017;41(7). https://doi.org/10.1007/s10916-017-0760-1.
8. Banerjee S(Sy), Hemphill T, Longstreet P. Wearable devices and healthcare: data sharing and privacy. Inform Soc. 2018;34(1):49–57. https://doi.org/10.1080/01972243.2017.1391912.
9. Böttcher S, Vieluf S, Bruno E, Joseph B, Epitashvili N, Biondi A, Zabler N, Glasstetter M, Dümpelmann M, Van Laerhoven K, Nasseri M, Brinkman BH, Richardson MP, Schulze-Bonhage A, Loddenkemper T. Data quality evaluation in wearable monitoring. Sci Rep. 2022;12(1). https://doi.org/10.1038/s41598-022-25949-x.
10. Brophy K, Davies S, Olenik S, Çotur Y, Ming D, Van Zalk N, O'hare D, Güder F, Yetisen AK. The future of wearable technologies. 2021. https://doi.org/10.25561/88893.
11. Buke A, Gaoli F, Yongcia W, Lei S, Zhiqi Y. Healthcare algorithms by wearable inertial sensors: a survey. China Communications. 2015;12(4);1–12.
12. Canali S, Schiaffonati V, Aliverti A. Challenges and recommendations for wearable devices in digital health: data quality, interoperability, health equity, fairness. PLOS Digit Health. 2022;1(10). Public Library of Science. https://doi.org/10.1371/journal.pdig.0000104.

13. Celik Y, Godfrey A. Bringing it all together: wearable data fusion. npj Digit Med. 2023;6(149):1–3.
14. Chan M, Estève D, Fourniols JY, Escriba C, Campo E. Smart wearable systems: current status and future challenges. Artif Intell Med. 2012;56(3):137–56. https://doi.org/10.1016/j.artmed.2012.09.003.
15. Chen L, Hoey J, Nugent CD, Cook DJ, Yu Z. Sensor-based activity recognition. IEEE Trans Syst Man Cybern Part C Appl Rev. 2012;42(6):790–808. https://doi.org/10.1109/TSMCC.2012.2198883.
16. Central Drugs Standard Control Organization (CDSCO). Medical devices rules, 2017/ (updated February 2023 version). Ministry of health and family welfare. Government of India. 2003.
17. Cheong IY, An SY, Cha WC, Rha MY, Kim ST, Chang DK, Hwang JH. Efficacy of mobile health care application and wearable device in improvement of physical performance in colorectal cancer patients undergoing chemotherapy. Clin Colorectal Cancer. 2018;17(2):e353–62. https://doi.org/10.1016/j.clcc.2018.02.002.
18. Cho S, Ensari I, Weng C, Kahn MG, Natarajan K. Factors affecting the quality of person-generated wearable device data and associated challenges: rapid systematic review. JMIR Mhealth Uhealth. 2021;9(3). JMIR Publications Inc. https://doi.org/10.2196/20738.
19. Chow R, Drkulec H, Im JHB, Tsai J, Nafees A, Kumar S, Hou T, Fazelzad R, Leighl NB, Krzyzanowska M, Wong P, Raman S. The use of wearable devices in oncology patients: a systematic review. Oncologist. 2024;29(4):e419–30. Oxford University Press. https://doi.org/10.1093/oncolo/oyad305.
20. Cilliers L. Wearable devices in healthcare: privacy and information security issues. Health Inf Manag J. 2020;49(2–3):150–6. https://doi.org/10.1177/1833358319851684.
21. Clarke M, De Folter J, Verma V, Gokalp H. Interoperable end-to-end remote patient monitoring platform based on IEEE 11073 PHD and ZigBee Health Care Profile. IEEE Trans Biomed Eng. 2018;65(5):1014–25. https://doi.org/10.1109/TBME.2017.2732501.
22. Collins FS, Varmus H. A new initiative on precision medicine. N Engl J Med. 2015;372(9):793–5. https://doi.org/10.1056/nejmp1500523.
23. Contreras I, Vehi J. Artificial intelligence for diabetes management and decision support: Literature review. J Med Internet Res. 2018;20(5).
24. Deshpande P, Bhatt MW, Shinde SK, Labhade-Kumar N, Ashokkumar N, Venkatesan KGS, Shadrach FD. Combining handcrafted features and deep learning for automatic classification of lung cancer on CT scans. J Artif Intell Technol. 2024;4(2):102–13. https://doi.org/10.37965/jait.2023.0388.
25. Dinh-Le C, Chuang R, Chokshi S, Mann D. Wearable health technology and electronic health record integration: scoping review and future directions. JMIR Mhealth Uhealth. 2019;7(9). JMIR Publications Inc. https://doi.org/10.2196/12861.
26. Eappen P, Gunn V, Brar HS, Stedman I. Capitalizing on the transformative role of AI and human capital to strengthen cybersecurity in healthcare. In: Martiri E, Vajjhala NR, Dalipi F, editors. AI-enabled threat intelligence and cyber risk assessment. CRC Press; 2025. p. 112–25. https://doi.org/10.1201/9781003504979-7.
27. Ghazizadeh E, Naseri Z, Deigner HP, Rahimi H, Altintas Z. Approaches of wearable and implantable biosensor towards of developing in precision medicine. Front Med. 2024;11. Frontiers Media SA. https://doi.org/10.3389/fmed.2024.1390634.
28. Glaros C, Fotiadis DI. Wearable devices in healthcare. StudFuz. 2005;184:237–64. www.springerlink.com.
29. Gross AS. Best practice in therapeutic drug monitoring. Br J Clin Pharmacol. 2001;52(S1):5–9. https://doi.org/10.1111/j.1365-2125.2001.00770.x.
30. Gunn V, Eappen P, Brar HS, Brulin E, Muntaner C. Integration of wearable devices in healthcare: the need to examine their implications for health workers. In: Eappen P, Vajjhala NR, Zikos D, Davidson KP, editors. Remote monitoring and wearable devices in healthcare. Information systems engineering and management, vol. 63. Cham: Springer; 2025. https://doi.org/10.1007/978-3-031-98897-4_6.

31. Guo Y, Liu X, Peng S, Jiang X, Xu K, Chen C, Wang Z, Dai C, Chen W. A review of wearable and unobtrusive sensing technologies for chronic disease management. Comput Biol Med. 2021;129. Elsevier Ltd. https://doi.org/10.1016/j.compbiomed.2020.104163.
32. Hasanzad M, Sarhangi N, Ehsani Chimeh S, Ayati N, Afzali M, Khatami F, Nikfar S, Aghaei Meybodi HR. Precision medicine journey through omics approach. J Diabetes Metab Disord. 2022;21(1):881–8. Springer Science and Business Media Deutschland GmbH. https://doi.org/10.1007/s40200-021-00913-0.
33. Health Canada. Exploring precision medicine in Canada: Opportunities and challenges. Government of Canada. 2022.
34. Heintzman ND. A Digital Ecosystem of Diabetes Data and Technology: Services, Systems, and Tools Enabled by Wearables, Sensors, and Apps. J Diabetes Sci Technol. 2015;20;10(1):35–41. https://doi.org/10.1177/1932296815622453. PMID: 26685994; PMCID: PMC4738231.
35. Hicks JL, Althoff T, Sosic R, Kuhar P, Bostjancic B, King AC, Leskovec J, Delp SL. Best practices for analyzing large-scale health data from wearables and smartphone apps. npj Digit Med. 2019;2(1). Nature Publishing Group. https://doi.org/10.1038/s41746-019-0121-1.
36. Hulshof P, Kortbeek N, Boucherie R, Hans E, Bakker P. Taxonomic classification of planning decisions in health care: a structured review of the state of the art in OR/MS. Health Syst. 2012;1(2):129–75. https://doi.org/10.1057/hs.2012.18.
37. Humburg MA, Collins FS. The path to personalized medicine. N Engl J Med. 2010;4(363):301–4.
38. Iqbal SMA, Mahgoub I, Du E, Leavitt MA, Asghar W. Advances in healthcare wearable devices. npj Flex Electron. 2021;5(1). Nature Research. https://doi.org/10.1038/s41528-021-00107-x.
39. Jacoba CMP, Celi LA, Silva PS. Biomarkers for progression in diabetic retinopathy: expanding personalized medicine through integration of AI with electronic health records. Semin Ophthalmol. 2021;36(4):250–7. Taylor and Francis Ltd. https://doi.org/10.1080/08820538.2021.1893351.
40. Johnson KB, Wei WQ, Weeraratne D, Frisse ME, Misulis K, Rhee K, Zhao J, Snowdon JL. Precision medicine, AI, and the future of personalized health care. Clin Transl Sci. 2021;14(1):86–93. https://doi.org/10.1111/cts.12884.
41. John JS, Prathap BR, Gupta G, Melanaturu J. Categorizing mental stress: A consistency-focused benchmarking of ML and DL models for multi-label, multi-class classification via taxonomy-driven NLP techniques. Nat Lang Process J. 2025;11:100162.
42. Joyner MJ, Paneth N. Promises, promises, and precision medicine. J Clin Invest. 2019;129(3):946–8. American Society for Clinical Investigation. https://doi.org/10.1172/JCI126119.
43. Kakria P, Tripathi NK, Kitipawang P. A real-time health monitoring system for remote cardiac patients using smartphone and wearable sensors. Int J Telemed Appl. 2015;2015. https://doi.org/10.1155/2015/373474.
44. Kang HS, Exworthy M. Wearing the future-wearables to empower users to take greater responsibility for their health and care: scoping review. JMIR Mhealth Uhealth. 2022;10(7). JMIR Publications Inc. https://doi.org/10.2196/35684.
45. Kapoor V, Singh R, Reddy R, Churi P. Privacy issues in wearable technology: an intrinsic review. SSRN Electron J. 2020. https://doi.org/10.2139/ssrn.3566918.
46. Katurura MC, Cilliers L. Electronic health record system in the public health care sector of South Africa: a systematic literature review. Afr J Prim Health Care Fam Med. 2018;10(1). https://doi.org/10.4102/phcfm.v10i1.1746.
47. Kaur R, Shahrestani S, Ruan C. Security and privacy of wearable wireless sensors in healthcare: a systematic review. Comput Netw Commun. 2024. https://doi.org/10.37256/cnc.2120243852.
48. Khan Y, Ostfeld AE, Lochner CM, Pierre A, Arias AC. Monitoring of vital signs with flexible and wearable medical devices. Adv Mater. 2016;28(22):4373–95. Wiley-VCH Verlag. https://doi.org/10.1002/adma.201504366.

49. Kharb S. Future directions: what LIES ahead for smart biochemical wearables in health monitoring? Front Anal Sci. 2024;4. https://doi.org/10.3389/frans.2024.1509815.
50. Kothinti RR. Artificial intelligence in healthcare: revolutionizing precision medicine, predictive analytics, and ethical considerations in autonomous diagnostics. World J Adv Res Rev. 2024;24(3):3394–406. https://doi.org/10.30574/wjarr.2024.24.3.3675.
51. Krzyszczyk P, Acevedo A, Davidoff EJ, Timmins LM, Marrero-Berrios I, Patel M, White C, Lowe C, Sherba JJ, Hartmanshenn C, O'Neill KM, Balter ML, Fritz ZR, Androulakis IP, Schloss RS, Yarmush ML. The growing role of precision and personalized medicine for cancer treatment. Technology. 2018;06(03n04):79–100. https://doi.org/10.1142/s2339547818300020.
52. Lander S, Linton LM, Birren B, Nusbaum C, Zody MC, Baldwin J, Devon K, Dewar K, Doyle M, FitzHugh W, Funke R, Gage D, Harris K, Heaford A, Howland J, Kann L, Lehoczky J, LeVine R, McEwan P, et al. Initial sequencing and analysis of the human genome International Human Genome Sequencing Consortium*. The Sanger Centre: Beijing Genomics Institute/ Human Genome Center. Nature. 2001;409. www.nature.com.
53. Lehne M, Sass J, Essenwanger A, Schepers J, Thun S. Why digital medicine depends on interoperability. npj Digit Med. 2019;2(1). Nature Publishing Group. https://doi.org/10.1038/s41746-019-0158-1.
54. Liang WS, Beaulieu-Jones B, Smalley S, Snyder M, Goetz LH, Schork NJ. Emerging therapeutic drug monitoring technologies: considerations and opportunities in precision medicine. Front Pharmacol. 2024;15. Frontiers Media SA. https://doi.org/10.3389/fphar.2024.1348112.
55. Liao Y, Thompson C, Peterson S, Mandrola J, Beg MS. The future of wearable technologies and remote monitoring in health care. Am Soc Clin Oncol Educ Book. 2019;39:115–21. https://doi.org/10.1200/edbk_238919.
56. Linh VTN, Han S, Koh E, Kim S, Jung HS, Koo J. Advances in wearable electronics for monitoring human organs: bridging external and internal health assessments. Biomaterials. 2025;314. https://doi.org/10.1016/j.biomaterials.2024.122865.
57. Linh VTN, Han S, Koh E, Kim S, Jung HS, Koo J. Advances in wearable electronics for monitoring human organs: Bridging external and internal health assessments. Biomaterials. 2025;314:122865
58. Lötvall J, Akdis CA, Bacharier LB, Bjermer L, Casale TB, Custovic A, et al. Asthma endotypes: A new approach to classification of disease entities within the asthma syndrome. J Allergy Clin Immunol. 2011;127(2):355–60.
59. Love-Koh J, Peel A, Rejon-Parrilla JC, Ennis K, Lovett R, Manca A, Chalkidou A, Wood H, Taylor M. The future of precision medicine: potential impacts for health technology assessment. PharmacoEconomics. 2018;36(12):1439–51. https://doi.org/10.1007/s40273-018-0686-6.
60. Lu L, Zhang J, Xie Y, Gao F, Xu S, Wu X, Ye Z. Wearable health devices in health care: narrative systematic review. JMIR Mhealth Uhealth. 2020;8(11). JMIR Publications Inc. https://doi.org/10.2196/18907.
61. Mahajan A, Heydari K, Powell D. Wearable AI to enhance patient safety and clinical decision-making. npj Digit Med. 2025;8(1). Nature Research. https://doi.org/10.1038/s41746-025-01554-w.
62. Manne R, Kantheti SC. Application of artificial intelligence in healthcare: chances and challenges. Curr J Appl Sci Technol. 2021:78–89. https://doi.org/10.9734/cjast/2021/v40i631320.
63. Martin T, Jovanov E, Raskovic D. Issues in wearable computing for medical monitoring applications: a case study of a wearable ECG monitoring device. 2020. https://doi.org/10.1109/ISWC.2000.888463.
64. Mihovska A, Kyriazakos SA, Mihaylov M, Prasad R. Standardization and innovation for smart e-health monitoring devices. In: Biodevices 2015 – 8th international conference on biomedical electronics and devices, proceedings; part of 8th international joint conference on biomedical engineering systems and technologies, BIOSTEC 2015; 2015. p. 283–90. https://doi.org/10.5220/0005318502830290.

65. Miller NA, Farrow EG, Gibson M, Willig LK, Twist G, Yoo B, Marrs T, Corder S, Krivohlavek L, Walter A, Petrikin JE, Saunders CJ, Thiffault I, Soden SE, Smith LD, Dinwiddie DL, Herd S, Cakici JA, Catreux S, et al. A 26-hour system of highly sensitive whole genome sequencing for emergency management of genetic diseases. Genome Med. 2015;7(1). https://doi.org/10.1186/s13073-015-0221-8.
66. Mukhopadhyay SC. Wearable sensors for human activity monitoring: a review. IEEE Sensors J. 2015;15(3):1321–30. Institute of Electrical and Electronics Engineers Inc. https://doi.org/10.1109/JSEN.2014.2370945.
67. Naithani N, Sinha S, Misra P, Vasudevan B, Sahu R. Precision medicine: concept and tools. Med J Armed Forces India. 2021;77(3):249–57. Elsevier B.V. https://doi.org/10.1016/j.mjafi.2021.06.021.
68. Ngueleu AM, Barthod C, Best KL, Routhier F, Otis M, Batcho CS. Criterion validity of ActiGraph monitoring devices for step counting and distance measurement in adults and older adults: a systematic review. J Neuroeng Rehabil. 2022;19(1). BioMed Central Ltd. https://doi.org/10.1186/s12984-022-01085-5.
69. Niknejad N, Ismail WB, Mardani A, Liao H, Ghani I. A comprehensive overview of smart wearables: the state of the art literature, recent advances, and future challenges. Eng Appl Artif Intell. 2020;90. https://doi.org/10.1016/j.engappai.2020.103529.
70. Obermeyer Z, Powers B, Vogeli C, Mullainathan S. Dissecting racial bias in an algorithm used to manage the health of populations. Science. 2019;366(6464):447–53. https://doi.org/10.1126/science.aax2342.
71. Oh YS, Kim JH, Xie Z, Cho S, Han H, Jeon SW, Park M, Namkoong M, Avila R, Song Z, Lee SU, Ko K, Lee J, Lee JS, Min WG, Lee BJ, Choi M, Chung HU, Kim J, et al. Battery-free, wireless soft sensors for continuous multi-site measurements of pressure and temperature from patients at risk for pressure injuries. Nat Commun. 2021;12(1). https://doi.org/10.1038/s41467-021-25324-w.
72. Pantelopoulos A, Bourbakis NG. A survey on wearable biosensor systems for health monitoring. Annu Int Conf IEEE Eng Med Biol Soc. 2008:4887–90.
73. Palmerini L, Reggi L, Bonci T, Del Din S, Micó-Amigo ME, Salis F, Bertuletti S, Caruso M, Cereatti A, Gazit E, Paraschiv-Ionescu A, Soltani A, Kluge F, Küderle A, Ullrich M, Kirk C, Hiden H, D'Ascanio I, Hansen C, et al. Mobility recorded by wearable devices and gold standards: the Mobilise-D procedure for data standardization. Sci Data. 2023;10(1). https://doi.org/10.1038/s41597-023-01930-9.
74. Perry B, Uuk R. Ai governance and the policymaking process: key considerations for reducing ai risk. Big Data Cogn Comput. 2019;3(2):1–17. https://doi.org/10.3390/bdcc3020026.
75. Priyadharshini S, Sivaranjani PS, Nagalakshmi S. The Registration of Medical Device in FDA EU and CDSCO: Overview Journal of Advances in Medical and Pharmaceutical Sciences. 2024;26(8):76–88. https://doi.org/10.9734/jamps/2024/v26i8709.
76. Ramalingam A, Eraiarasan A. The future of wearable technology and its impact on healthcare. Quing Int J Innov Res Sci Eng. 2023;2(2):110–6. https://doi.org/10.54368/qijirse.2.2.0012.
77. Ramaswami R, Bayer R, Galea S. Precision medicine from a public health perspective. On Sat. 2025;29:58. https://doi.org/10.1146/annurev-publhealth.
78. Ristevski B, Chen M. Big data analytics in medicine and healthcare. J Integr Bioinform. 2018;15(3). https://doi.org/10.1515/jib-2017-0030.
79. Ritz D. Connecting health information systems for better health leveraging interoperability standards to link. JLN. 13–25 Sept 2014.
80. Saad HS, Zaki JFW, Abdelsalam MM. Employing of machine learning and wearable devices in healthcare system: tasks and challenges. Neural Comput & Applic. 2024. Springer Science and Business Media Deutschland GmbH. https://doi.org/10.1007/s00521-024-10197-z.
81. Sabry F, Eltaras T, Labda W, Alzoubi K, Malluhi Q. Machine learning for healthcare wearable devices: the big picture. J Healthc Eng. 2022;2022. Hindawi Limited. https://doi.org/10.1155/2022/4653923.

82. Seymour CW, Gomez H, Chang CCH, Clermont G, Kellum JA, Kennedy J, Yende S, Angus DC. Precision medicine for all? Challenges and opportunities for a precision medicine approach to critical illness. Crit Care. 2017;21(1). BioMed Central Ltd. https://doi.org/10.1186/s13054-017-1836-5.
83. Smirnov VV. A generalized addressing concept for correlative memory and neural networks. Neurocomputing. 2006;69(13–15):1637–44. https://doi.org/10.1016/j.neucom.2005.05.014.
84. Smuck M, Odonkor CA, Wilt JK, Schmidt N, Swiernik MA. The emerging clinical role of wearables: factors for successful implementation in healthcare. npj Digit Med. 2021;4(1). Nature Research. https://doi.org/10.1038/s41746-021-00418-3.
85. Someya T, Bao Z, Malliaras GG. The rise of plastic bioelectronics. Nature. 2016;540(7633):379–85. Nature Publishing Group. https://doi.org/10.1038/nature21004.
86. Stepleton T, Pascanu R, Dabney W, Jayakumar SM, Soyer H, Munos R. Low-pass recurrent neural networks – a memory architecture for longer-term correlation discovery. 2018. http://arxiv.org/abs/1805.04955.
87. Sun W, Lee J, Zhang S, Benyshek C, Dokmeci MR, Khademhosseini A. Engineering precision medicine. Adv Sci. 2019;6(1). John Wiley and Sons Inc. https://doi.org/10.1002/advs.201801039.
88. Tu J, Gao W. Ethical considerations of wearable technologies in human research. Adv Healthc Mater. 2021;10(17). https://doi.org/10.1002/adhm.202100127.
89. Vijayan V, Connolly J, Condell J, McKelvey N, Gardiner P. Review of wearable devices and data collection considerations for connected health. Sensors. 2021;21(16). MDPI AG. https://doi.org/10.3390/s21165589.
90. Wang X, Wang C. How does health status affect marginal utility of consumption? Evidence from China. Int J Environ Res Public Health. 2020;17(7). https://doi.org/10.3390/ijerph17072234.
91. World Health Organization. Global strategy on digital health 2020-2025. Geneva: World Health Organization. 2020.
92. Yan Y, Ivanov K, Omisore OM, Igbe T, Liu Q, Nie Z, Wang L. Gait rhythm dynamics for neuro-degenerative disease classification via persistence landscape-based topological representation. Sensors (Switzerland). 2020;20(7). https://doi.org/10.3390/s20072006.
93. Yasini M, Marchand G. Mobile health applications, in the absence of an authentic regulation, does the usability score correlate with a better medical reliability? Stud Health Technol Inform. 2015;216:127–31. https://doi.org/10.3233/978-1-61499-564-7-127.
94. Yuqiao L, Junmin L, Shenghao L, Yanhui X, Mingxia L, Lixiu B, Jiaqian G, Dajing Z, Chen Y. Revolutionizing precision medicine: Exploring wearable sensors for therapeutic drug monitoring and personalized therapy. Biosensors (Basel). 2023;13(7):726
95. Jiang F, Jiang Y, Zhi H, Dong Y, Li H, Ma S, et al. Artificial intelligence in healthcare: Past, present and future. Stroke Vasc Neurol. 2017;2(4):230–43.
96. Zhao A, Li J, Dong J, Qi L, Zhang Q, Li N, Wang X, Zhou H. Multimodal gait recognition for neurodegenerative diseases. 2021. http://arxiv.org/abs/2101.02469.
97. Zikos D, Eappen P, Brockman M. Wearable devices in healthcare: machine learning methods to transform data streams to insights. In: Eappen P, Vajjhala NR, Zikos D, Davidson KP, editors. Remote monitoring and wearable devices in healthcare. Information systems engineering and management. Cham: Springer. 2025;63. https://doi.org/10.1007/978-3-031-98897-4_4.

Chapter 13
Smart Living for Seniors: Bridging Technology and Elderly Well-Being

Mohammad Salah Uddin

Introduction

The world's population is aging rapidly. More people are living longer than ever before. This is driving a growing demand for better ways to maintain health, safety, and independence in everyday life. The Internet of Things (IoT) is improving elder care in many ways. It provides smart systems to meet the growing demands of the elderly. IoT works through connected devices and sensors. These devices continuously receive and share data. IoT supports health monitoring, daily care, and routine tasks. It creates a strong connection between older adults, caregivers, and healthcare professionals. It also helps manage common age-related challenges. These include chronic illnesses, regular medications, risk of falls, and social isolation. Many older adults face multiple health problems at the same time. Regular monitoring helps to identify problems promptly. This allows for faster treatment and better outcomes. Smart devices such as medication reminders provide reminders to take medications on time.

Fall detection technology sends quick alerts when accidents occur. These devices improve safety and reduce the need of manual supervision. Smart home technology provides additional assistance in everyday life. Automated lighting, thermostats, and appliances make it easier to manage the home. Voice assistant systems include voice commands to control household appliances. It improves comfort and supports independent living.

Environmentally sensitive devices monitor air quality, temperature, and humidity. These devices are helpful in maintaining a healthy and safe living environment. IoT also supports mental well-being. Video calling systems help seniors stay connected with family and friends. Social chatbots provide communication and daily

M. S. Uddin (✉)
Department of Computer Science and Engineering, East West University, Dhaka, Bangladesh
e-mail: uddin@ewubd.edu

P. Eappen et al. (eds.), *Advancing Healthcare with the Medical Internet of Things*, Health Informatics, https://doi.org/10.1007/978-3-032-23933-4_13

reminders to seniors. They reduce feelings of loneliness. GPS trackers and geo-fencing protect people with short-term memory loss. Alerts are sent when someone moves outside a safe area. Emergency response systems provide quick assistance.

Smart kitchen technology is helpful for cooking and food management. Nutrition trackers record healthy eating habits. Memory and task assistants help manage daily routines efficiently. These tools support brain health and encourage independent living.

This chapter covers various applications of Internet of Things (IoT) such as remote health monitoring, fall detection, smart home, air and temperature monitoring, GPS tracking, emergency systems, and nutrition tracking along with their benefits. It also discusses implementation challenges as well as positive impact analysis based on several research works. These technologies improve the quality of life of older people.

Remote Health Monitoring

Remote health monitoring systems track health conditions remotely. The system uses wearable devices and sensors for collecting health parameters. These parameters include heart rate, blood pressure, oxygen levels, and body temperature. The collected data is sent to the cloud for analysis. Doctors, caregivers, or family members can also access that information via mobile devices. This helps to respond quickly if a measurement goes outside the normal range. Early diagnosis helps prevent serious health problems. It reduces hospital visits and avoids emergency situations. This helps with long-term care planning and treatment coordination. It also reduces the need for frequent in-person checkups. Elders can stay at home and still receive proper care. Remote monitoring gives peace of mind to both patients and caregivers. It makes healthcare more proactive, efficient, and accessible. Uddin et al. [1] have developed a remote patient monitoring system specifically for continuous observation of critically ill patients. The system uses multiple sensors to collect health parameters. Those parameters are then displayed in real time through a mobile application. If a patient's condition becomes unstable, the system automatically sends push notifications to alert caregivers. In reference [2, 3], a variety of wearable health devices are highlighted.

Wearable Health Devices

Wearable devices include smartwatches, fitness bands, and biosensors. These devices track heart rate, blood pressure, body temperature, oxygen levels, and sleep patterns. The information is sent to the care platform or cloud in real time. Continuous tracking helps in early detection of warning signs and supports quick medical action. Several benefits are listed in Table 13.1.

Table 13.1 Remote health monitoring benefits

Benefit	Description
Early detection of health changes	Health issues can be identified early before becoming severe
Simple, non-intrusive tracking during daily routines	Wearables and sensors track vital signs without interrupting daily activities
Reduced emergency visits and hospitalizations	Collected data helps create personalized care plans tailored to individual needs
Custom care plans based on real-time data	Monitoring and alerts help prevent severe incidents and reduce hospital trips
Better coordination between caregivers and healthcare providers	IoT platforms share data across care teams for faster, informed decisions

Note: Remote health monitoring systems enhance patient safety and reduce medical emergencies by enabling real-time tracking and communication between care teams

Table 13.2 Benefits of medication management

Benefit	Description
Better medication adherence	Smart pill dispensers and reminders help ensure medications are taken on time
Fewer errors in dosage or timing	Automated systems help prevent missed doses or wrong timing
Real-time updates for caregiver support	Caregivers get instant alerts and updates on how medications are being taken

Note. These tools help people take their medications correctly and keep caregivers in the loop

Smart Pill Dispensers

Smart pill dispensers help manage medication schedules. These devices release the correct dose at the right time. Reminders reduce missed doses. If a dose is skipped, alerts are sent to caregivers. This helps avoid serious health risks from missed or incorrect medication. The benefits are listed in Table 13.2. Several researchers have introduced their own pill dispenser designs, detailed in references [4, 5].

Health Monitoring Apps

Health apps connect data from all IoT health tools. These platforms track progress, set goals, and offer health tips. Apps show all health data in one place for easier understanding. Many apps also allow direct communication between healthcare teams and care recipients. Several benefits of health monitoring apps are shown in Table 13.3. Welltory [6], a digital health company, offers a health monitoring application. It uses smartphone sensors and wearable devices to track heart rate, stress, and energy. Real-time analysis provides personalized insights and recommendations. This approach promotes better well-being and stress management.

Table 13.3 Benefits of health monitoring apps

Benefit	Description
Centralized inspection of health data	These apps combine data from different IoT devices to give a full picture of someone's health
Better engagement in daily health management	People can track their progress, set goals, and stay involved in their health routines
Easier coordination between doctors and caregivers	Shared data and chat tools help caregivers, doctors, and families work together more easily

Note: Health monitoring apps bring together useful data and tools that make daily care and teamwork much easier

Fall Detection and Prevention

Fall detection and prevention systems are important components in elderly care. Falls are a major cause of injury among older adults. IoT technology helps detect falls early and prevent accidents before they happen.

Fall Detection Systems

Sensors are placed on wearables, furniture, walls or floors. They continuously track movement and body position. These sensors detect walking patterns, sitting, standing or lying down. If there is a sudden change, such as a fall or injury, the system responds immediately. It triggers an automatic alert without any manual action. Alerts are sent to caregivers, family members, or emergency services in real time. This rapid response can prevent serious injuries or delays in treatment. Fall detection systems help ensure safety, especially for people living alone. Some of the benefits of this system are given in Table 13.4.

Fall Prevention Systems

IoT systems also help prevent falls before it happens. Fall prevention systems do more than just send alerts after a fall. Smart flooring and motion sensors track daily movement patterns. Predictive analytics study walking speed, posture, and balance. If the system notices unusual movement or unsteadiness, it sends an early warning. Lights can automatically turn on when movement is detected at night. This reduces the risk of tripping or stumbling in the dark. Fall prevention features improve safety and support independent living. Table 13.5 lists several advances of fall prevention systems.

Devices like Life Alert [7] and Medical Guardian [8] provide wearable fall detection that alerts in-charge personnel when a fall occurs. Apple Watch and other smartwatches with built-in fall detection method notify emergency contacts when a hard fall is detected.

Table 13.4 Fall detection system benefits

Benefit	Description
Faster response after a fall	Fall detection systems send immediate alerts to caregivers or emergency services, reducing response time
Lower risk of serious injury or delayed help	Early alerts prevent complications by ensuring timely medical attention
Peace of mind for caregivers and family members	Real-time monitoring and notifications provide assurance to those responsible for elder care

Note: Fall detection system is helpful for improving safety and reduce stress for caregivers and family members

Table 13.5 Fall prevention systems advantages

Benefit	Description
Fewer accidents through early risk detection	Predictive analytics and motion sensors detect irregular movement patterns to prevent falls before occur
Safer navigation at home, especially at night	Smart lighting and environmental adjustments reduce fall risk during nighttime activity
More confidence in everyday movement	Reliable support systems help individuals feel more secure and stable during daily activities

Note: Fall prevention systems help reduce risks and enables safer, more confident movement at home

Smart Home Integration

An important part of IoT in elderly care is smart home technology. It automates tasks such as turning lights on or off, adjusting room temperature, and securing doors [9]. It brings greater comfort and security to everyday life. The devices work together and can be managed via a mobile app. They reduce manual effort and continuous observation for unusual changes. Sensors detect doors opening/closing or sudden changes in temperature/humidity. Alerts are issued if measurement patterns change or indicate health problems. This extra support helps older adults remain independent and feel safe in their own homes.

Automated Lighting

Automatic lighting systems respond to movement, time of day, or voice commands. They turn on automatically when someone enters the room. Night lighting increases visibility and reduces the risk of falls. This technology also supports scheduled switching methods. Table 13.6 highlights some of the key benefits of automated lighting.

Table 13.6 Advantages of using automated lighting

Benefit	Description
Safer movement during nighttime	Motion-activated lighting reduces the risk of falls or injuries by providing automatic illumination in dark areas
Easier access to lighting without physical switches	Voice-controlled or sensor-based lighting allows hands-free operation, reducing the need for physical effort
Improved visibility for daily activities	Consistent lighting enhances visibility and supports safer completion of routine tasks

Note: In home environment, automated lighting helps improve safety, comfort, and ease of use

Smart Thermostats

Temperature control is important for comfort and health. Smart thermostats automatically adjust settings based on room conditions or user preferences. Some cloud-connected systems allow caregivers to adjust temperatures remotely. The benefits of smart thermostats are listed in Table 13.7. One example of a smart thermostat is the Google Nest Thermostat [10].

Voice-Controlled Devices

Voice assistants like Amazon Alexa and Google Assistance [11] make it easy to control appliances, lights, and other home devices. Simple voice commands can turn off lights, adjust the thermostat, or play music. These tools allow hands-free living and make everyday tasks simpler. Several advantages are shown in Table 13.8. The workflow diagram of voice-controlled devices is illustrated in Fig. 13.1.

Smart Appliances

Smart kitchen devices offer safety and convenience. They monitor cooking times, detect stove usage, and send alerts if appliances are left on for a long time. Some smart systems even provide step-by-step cooking instructions. Some of the key benefits are listed in Table 13.9. A grocery item tracking system was developed by a group of researchers from East West University in Bangladesh. Their solution monitors various items, including cooking oil, eggs, and salt stored in kitchen [12].

Table 13.7 Smart thermostats system benefits

Benefit	Description
Stable indoor climate	Smart thermostats automatically adjust temperature settings to maintain consistent comfort levels
Reduced risk of overheating or exposure to cold	Temperature control systems prevent extreme indoor temperatures that can affect health and safety
Energy savings through efficient use	Energy-efficient operation reduces power usage and lowers utility costs without compromising comfort

Note: Smart thermostats support both comfort and safety while minimizing energy costs

Table 13.8 Advantages of using smart/voice-controlled devices

Benefit	Description
Safer movement during nighttime	Motion-activated lighting reduces the risk of falls by providing automatic illumination in dark areas
Easier access to lighting without physical switches	Voice-controlled or sensor-based lighting allows hands-free operation, reducing the need for physical effort
Improved visibility for daily activities	Consistent lighting enhances visibility and supports safer completion of routine tasks

Note: Smart devices improve safety and make home routines more comfortable and accessible

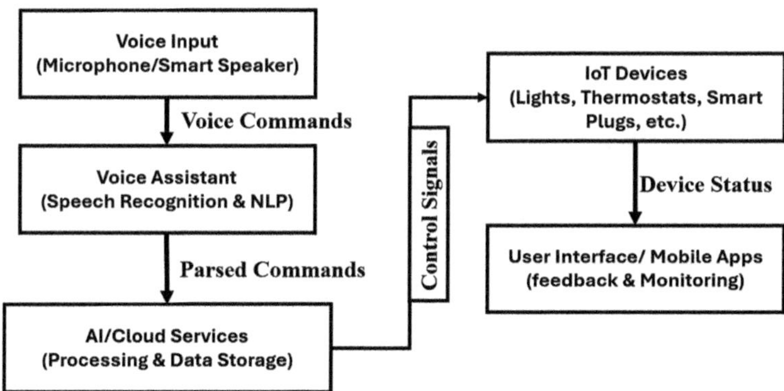

Fig. 13.1 Voice controlled device workflow

Table 13.9 Advantages of smart appliances

Benefit	Description
Safer use of kitchen equipment	Smart kitchen devices include safety features that help prevent burns, fires, or mishandling of equipment
Fewer accidents from unattended appliances	Sensors and automatic shut-off features reduce the risk of accidents from forgotten appliances
Better support for daily meal preparation	Guided cooking tools and timers assist with meal preparation, improving confidence and safety in the kitchen

Note: Smart kitchen appliances have several safety features. It makes cooking more manageable and less stressful

Home Security Systems

IoT-based security systems keep an eye on doors, windows, and activity around the home. Motion sensors and cameras send alerts when they detect unusual movement or potential intrusions. They help ensure a safe and secure living environment. Table 13.10 shows several advantages of home security systems.

Diet, Nutrition, and Meal Support

Nutrition plays a major role in maintaining health of elderly people. IoT tools help manage diet, offer healthy eating habits, and improve food safety. Smart systems make meal planning and food tracking easier and accurate.

Smart Kitchen Devices

IoT-enabled kitchen tools assist with cooking, timing, and safety. Devices include smart ovens, induction cooktops, and automated timers. Some systems detect overheating, alert when food is ready, or shut off appliances if left unattended. Some advantages are shown in Table 13.11.

Food Storage Monitoring

Smart refrigerators with sensors track temperature, humidity, and expiration dates. Notification is generated when food is spoiled or needs to be replaced. Systems can suggest grocery lists based on stock levels. Several benefits are listed in Table 13.12.

Table 13.10 Advantages of home security systems

Benefit	Description
Increased protection against break-ins or unwanted access	IoT-enabled security systems monitor doors, windows, and movements to prevent unauthorized entry
Real-time notifications for caregivers or family members	Sensors and cameras send instant alerts when suspicious activity is detected
Greater peace of mind at home	Constant surveillance and quick response features enhance the feeling of safety and security at home

Note: Home security systems improve safety, generate quick alert, and provide peace of mind through continuous monitoring

Table 13.11 Advantages of smart kitchen devices

Benefit	Description
Safer cooking processes	Smart stoves, ovens, and induction cooktops include automatic shut-off features to prevent fires and overheating
Reduced risk of kitchen accidents	Sensors detect unattended cooking and send alerts to users or caregivers to avoid potential hazards
More support for independent meal preparation	Guided cooking systems provide step-by-step instructions, timers, and temperature control for easier meal preparation

Note: Smart kitchen devices improve kitchen safety and help users cook more confidently and independently

Table 13.12 Benefits of food storage monitoring

Benefit	Description
Better food safety and freshness	Smart refrigerators and storage sensors monitor temperature and humidity to preserve food quality
Fewer risks of consuming expired items	IoT systems track expiration dates and send alerts to avoid consumption of spoiled items
Improved kitchen management and organization	Inventory tracking features help manage supplies and reduce food waste through timely restocking

Note: Food storage monitoring systems help reduce wastage and keep kitchens more organized

Nutrition Tracking Tools

Wearable devices and health apps record calorie intake, hydration levels, and nutrient balance. Data can be synced with health platforms to monitor diet goals and nutritional needs. Key benefits of these tools are presented in Table 13.13.

Table 13.13 Key benefits of nutrition tackers

Benefit	Description
Personalized nutrition management	Nutrition trackers monitor calorie intake, hydration levels, and nutrient balance to tailor diet plans
Early detection of undernutrition or dehydration	Real-time data from IoT devices helps identify signs of nutritional deficiencies or fluid imbalance
Stronger support for chronic condition diets (e.g., diabetes, hypertension)	Customized diet recommendations help manage specific health conditions and improve overall well-being

Note: Nutrition trackers help people eat better, stay hydrated, and manage health conditions more effectively

Table 13.14 Benefits of meal planning systems

Benefit	Description
Consistent and balanced meal routines	Smart meal planning tools help schedule regular, well-balanced meals tailored to nutritional needs
Easier management of special diets	IoT systems support dietary restrictions by suggesting appropriate food options and recipes
Increased engagement in healthy food choices	Interactive meal planning apps encourage user participation and promote healthier eating habits

Note: The meal planning system supports healthy eating, making it easy to organize, customize, and enjoy daily meals

Meal Planning Systems

Digital tools assist with weekly meal planning and dietary adjustments. Systems suggest recipes based on health goals, dietary restrictions, and available ingredients. Table 13.14 includes some benefits of meal planning systems.

Environmental Monitoring

Environmental monitoring systems share data with caregivers and facility managers. Notifications are sent in real time if conditions change suddenly or reach unsafe levels.

Air Quality Monitoring

Air quality sensors detect harmful substances in the air. These include pollutants, allergens, smoke, and carbon monoxide. High levels of these can be harmful to health, especially for the elderly. The sensors continuously monitor the air. If levels exceed safe limits, an alert is sent immediately. Caregivers are notified via

Table 13.15 Role of air quality monitoring system for healthy indoor environment

Benefit	Description
Reduced exposure to harmful pollutants	Air quality sensors detect pollutants such as smoke, allergens, and carbon monoxide, helping maintain a safer environment
Better respiratory health	Cleaner air supports lung function and reduces respiratory problems, especially for individuals with chronic conditions
Immediate response to indoor air risks	Real-time alerts notify caregivers or users when indoor air quality drops, allowing quick action to restore safety

Note: Air quality monitoring systems help create a safer indoor space by tracking pollutants and supporting respiratory health

app or alarm. Some systems also send alerts to emergency services. In some homes, the ventilation system works with the help of sensors. It turns on automatically to improve air circulation. It helps remove harmful particles from the air. This keeps the house fresh and safe to breathe. Monitoring air quality reduces health risks. It also supports a healthier and more comfortable living environment. The role of air quality system for maintaining a healthy indoor environment is listed in Table 13.15.

Temperature Monitoring

Temperature sensors keep track of room conditions throughout the day. Systems adjust heating or cooling automatically when temperatures go outside safe ranges. Caregivers can also monitor temperature remotely. The key benefits of temperature monitoring are listed in Table 13.16.

Humidity Monitoring

Humidity sensors help maintain balanced indoor moisture levels. Excess humidity can cause mold, while low humidity can lead to dry air and respiratory issues. Systems adjust humidifiers or dehumidifiers as needed. Several benefits of humidity monitoring are shown in Table 13.17.

Geolocation and Safety Tracking

Geolocation and safety tracking are crucial in IoT-based elder care. These technologies protect individuals with memory loss or cognitive impairments. Real-time location tracking helps prevent wandering and speeds up emergency responses.

Table 13.16 Benefits of temperature monitoring

Benefit	Description
Protection from extreme heat or cold	IoT sensors maintain safe indoor temperatures by automatically adjusting heating or cooling systems
Greater comfort and energy efficiency	Smart control systems optimize temperature settings for consistent comfort and reduced energy use
Early detection of equipment malfunction	Monitoring systems detects irregular temperature changes and alert users or in-charge personnel to possible HVAC system failures

Note: Temperature monitoring helps keep indoor spaces safe, comfortable, and energy-efficient by catching problems in advance

Table 13.17 Benefits of humidity monitoring

Benefit	Description
Healthier air quality	Humidity sensors help maintain optimal moisture levels, contributing to overall indoor air health
Reduced risk of mold or dryness-related issues	Balanced humidity prevents mold growth and reduces respiratory discomfort from dry air
More stable indoor environment	Automatic adjustments by humidifiers or dehumidifiers ensure consistent indoor climate conditions

Note: Monitoring humidity supports better air quality, helps prevent health issues, and keeps indoor spaces more comfortable

GPS Tracking Devices

GPS-enabled wearables or mobile devices provide constant location updates. These tools allow caregivers to monitor movement and travel routes. Location data is stored and shared through connected apps or platforms. Benefits of GPS tacking devices are given below:

- Real-time tracking for enhanced safety
- Faster response in case of disorientation or getting lost
- Peace of mind for care teams and family members

Geo-Fencing Technology

Geo-fencing systems create virtual boundaries around safe areas, such as homes or nearby neighborhoods. When a person crosses the boundary, automatic alerts are sent to caregivers or monitoring centers. The benefits of geo-fencing technology are listed in Table 13.18.

Table 13.18 Advantages of geo-fencing technology

Benefit	Description
Early warning when someone leaves a safe area	Geo-fencing systems set digital boundaries and send alerts when those boundaries are crossed
Prevention of wandering-related incidents	Virtual zones reduce the risk of disorientation and help keep individuals within safe areas
Automated notifications for faster intervention	Automatic alerts notify caregivers or emergency contacts for quick response and recovery

Note: Geo-fencing technology improves safety and enables timely support by alerting caregivers when someone leaves a secure area

Table 13.19 Advantages emergency response system

Benefit	Description
Fast access to help during emergencies	Wearable emergency devices allow immediate alerting caregivers or emergency services with a single press
Reduced delay in medical response	Quick alerts ensure faster intervention and reduce the risk of complications during health incidents
Greater safety during daily activities	Continuous monitoring and easy access to assistance enhance safety throughout the day

Note: Emergency response systems provide quick help, reduce risks, and support safer daily living—especially for vulnerable individuals

Emergency Response Systems

An important part of Internet of things in elder care is emergency response systems. These devices provide immediate assistance during medical incidents, accidents, or sudden health changes. Rapid alerts and automated communication help reduce response times and improve outcomes. Wearable devices include panic buttons, fall sensors, and health monitors. The devices are worn as bracelets, pendants, or smartwatches. A single press or automatic trigger sends an alert to caregivers, emergency services, or monitoring centers. The benefits of emergency response systems are presented in Table 13.19.

Challenges in Implementing IoT in Elder Care

Privacy and Data Security

- IoT devices collect vast amounts of sensitive health and personal data. Without strong encryption and secure data storage protocols, this information is vulnerable to breaches.

- A lack of standardized privacy regulations across manufacturers and systems exacerbates the risk, leaving elder care facilities unsure of compliance requirements.
- Older adults may also feel uneasy about how their data is collected, shared, and used, potentially eroding trust in the system.

Cost and Affordability

- The upfront cost of IoT devices such as smart sensors, wearables, and home automation systems can be prohibitive, particularly for smaller care facilities or low-income households.
- Ongoing expenses, including device maintenance, software subscriptions, and infrastructure upgrades (e.g., high-speed Internet), add to the financial burden.
- Public funding and insurance coverage for such technology are often limited, delaying broader adoption.

Technical Complexity and Usability

- Many IoT devices are not designed with elderly users in mind. Complicated user interfaces, touchscreens, or voice-activated systems can be confusing and frustrating.
- Regular technical support is essential, yet often unavailable, leaving both caregivers and older adults struggling with setup and troubleshooting.
- The digital divide—limited tech literacy among older generations—can lead to underutilization or complete avoidance of the technology.

Integration and Interoperability

- Different devices and platforms often fail to communicate effectively, creating fragmented systems that do not sync or share data properly.
- This lack of interoperability makes it difficult to integrate IoT tools with electronic health records (EHRs) or other healthcare management systems.
- As a result, caregivers may end up managing multiple dashboards or manually transferring information, reducing efficiency.

Reliability and Infrastructure Dependence

- IoT systems depend on stable Internet connectivity and consistent power supply—both of which can be unreliable in rural areas.
- Device malfunctions or software bugs can disrupt monitoring, leading to missed alerts or false alarms.
- Environmental factors, like humidity or temperature fluctuations, may affect device performance and durability.

Resistance to Adoption

- Fear of the unknown, distrust in technology, and generational skepticism often hinder acceptance among older adults.
- Some caregivers also resist due to perceived complexity or concerns about being replaced by machines.
- Education, training, and user-friendly designs are key to overcoming this psychological barrier.

Maintenance

- IoT devices and sensors require periodic updates, battery replacements, and technical inspections to function properly.
- Access to timely and affordable technical support is often limited, especially in remote area.
- Equipment breakdowns or outdated firmware can compromise the continuity and safety.

Impact Assessment of IoT Technologies in Elderly Well-Being

This section aims to measure the positive impact of various IoT-based technologies on the well-being of the elderly. The analysis is based on peer-reviewed literature, caregiver and clinician surveys, and implementation case reports.

Fall Detection (95%)

AI-based systems detect falls with nearly 100% accuracy. Alharbi et al. [13] observed that they reduced fall-related hospitalizations by 63%. Users accepted the systems well. Cost and privacy needed to be addressed first [14].

Smart Kitchen (60%)

According to Kaczor et al. [15], kitchen automation reduced injuries by 40–60%. Surveys showed concerns about usability and cost [16].

Smart Dieting (72%)

Gouda et al. [17] found that about 72% of caregivers reported improved dietary adherence using voice-assisted meal tracking systems.

Medication Management (88%)

Smart pill dispensers and reminders led to an 88% boost in medication adherence [18].

Clinician/Caregiver Views (80%)

Around 80% of clinicians valued smart health systems but noted challenges with data ethics, training, and workflow integration [19].

A graphical representation of those effects is presented in Fig. 13.2. In addition, the estimated effects are depicted in Table 13.20.

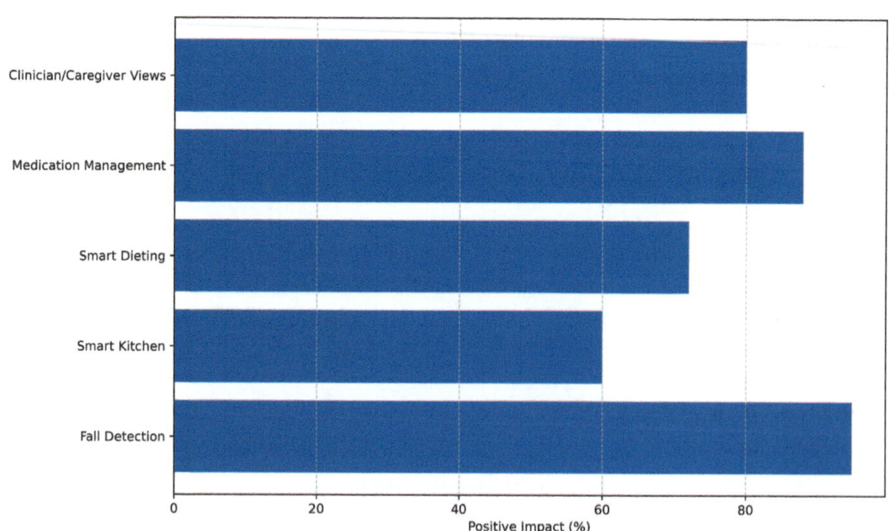

Fig. 13.2 Estimated positive impact of IoT technologies in elderly care

Table 13.20 The key barriers identified in survey analyses for IoT technologies in elderly well-being

Technology	Positive impact (%)	Key barriers
Fall detection	95	Cost, privacy
Smart kitchen	60	Usability, cost
Smart dieting	72	Tech literacy, trust
Medication management	88	Complexity, training
Clinician or caregiver views	80	Ethical, workflow

Note: This table summarizes the primary barriers perceived in IoT-based solutions for elderly care, as reported in survey analyses

Conclusion

IoT technology is reshaping elder care. Connected devices and smart systems support health, safety, and independence in daily life. From wearable health monitors to fall detection systems, smart home tools, nutrition support, and emergency responses, IoT is transforming elder care. IoT reduces risks, improves care response, and eases the workload on caregivers. Real-time data, automation, and personalized tools create a more proactive care environment. Older adults can stay in familiar settings longer, with greater comfort and safety. As adoption grows, IoT will continue to improve care quality, lower costs, and expand access. Technology is not replacing human care—it is making care stronger, safer, and more responsive. IoT offers a clear path forward for aging with dignity, independence, and better quality of life.

References

1. Uddin MS, Alam JB, Banu S. Real time patient monitoring system based on Internet of Things. In: 2017 4th international conference on advances in electrical engineering (ICAEE). IEEE; 2017. p. 516–21.
2. Lu L, Zhang J, Xie Y, Gao F, Xu S, Wu X, Ye Z. Wearable health devices in health care: narrative systematic review. JMIR Mhealth Uhealth. 2020;8(11):e18907.
3. Iqbal SM, Mahgoub I, Du E, Leavitt MA, Asghar W. Advances in healthcare wearable devices. NPJ Flexible Electron. 2021;5(1):9.
4. Rosdi WMFWM, Suhaimi SA, Lazam NM, Alias AJ, Abdullah F, Azemi SN. Smart pill dispenser with monitoring system. In: 2021 IEEE symposium on Wireless Technology & Applications (ISWTA). IEEE; 2021. p. 58–62.
5. Viana ÓT, Lima O, Terroso M, Vilaça JL. Developing a smart pill dispenser to support aging individuals. In: Perspectives on design and digital communication V: research, innovations and best practices. Springer Nature Switzerland: Cham; 2024. p. 39–60.
6. Inc WT. Health monitor app. Retrieved from. 2024; https://welltory.com/devices/health-monitor-app/
7. Ahn B. Life alert system for vulnerable adults who live alone. 2016.
8. Inc.com. Inc. 5000 2021: America's fastest-growing private companies. 2021. Retrieved from https://www.inc.com/inc5000/2021

9. Vardakis G, Hatzivasilis G, Koutsaki E, Papadakis N. Review of smart-home security using the Internet of Things. Electronics. 2024;13(16):3343.
10. Google Store. Nest thermostat from Google. 2024. Retrieved from https://store.google.com/us/product/nest_thermostat
11. Susmitha MM, Babu ND, Sri VT, Deepika S, Krishna KV, Koteswararao KV. Home automation using Google assistance. Int J Eng Res Sci Technol. 2024;20(2):51–7.
12. Uddin MS, Khan MDA, Khan MN. Kitchen grocery items monitoring system based on Internet of Things. Int J Comput Netw Technol. 2019;7(2). https://hdl.handle.net/20.500.14536/3739.
13. Alharbi HA, Alharbi KK, Hassan CAU. Enhancing elderly fall detection through IoT-enabled smart flooring and AI for independent living sustainability. Sustainability. 2023;15(22):15695. https://doi.org/10.3390/su152215695.
14. Wang C-Y, Lin F-S. AI-driven privacy in elderly care: developing a comprehensive solution for camera-based monitoring of older adults. Appl Sci. 2024;14(10):4150. https://doi.org/10.3390/app14104150.
15. Kaczor J, Fabisiak B, Bartuzel M, Domański P, Marciniak O, Wiktorski T. Universal design in kitchen furniture: a case study on enhancing accessibility and safety for the elderly and people with mobility challenges. Annals of Warsaw University of Life Sciences-SGGW. Forestry and Wood Technology; 2023.
16. Yaddaden A, Bottari C, Lussier M, Kenfack-Ngankam H, Couture M, Giroux S, et al. The COOK assistive technology for cognition for older adults with cognitive deficits: a usability study. Disability and Rehabilitation: Assistive Technology; 2025. p. 1–15.
17. Gouda P, Ganni E, Chung P, Randhawa VK, Marquis-Gravel G, Avram R, et al. Feasibility of incorporating voice technology and virtual assistants in cardiovascular care and clinical trials. Curr Cardiovasc Risk Rep. 2021;15:1–8.
18. Ghosh M. Digital era of well-being. In: India's silver surfers: transforming the digital inequalities/diversities. Springer Nature Switzerland: Cham; 2024. p. 55–68.
19. Montellato M. The impact of digital health on healthcare professionals: a case study. 2023.

GPSR Compliance

The European Union's (EU) General Product Safety Regulation (GPSR) is a set of rules that requires consumer products to be safe and our obligations to ensure this.

If you have any concerns about our products, you can contact us on ProductSafety@springernature.com

In case Publisher is established outside the EU, the EU authorized representative is:

Springer Nature Customer Service Center GmbH
Europaplatz 3
69115 Heidelberg, Germany

Batch number: 10370736

Printed by Printforce, the Netherlands